Emergency Medical Technician Exam Review

D1500966

Emergency Medical Technician Exam Review

Second Edition

Kirsten M. Elling, BS, EMT-P

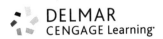

DELMAR
CENGAGE Learning·

Australia • Brazil • Japan • Korea • Mexico • Singapore • Spain • United Kingdom • United States

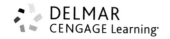

**Emergency Medical Technician Exam Review,
Second Edition**
Kirsten M. Elling

Vice President, Career and Professional
Editorial: Dave Garza

Director of Learning Solutions: Sandy Clark

Senior Acquisitions Editor: Janet E. Maker

Managing Editor: Larry Main

Senior Product Manager: Jennifer Starr

Editorial Assistant: Leah Costakis

Vice President, Career and Professional
Marketing: Jennifer Baker

Marketing Director: Deborah Yarnell

Associate Marketing Manager: Erica Glisson

Senior Production Director: Wendy Troeger

Production Manager: Mark Bernard

Content Project Management: PreMediaGlobal

Cover Design: PreMediaGlobal

For product information and technology assistance, contact us at
Cengage Learning Customer & Sales Support, 1-800-354-9706

For permission to use material from this text or product,
submit all requests online at **cengage.com/permissions**
Further permissions questions can be emailed to
permissionrequest@cengage.com

Library of Congress Control Number: 2012931396

ISBN-13: 978-1-133-13126-7

ISBN-10: 1-133-13126-3

Delmar
5 Maxwell Drive
Clifton Park, NY 12065-2919
USA

Cengage Learning is a leading provider of customized learning solutions with office locations around the globe, including Singapore, the United Kingdom, Australia, Mexico, Brazil, and Japan. Locate your local office at:
international.cengage.com/region

Cengage Learning products are represented in Canada by Nelson Education, Ltd.

To learn more about Delmar, visit **www.cengage.com/delmar**

Purchase any of our products at your local college store or at our preferred online store **www.CengageBrain.com**

Notice to the Reader
Publisher does not warrant or guarantee any of the products described herein or perform any independent analysis in connection with any of the product information contained herein. Publisher does not assume, and expressly disclaims, any obligation to obtain and include information other than that provided to it by the manufacturer. The reader is expressly warned to consider and adopt all safety precautions that might be indicated by the activities described herein and to avoid all potential hazards. By following the instructions contained herein, the reader willingly assumes all risks in connection with such instructions. The publisher makes no representations or warranties of any kind, including but not limited to, the warranties of fitness for particular purpose or merchantability, nor are any such representations implied with respect to the material set forth herein, and the publisher takes no responsibility with respect to such material. The publisher shall not be liable for any special, consequential, or exemplary damages resulting, in whole or part, from the readers' use of, or reliance upon, this material.

Printed in the United States of America
1 2 3 4 5 6 7 16 15 14 13 12

Dedication

*This work is dedicated to my three grandchildren, Destinee, Devon, and Darren, because
I am so proud of you.*

—

Special Thanks

*My deepest thanks to my close friend and colleague Mikel A. Rothenberg, M.D.,
for all his hard work, insight, and guidance during the development of
the companion text,* Why-Driven EMS Review.

Contents

Preface

Intent of This Book

The *Emergency Medical Technician Exam Review,* Second Edition, is a comprehensive resource for preparing for state and national EMT exams. This book is a valuable tool to help practice and review your knowledge of the EMT requirements in order to build confidence for the actual exam. It is designed to follow the National EMS Education Standards for the Emergency Medical Technician, and is updated to the 2010 American Heart Association Guidelines.

Approach of This Book

Early in this project we decided that the questions would only be the multiple-choice style, with the standard format of three "distracters" (incorrect or less than optimal answers) and one correct answer to each question. Because this book will be used to prepare for both state and national EMT examinations, it makes the most sense to use the format and style of questions used on these types of exams.

For each question there is only one correct answer. When you have difficulty narrowing the choice down, always read through all four choices and select the best answer. This book has more than 1,500 questions and another 300 on the CD. I suggest that you tackle a chapter at a time; then, after taking each exam, check the answer key and mark the areas where you need to review the material.

I sincerely hope you will enjoy *The EMT Exam Review* and benefit from the test-taking review to expand your knowledge base. After all, the real test occurs in the field, where our patients rely on us to be prepared.

See you in the streets!

—*Kirt*

Features of This Book

- *Aligns with the National EMS Education Standards* consisting of multiple-choice questions covering all topics and objectives (cognitive and affective) in the current National EMS Education Standards for the Emergency Medical Technician level.

- *Current to the 2010 American Heart Association Guidelines* to keep you informed of the latest requirements.

- *Answers and Rationale* are provided in the Appendices, offering validation and explanation for the correct response.

- *Basic Life Support Review* is included in the Appendices, ensuring the necessary review of BLS skills.

- *NREMT Skill Sheets* are provided in the Appendices, offering the necessary knowledge of the requirements for those preparing for the National Registry EMT certification exam.

- *An interactive CD offers further practice and review* including two full-length simulated practice exams, games, plus more!

New to This Edition

- *Thoroughly revised to reflect the National EMS Education Standards and 2010 AHA Guidelines* to properly prepare you for the certification exam and beyond. This includes revised terminology, reorganized information, and new questions to align with current requirements and an all-important BLS review.

- *Accompanying CD includes interactive practice exams, games, and more,* all reflecting current information of the National EMS Education Standards and the 2010 AHA Guidelines and offering additional review for the exam.

Also Available

Elling, Elling & Rothenburg/*Why Driven EMS Review*, Second Edition
(978-1-4180-3817-5)

Elling, Kirsten/*Emergency Medical Responder*, First Edition
(978-1-4180-7286-5)

Elling, Elling/*Advanced EMT Review*, Second Edition
(978-1-1336-8702-3)

Elling, Elling/*Paramedic Exam Review*, Third Edition
(978-1-1331-3129-8)

About the Author

Kirsten M. Elling, BS, EMT-P

Kirsten (Kirt) Elling is a career paramedic who works for Colonie EMS and Whiteface Mountain in upstate New York. She began EMS work in 1988 as an EMT/firefighter and has been an EMS educator since 1990, teaching basic and advanced EMS programs at the Institute of Prehospital Emergency Medicine in Troy, New York. Kirt serves as Regional Faculty for the New York State Department of Health, Bureau of EMS, and Regional Faculty for the American Heart Association. She has written *The Emergency Medical Responder Exam Review, The Emergency Medical Technician Exam Review,* and numerous scripts for the EMS training video series *PULSE: Emergency Medical Update.* She is a co-author of *Why-Driven EMS Review, The Paramedic Exam Review, The Advanced EMT Exam Review, Principles of Assessment, Paramedic: Anatomy & Physiology, Paramedic: Pharmacology Applications,* and *Paramedic: Pathophysiology*; a contributing author of the IPEM *Paramedic Lab Manual*; and an adjunct writer for the 1998 revision of the National Highway Traffic Safety Administration, EMT-Paramedic, and EMT-Intermediate: and National Education Standard Curricula.

Acknowledgments

Thank you to the editorial and production team at Delmar Cengage Learning who contributed to this new edition, especially Janet Maker, Jennifer Starr, Jim Zayicek, and Jennifer Hanley, as well as the project team at PreMediaGlobal.

And thank you to our reviewers:

J. Alan Baker, AS, NREMT-P, LP
Assistant Director of EMSP
Victoria College
Victoria, TX

Tom Chartier, BAE, EMT-I
Western Iowa Tech Community College
Sioux City, IA
Woodbury Central High School
Moville, IA

Kevin Costa, Captain II
EMS Coordinator
Pasadena Fire Department
Pasadena, CA

Michael Dant
EMT Program Supervisor
Health Careers & Public Services
Illinois Central College
Peoria, IL

Loren Deichman, NREMT-P, CCEMT-P, I/C
Clinical Coordinator
ENMU-R EMS Program
Roswell, NM

Ken Davis, NR/CCEMT-P, FP-C, I/C
Paramedic Coordinator
Eastern New Mexico University—Roswell
Roswell, NM

Bruce Evans, MPA, NREMT-P
Fire Captain, Fire Program Coordinator
Community College of Southern Nevada
Henderson, NV

Lynda Goerisch, MA, NREMT-P
EMT Coordinator/Instructor
Century College
White Bear Lake, MN

Michael Hastings, MS, NREMT-P
EMS Program Director
Central Piedmont Community College
Charlotte, NC

Robbie Murray, NREMT-P, A.A.S.
Training Coordinator
Sussex County Emergency Medical Services
Georgetown, DE

M. Jane Pollock, EMT-P, CEN, Level II, EMD
Adjunct Clinical Instructor
Education and Training Specialist
Brody School of Medicine, East Carolina University
Department of Emergency Medicine,
Division of EMS
Greenville, NC

J. Penny Shutts, AEMT, NREMT-B, CIC
Educator
Sandy Creek, NY

Sandy Waggoner, EMT-P, FF, EMSI
Public Safety Coordinator
EHOVE Ghrist Adult Career Center
Milan, OH

Jean B. Will, Ed.D., RN, MSN, CED, EMT-P
Director of EMS Programs
Drexel University
Philadelphia, PA

SECTION

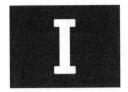

PREPARATORY

CHAPTER

Introduction to Emergency Medical Care

1. Emergency medical service (EMS) system is defined as:
   a. a continuum of patient care that extends until discharge.
   b. everything that happens to an injured person before he reaches the hospital.
   c. a public service capable of transporting the disabled.
   d. patient care that begins at the scene of an injury or illness.

2. The emergency access telephone number 9-1-1 does not permit which of the following functions?
   a. reduced time for the caller to access EMS
   b. access to police, fire, and EMS with one number
   c. accelerated access to EMS with the use of cell phones
   d. instructions for life-saving emergency care over the phone

3. As an EMT, one of your responsibilities is to tell the hospital staff of any concerns your patient expressed to you during your time caring for him. This role is called:
   a. patient safety.
   b. transfer of care.
   c. patient advocate.
   d. medical transcriptionist.

4. The emergency medical dispatcher (EMD) is trained to receive emergency calls, dispatch emergency services, and:
   a. determine when the caller is a minor.
   b. transcribe medical terminology.
   c. provide instructions for immediate emergency care.
   d. provide instruction for obtaining vital signs, including a blood pressure reading.

5. A respiratory therapist, a dental technician, and an oncology specialist are all examples of:
   a. EMDs.
   b. allied health personnel.
   c. bystanders.
   d. emergency department staff.

6. The health care provider who is typically the first person on the scene of an acute illness or injury in a non-health-care-related workplace is a:
   a. licensed practical nurse (LPN).
   b. first responder.
   c. paramedic.
   d. physician's assistant (PA).

7. During the transport of a patient, the EMT learns that the patient has some very specific concerns about possible treatment options for his present condition. Upon arrival at the hospital, the EMT conveys the patient's concerns to the nurse. This is an example of:
   a. patient advocacy.
   b. patient assessment.
   c. a Good Samaritan act.
   d. quality improvement.

8. An EMT should have good color vision because it can be critical to patient assessment, as well as:
   a. taking the EMT certification exam.
   b. maintaining emergency equipment.
   c. keeping good documentation.
   d. operating an emergency vehicle.

9. The responsibilities of an EMT include:
   a. transferring patient care.
   b. activating the EMS system.
   c. issuing standing orders.
   d. registering with the National Association of EMTs.

10. In the field of emergency medicine, having _____ means identifying with and understanding the feelings, situations, and motives of your patients.
    a. integrity
    b. sympathy
    c. empathy
    d. honesty

11. Your ambulance is dispatched to stand by at the scene of a house fire. Upon arrival at the scene, your first priority is to:
    a. notify dispatch that your unit is the first on the scene.
    b. notify incoming emergency units of smoke or fire conditions.
    c. protect your own safety.
    d. establish EMS command and request additional resources.

12. The EMT who keeps his or her immunizations up to date is demonstrating:
    a. compliance with standing orders.
    b. personal safety.
    c. the use of personal protective equipment (PPE).
    d. continuous quality improvement.

13. As an EMT, which of the following topics might you present to the community on a public health information day?
    a. global warming
    b. injury prevention
    c. clean drinking water
    d. radiation poisoning from nuclear fallout

14. When an EMT relocates to another region, state, or territory, the process of obtaining the same certification is known as:
    a. reentrance.
    b. reciprocity.
    c. occupation barter.
    d. reactivation.

15. Which of the following is an example of an EMT advocating for a patient?
    a. ensuring a rapid response time and establishing a safe scene
    b. thoroughly documenting a refusal of medical attention (RMA)
    c. allowing a family member to ride in the ambulance with the patient when the patient does not want that
    d. collecting and safeguarding a patient's medical information while the patient is in the EMT's care

16. The practice of reviewing and auditing calls within an EMS system to ensure a high quality of care is referred to as:
    a. quality improvement.
    b. medical review.
    c. the National Highway Safety Act.
    d. medical direction.

17. The patient care guidelines under which EMS personnel function are referred to as:
    a. protocols.
    b. quality control.
    c. online medical direction.
    d. state and local ordinances.

18. The EMT can help improve the quality of patient care by:
    a. participating in continuing education.
    b. washing his hands after each patient contact.
    c. carrying a portable radio whenever possible.
    d. avoiding direct contact with infectious patients.

19. Every EMS system has a/an _____ who assumes definitive responsibility for oversight of the patient care aspects of the EMS system.
    a. EMS supervisor
    b. medical director
    c. senior paramedic
    d. paramedic supervisor

20. An EMT who gives oral glucose to a patient who has signs and symptoms of hypoglycemia, per standing-orders protocol, is using:
    a. Red Cross guidelines.
    b. online medical direction.
    c. offline medical direction.
    d. national care standards.

21. An example of online (direct) medical control is:
    a. assisting a patient to take nitroglycerin per standing orders.
    b. contacting a physician by radio prior to performing a skill.
    c. obtaining feedback from the hospital staff after caring for a patient.
    d. administering a medication to a patient, and then notifying the hospital to advise of the incoming patient and his status.

22. An on-duty EMT is working _____ of the medical director for the EMS system.
    a. on Good Samaritan extension
    b. on advance directives
    c. as a designated agent
    d. for the scope of practice

23. The EMT is responsible for completing the prehospital care report (PCR), which contains two types of information: _____ and _____.
    a. regional, national
    b. behavioral, characteristic
    c. technical, supportive
    d. patient, administrative

24. The policies and procedures used by an EMS system may be authorized by a _____ agency.
    a. state
    b. regional
    c. local
    d. all of the above

25. After becoming an EMT you will need to _____ in order to recertify and stay an EMT.
    a. participate in continuing education
    b. make a commitment to ongoing research
    c. join the quality improvement committee
    d. become a member of the National Registry of EMTs

Chapter 1 Answer Form

	A	B	C	D			A	B	C	D
1.	❑	❑	❑	❑		14.	❑	❑	❑	❑
2.	❑	❑	❑	❑		15.	❑	❑	❑	❑
3.	❑	❑	❑	❑		16.	❑	❑	❑	❑
4.	❑	❑	❑	❑		17.	❑	❑	❑	❑
5.	❑	❑	❑	❑		18.	❑	❑	❑	❑
6.	❑	❑	❑	❑		19.	❑	❑	❑	❑
7.	❑	❑	❑	❑		20.	❑	❑	❑	❑
8.	❑	❑	❑	❑		21.	❑	❑	❑	❑
9.	❑	❑	❑	❑		22.	❑	❑	❑	❑
10.	❑	❑	❑	❑		23.	❑	❑	❑	❑
11.	❑	❑	❑	❑		24.	❑	❑	❑	❑
12.	❑	❑	❑	❑		25.	❑	❑	❑	❑
13.	❑	❑	❑	❑						

CHAPTER

2

Well-Being of the EMT

1. Which of the following statements is most accurate about dealing with the stress in EMS?
   a. There are limited ways for EMTs to deal with stress.
   b. EMTs become desensitized to stress after working on the job for one year.
   c. A single critical incident can produce different reactions in different EMTs.
   d. Good lifestyle habits will eliminate any stress associated with being an EMT.

2. After returning from a cardiac arrest call, which involved the unexpected death of a young patient, it would be normal and mentally healthy for the EMT to:
   a. talk about the call with crew members.
   b. become depressed.
   c. indulge in the use of alcohol.
   d. request more work hours or overtime.

3. Cumulative stress brought on by repeated exposure to critical emergency care situations can cause the EMT to:
   a. burn out.
   b. become bored.
   c. work longer hours.
   d. take a paramedic course.

4. The family of a woman in cardiac arrest is waiting at the emergency department (ED) when you arrive. After you turn the patient over to the staff, you realize that the family is looking at you and it is obvious that they want to talk to you. At this point you:
   a. avoid them until the ED physician has talked to them first.
   b. assume that they will be angry and prepare for the worst.
   c. listen to what they have to say, but do not give them any false hopes.
   d. tell them that you have no good news at this time and to wait to speak to the ED physician.

5. During a career in EMS, the EMT may have to help patients, or patients' family members, or even coworkers with the various stages of:
   a. confidentiality.
   b. working out a living will.
   c. developing a do not resuscitate order (DNR).
   d. the grieving process.

6. After being on the scene for 10 minutes with another crew that is working on a patient in cardiac arrest, you are getting ready to move the patient into the ambulance. Just then the patient's daughter arrives. She is very upset and appears to be in shock about her father. She keeps repeating that there is nothing wrong with him. What emotional stage of the death and dying process is she exhibiting?
   a. anger
   b. bargaining
   c. denial
   d. depression

7. The fire department was the first to respond to the scene of a cardiac arrest. When you arrive, they are performing CPR, although the patient appears to have obvious signs of lividity. The family is very upset and requests that you do everything possible to save the patient. What steps do you take in the approach to this family that is confronted with death and dying?
   a. Stop CPR and tell them that nothing else can be done.
   b. Keep doing CPR and begin transport of the patient.
   c. Stop CPR and show them the signs of irreversible death found on the patient.
   d. Keep doing CPR until the coroner arrives to convince the family that the patient is dead.

8. After being dispatched to a home on a cardiac arrest call, you arrive to find that the resident appears to have been dead for several hours. You notify dispatch that this is an unattended death and turn your attention to the family member who discovered the body. The relative tells you that the patient has been sick for a long time but has refused any help. The relative does not appear to be too upset. What stage of grieving does this represent?

    a. acceptance
    b. bargaining
    c. denial
    d. depression

9. Dispatch has sent you to a call for a sick person. When you arrive, the family tells you that the patient is terminally ill with lung cancer and that they need her transported to the hospital for a test. The approach to take with this patient is to:

    a. expect that the patient will be angry with you and verbally abuse you.
    b. let the family and patient know that the patient will not die on this transport.
    c. make the patient comfortable, maintain her dignity, and be respectful.
    d. call an ALS unit to do the transport, because the patient is medicated.

10. Your family is always complaining that your work takes all your time and that your job seems more important to you than they are. This reaction from your family is:

    a. a nuisance.
    b. uncommon and can be disregarded.
    c. a form of distrust.
    d. something you need to give priority attention to.

11. You are stuck on a late call again and have called your friends to tell them that you will not be able to go to the movies with them as planned. In the past they have been disappointed when this has happened, and this time they sound angry. How can you reasonably prevent this from occurring in the future?

    a. Avoid making any plans with your friends.
    b. Do not make plans for times near the end of your shift.
    c. Explain to your friends that this is the way it has to be.
    d. Consider quitting EMS and going into another type of work.

12. You and your crew have returned to the station after responding to a successful suicide by gunshot. The supervisor was present as well and has made arrangements for debriefing the incident. Which statement about stress debriefing is most accurate?

    a. No one should be forced or compelled to attend.
    b. Everyone must attend for a successful debriefing.
    c. The medical director must attend for a successful debriefing.
    d. Police and other responders should attend a similar debriefing, but separate from EMS.

13. The EMT's possible reactions to critical-incident stress:

    a. are initially the same for everyone.
    b. always affect the EMT's family.
    c. are usually healthy and not a problem.
    d. are individual and are affected by previous exposures.

14. You are back at work after a two-week vacation. It does not take you long to see that your partner is acting different. She complains of a headache and nausea and tells you that she has not been sleeping well and has distressing dreams. You recognize that these may be signs of:

    a. the flu.
    b. substance abuse or withdrawal.
    c. a stress reaction.
    d. feelings of incompetence.

15. Signs and symptoms of a crisis-induced stress reaction can:

    a. be avoided altogether.
    b. produce feelings of euphoria.
    c. occur during or after an incident.
    d. occur before, during, or after an incident.

16. Each of the following is a recommended technique that the EMT can use for reducing or minimizing stress, *except:*

    a. coping.
    b. self-medication.
    c. problem solving.
    d. adaptation.

17. On a call for an unattended obvious death, the daughter arrived after the ambulance. She is overwhelmed by the unexpected death of her mother and appears very angry. How can you best be helpful to her?

    a. Leave the scene as soon as possible.
    b. Be understanding and listen without returning anger.
    c. Give her the phone number to your favorite funeral home.
    d. Invite her to attend a critical stress management debriefing.

18. This week you have decided to join a gym and begin an exercise program to help alleviate some of the stress in your life. Exercise is a great stress reliever because:
    a. finding time for yourself relieves stress.
    b. it provides a physical release of pent-up energy.
    c. it helps you focus on the positives.
    d. all of the above.

19. It is 2:00 a.m. and the house you have been dispatched to is completely dark. Why is this potentially a threat to the EMT?
    a. The patient may be blind.
    b. It may not be an actual EMS emergency.
    c. The patient may have fallen and been unable to turn on the lights.
    d. The patient may be unresponsive and alone.

20. A routine call for a sick person has suddenly become dangerous. The patient is refusing care and is threatening to take a swing at you. The safest way to handle this situation is to:
    a. quickly turn your back and run away.
    b. without raising your voice, state with authority that you will not allow any violence to occur here.
    c. call for the police and retreat if necessary.
    d. get the patient to sign a refusal-of-care form and leave.

21. Many scenes involve some type of possible hazard to the EMT, which can easily be controlled if recognized. Which of the following scenes should the EMT be able to control?
    a. an overturned motor vehicle that is leaking fuel
    b. a walkway to the house that is covered with ice
    c. a crime scene where the perpetrator is still present
    d. an ongoing domestic dispute between a mother and daughter

22. The efforts you take to protect yourself against disease transmission by bloodborne pathogens are:
    a. referred to as the scope of well-being.
    b. a form of sterilization.
    c. a low priority of the job.
    d. referred to as standard precautions.

23. The use of personal protective equipment (PPE) is of such paramount importance that EMS employers are required to have specific procedures in place and ensure that the necessary equipment is available. What component of standard precautions is the EMT responsible for?
    a. ensuring that gloves are available for use on every call
    b. developing a written exposure control plan
    c. ensuring that handwashing is done after each call
    d. developing and enforcing a written plan of action in case of an exposure

24. When you arrive at work, your designated officer tells you that two days ago you transported a patient with a potentially life-threatening airborne disease. What action must be taken at this point?
    a. Your employer must arrange for you to be evaluated by a health care professional.
    b. You must go home until you are evaluated and cleared by a health care professional.
    c. Nothing has to be done until 48 hours have passed.
    d. Nothing has to be done until 90 days have passed.

25. An example of an airborne pathogen that EMTs are at risk for exposure to during EMS calls is:
    a. hepatitis B.
    b. hepatitis C.
    c. German measles.
    d. staphylococcal skin infection.

26. Which of the following immunizations is not currently recommended for the EMT?
    a. polio
    b. tetanus
    c. hepatitis
    d. smallpox

27. In areas where tuberculosis is highly prevalent, TB screening for the EMT is recommended every _____ months.
    a. 6
    b. 12
    c. 18
    d. 24

28. Dispatch has sent you to a call for an assault. You are instructed to stand by one block from the address until the police call for you. While preparing for the call, you consider what PPE will be needed, and you:
    a. get out the bulletproof vests.
    b. decide that you will need gloves, at the very minimum.
    c. decide that you need nothing at this time without further information.
    d. put on your turnout jacket and helmet.

29. You have been assigned to perform a routine transport of a patient known to have bacterial meningitis. In preparation for the transport, which PPE and precautions will you need to take?
    a. gloves, eyewear, and surgical mask
    b. gloves, surgical mask, and handwashing after the call
    c. gloves, eye protection, and handwashing after the call
    d. gloves, HEPA respirator, and handwashing after the call

30. The county jail has requested transportation for an ill inmate, who is to be taken to the local hospital for evaluation of whooping cough. In preparation for this transport, which PPE and precautions will you need?
    a. gloves, eyewear, and surgical mask
    b. gloves, surgical mask, and handwashing after the call
    c. gloves, eye protection, and handwashing after the call
    d. gloves, HEPA respirator, and handwashing after the call

31. When responding to and working in a crime scene, the primary safety of the EMT is the responsibility of the:
    a. EMT.
    b. detective at the scene.
    c. safety officer.
    d. EMS supervisor.

32. During a severe thunderstorm, a loud burst of thunder and a lightning strike get your attention. When you look outside your station, you see that a power pole has been struck and wires are down on the road. You notify dispatch and request additional resources and then take which of the following safety precautions?
    a. Stay inside the building until the power company arrives.
    b. Put on rubber boots and investigate the area further.
    c. Stay inside the building until the fire department arrives.
    d. Establish a perimeter to keep people outside of the danger zone.

33. During the last call, blood from the patient dripped down onto a stretcher rail. Before putting the stretcher back into service, you make sure that the blood has been wiped off and the stretcher has been properly decontaminated. The reason for doing this right away is:
    a. that you will maintain the cleanest ambulance and equipment in the department.
    b. that your next patient might come into contact with the dried blood if you wait until later.
    c. because the longer you wait to clean the blood off, the harder it is to disinfect the stretcher.
    d. because the longer you wait to clean the blood off, the higher the risk of it drying and turning into airborne particles.

34. The supervisor has asked you to help train two new employees. She has most likely chosen you to be a field-training officer because of your experience and how you routinely demonstrate:
    a. that there is never a need to call in sick.
    b. the importance of not showing any signs of stress.
    c. how an EMS professional should dress.
    d. the importance of taking protective measures against infectious diseases.

35. Each fall semester you help teach labs in the EMT original course. The instructor likes your style and has told you that she likes the way you advocate the use of standard precautions against infectious diseases and other hazards in each lab. One of the ways you do this is to:
    a. tell the students about all the times they will need to wear PPE in the field.
    b. spend a great deal of time talking about the use of PPE in various situations, as well as in rescue operations.
    c. have the students practice wearing gloves, eyewear, and masks in lab sessions.
    d. have the students wash their hands before and after each lab session.

Chapter 2 Answer Form

	A	B	C	D		A	B	C	D
1.	❏	❏	❏	❏	19.	❏	❏	❏	❏
2.	❏	❏	❏	❏	20.	❏	❏	❏	❏
3.	❏	❏	❏	❏	21.	❏	❏	❏	❏
4.	❏	❏	❏	❏	22.	❏	❏	❏	❏
5.	❏	❏	❏	❏	23.	❏	❏	❏	❏
6.	❏	❏	❏	❏	24.	❏	❏	❏	❏
7.	❏	❏	❏	❏	25.	❏	❏	❏	❏
8.	❏	❏	❏	❏	26.	❏	❏	❏	❏
9.	❏	❏	❏	❏	27.	❏	❏	❏	❏
10.	❏	❏	❏	❏	28.	❏	❏	❏	❏
11.	❏	❏	❏	❏	29.	❏	❏	❏	❏
12.	❏	❏	❏	❏	30.	❏	❏	❏	❏
13.	❏	❏	❏	❏	31.	❏	❏	❏	❏
14.	❏	❏	❏	❏	32.	❏	❏	❏	❏
15.	❏	❏	❏	❏	33.	❏	❏	❏	❏
16.	❏	❏	❏	❏	34.	❏	❏	❏	❏
17.	❏	❏	❏	❏	35.	❏	❏	❏	❏
18.	❏	❏	❏	❏					

CHAPTER

3

Medical, Legal, and Ethical Issues

1. The collective set of regulations and ethical considerations that defines the capacity of an EMT's job is referred to as:
   a. protocols.
   b. certification.
   c. scope of practice.
   d. improvement.

2. When writing a patient care report (PCR), the EMT should document _____ findings that have been observed during the time with the patient.
   a. objective
   b. subjective
   c. personal
   d. weighted

3. When operating an emergency vehicle, the general rule for EMTs is to:
   a. assume that other drivers will yield to emergency traffic.
   b. let the most senior EMS provider drive when using lights and sirens.
   c. always use both lights and sirens when responding to a call.
   d. exercise due regard for the safety of others.

4. Which of the following is most accurate regarding prehospital certification and licensing?
   a. EMT is a certification granted by a state.
   b. Before a state grants a license to an EMT, that EMT must obtain state certification.
   c. Most states allow EMTs reciprocity for licensing only.
   d. Reciprocity is not applicable to EMTs who are certified.

5. A do not resuscitate order (DNR) is a legal document, typically signed by the _____, that states the patient has a terminal illness and does not wish to prolong his life with resuscitative measures.
   a. patient
   b. patient and his physician
   c. patient's legal guardian
   d. patient and his spouse

6. A do not resuscitate order is called a/an _____, because it is drawn up and signed prior to an event when resuscitation might be initiated.
   a. declaration
   b. advance directive
   c. proximate decree
   d. expressed consent

7. A legal document that allows a person to designate an agent to make decisions as to the type of life-saving medical treatment the person wants or does not want, if he is terminally ill and unable to decide for himself, in a coma, or in a persistent vegetative state, is a/an:
   a. DNR.
   b. living will.
   c. expressed consent.
   d. health care proxy.

8. Living wills and health care proxies usually relate to situations that occur in:
   a. a nursing home.
   b. the residence.
   c. the hospital setting.
   d. the prehospital setting.

9. Permission to treat a patient, or *consent*, is required:
   a. only if the patient is conscious and sober.
   b. in writing, using a standard EMS consent form.
   c. for any treatment or action performed by the EMT.
   d. for every patient the EMT establishes contact with.

10. Which of the following methods is acceptable for the EMT to use to obtain consent from a patient?
    a. Tell the patient you are there to help him, and ask if it is okay.
    b. Introduce yourself and ask the patient if you may take his vital signs.
    c. Tell the patient that you are an EMT and that you are willing to treat him, and ask him to sign your agency's consent form.
    d. All of the above.

11. Prior to treating an adult patient with severe mental disability, legally the EMT must:
    a. obtain consent from a guardian.
    b. notify dispatch before transporting.
    c. use local law enforcement.
    d. obtain consent from the patient's physician.

12. The EMT must obtain expressed consent:
    a. from intoxicated adults of legal age.
    b. from all nursing home residents who do not have a DNR.
    c. from conscious and mentally competent adults.
    d. prior to treatment and transportation of the unconscious patient.

13. When care for a patient is begun under implied consent, this type of consent remains in effect as long as the patient is mentally impaired and:
    a. as long as the patient is in protective custody.
    b. as long as the patient requires life-saving treatment.
    c. until the patient arrives at the emergency department.
    d. until the patient is discharged from the hospital.

14. An EMT is caring for an unresponsive patient who was found alone, and who is wearing a Medic Alert® tag with "Diabetic" written on it. The EMT may treat this patient under which type of consent?
    a. expressed
    b. informed
    c. involuntary
    d. emergency doctrine

15. An EMT is attempting to assess and treat a patient who is reported to have a low blood sugar reading. Initially the patient was conscious, but refused any intervention. During the interview, the patient became unconscious. Now the EMT may treat the patient under:
    a. medical control.
    b. implied consent.
    c. involuntary consent.
    d. protective custody.

16. You are called to care for a 22-year-old male who had openly stated that he wanted to harm himself, but now he has changed his mind. The patient is uninjured and is refusing care, so now you should:
    a. try to convince the patient to go to the hospital for evaluation.
    b. not leave the patient alone, but wait for family or a friend to arrive.
    c. transport the patient, as the threat to harm himself requires follow-up psychological care.
    d. allow the patient to refuse medical attention (RMA), as he is uninjured and has changed his mind about harming himself.

17. You have been called to a day care center for a 4-year-old child who is experiencing a severe allergic reaction after being stung by a bee. You may treat this child under which type of consent?
    a. implied
    b. informed
    c. expressed
    d. emergent

18. Under certain conditions, a minor may legally give consent for or refuse care. These minors are referred to as:
    a. liberated.
    b. adolescent.
    c. detached.
    d. emancipated.

19. A terminally ill patient tells you that he has a document that states he does not want to be placed on a ventilator if he goes into a coma. The document he is describing is a:
    a. living will.
    b. release of liability.
    c. comfort care order.
    d. do not resuscitate order.

20. After being dispatched to a grade school for a child with a hand laceration that will require sutures, what must occur before the EMT transports the child to the hospital?
    a. A parent or guardian must be contacted and consent obtained.
    b. The school nurse must provide consent for the EMT to treat the child.
    c. As the injury is minor, a parent or guardian must come to the school first.
    d. As the accident occurred on public property, the police must take a report.

21. You are treating a patient who sustained a possible spinal injury in a motor vehicle collision. The patient is willing to go to the hospital, but is adamantly refusing the application of a cervical collar. You should:
    a. carefully document the incident and refuse transport.
    b. tell the patient that without the cervical collar, he will become permanently crippled and have no recourse for a lawsuit.
    c. not transport the patient without the cervical collar and full spinal immobilization.
    d. document the refusal for the collar application, have the patient sign off on that matter, and then transport the patient to the hospital.

22. An EMT is assessing a 10-year-old child who has an ankle injury, but is refusing care and does not want to get into the ambulance. Which of the following statements is most accurate concerning this refusal of care?

    a. The EMT may treat the child under involuntary consent.
    b. Children may refuse care if they are given full disclosure by the EMT.
    c. The EMT may treat the child under expressed consent.
    d. Children cannot legally refuse care without a parent or guardian's agreement.

23. The EMT-B has the responsibility to be sure that all of the following conditions exist before allowing a patient to refuse care, except:

    a. the patient must be an adult.
    b. the patient must be mentally competent.
    c. all patients have a right to refuse care; no conditions can preclude that right.
    d. the patient must be fully informed and understand the risks of refusing care.

24. An EMT has responded to assist a 50-year-old male who has a deep laceration to the forearm. The wound was bandaged and bleeding has been controlled. Now the patient is refusing transport and states that he will drive himself to his doctor's office. It would now be appropriate for the EMT to:

    a. determine if the patient has a valid driver's license.
    b. try to get a family member or friend to take the patient to the doctor.
    c. ask the patient to take a breathalyzer test to reduce the liability for refusal of care.
    d. advise the patient not to call EMS again, as he cannot change his mind about help or transport once he has refused.

25. Which of the following statements regarding refusal of care is most accurate?

    a. A patient must sign a release-from-liability form.
    b. The patient cannot be left alone after refusing care.
    c. A competent adult patient can revoke consent at any time.
    d. An attempt to contact the patient's physician should be made before releasing the patient.

26. When harm occurs as a result of failure to exercise an acceptable degree of professional skill or competence while providing patient care, it is referred to as:

    a. negligence.
    b. consignment.
    c. discharge.
    d. obstruction.

27. An off-duty EMT stopped at the scene of a motor vehicle collision (MVC) to offer assistance, and began to triage patients. After several minutes, the EMT heard the siren of the ambulance in the distance and realized that he was late for work. Knowing that the patient was stable and that the ambulance would soon arrive, the EMT left to go to work. This is an example of:

    a. neglect.
    b. indifference.
    c. abandonment.
    d. leaving the scene of an accident.

28. During the transport of a patient with an altered mental status, the patient punches the EMT. Which of the following has occurred?

    a. The patient assaulted the EMT.
    b. The EMT is responsible for contributory negligence.
    c. The EMT failed to act with due regard for the patient.
    d. The patient is protected under governmental immunity because of the altered mental status.

29. When the EMT does not obtain consent from an oriented, competent adult prior to treatment and transport, his actions may be considered:

    a. false imprisonment.
    b. negligence.
    c. slander.
    d. libel.

30. Touching a competent adult patient without the patient's consent may be construed as:

    a. battery.
    b. an acceptable part of assessment.
    c. acceptable under the mental health laws.
    d. very serious if done in front of a child.

31. The EMT has a duty to act:

    a. only when he is paid to do so.
    b. when there is no threat to personal safety.
    c. only when his status is that of a volunteer.
    d. as soon as he receives state certification or licensure.

32. While on vacation in another state, you encounter a life-threatening medical emergency and quickly decide to help until the local EMS arrives at the patient's side. Legally, the safest approach is to:

    a. perform any actions necessary at the EMT level.
    b. identify yourself as a trained EMT and offer to ride to the hospital with the local EMS.
    c. stand by and intervene only if the patient requires CPR.
    d. limit your care to life-saving BLS treatment as a first responder.

33. While taking care of a patient within a crime scene, the primary responsibility of the EMT is:
    a. patient care.
    b. self-protection.
    c. preserving evidence.
    d. to document unusual findings.

34. The EMT's duty to act is not always clear because:
    a. there are no national standards for EMTs.
    b. when an EMT is on duty he has an obligation to provide service.
    c. state and local laws can vary significantly.
    d. there are multiple definitions of *duty to act*.

35. Confidentiality is a professional and legal responsibility that pertains to:
    a. a patient's privacy.
    b. censoring a patient's medical information.
    c. your experience level.
    d. safeguarding a patient's medical identification tag.

36. In which of the following manners may information about your patient legally be released to someone other than a health care provider?
    a. the information may be given to a spouse without a release
    b. over the phone if the patient has given verbal permission
    c. with a written release signed by the patient
    d. by fax with permission from the patient's family

37. A health care professional who spreads rumors that may injure the reputation of another is guilty of:
    a. libel.
    b. slander.
    c. false compliment.
    d. damaging etiquette.

38. The EMT must report which of the following observations in a patient's residence?
    a. untidiness
    b. suspected child abuse
    c. large sums of cash or coins
    d. excessive quantities of liquor bottles, both full and empty

39. On a recent call, you witnessed your paramedic partner make a medication error when dosing a sick patient. Later you observed your partner cover up the error on the patient care report. What your partner has done is:
    a. legal.
    b. immoral.
    c. unethical.
    d. exercising privileges during an emergency.

40. In which of the following ways could the EMT verify that a patient has consented to be an organ donor?
    a. A family member advises the EMT of the patient's wishes.
    b. The patient is carrying an organ donor card.
    c. The patient's driver's license indicates that the patient is an organ donor.
    d. All of the above.

41. When managing a critically injured patient who is a potential organ donor, the EMT should:
    a. provide comfort care only for the patient until arriving at the hospital.
    b. withhold treatment until the patient becomes pulseless, then begin CPR.
    c. care for the patient the same as for any other patient in need of emergency care.
    d. request police assistance, as the patient is now considered to be in protective custody.

42. The victim of a traumatic head injury is near death, and you are able to learn that he is an organ donor, but specifically for the eyes. During your assessment, you discover that the patient's eyes are badly damaged. You should now:
    a. care for the patient the same as for any other patient.
    b. attempt to contact a relative for modified donor instructions.
    c. terminate your resuscitative efforts because the eyes are not viable.
    d. call the patient's physician, report your findings, and inquire about advance directives.

43. You have been called to the scene of a hanging. The hanging is recent and you are going to attempt resuscitation. In helping to preserve the crime scene, you should avoid:
    a. untying the knot.
    b. cutting at least 6 inches above the knot.
    c. asking the police to manage the rope.
    d. using a sharp knife to make a clean cut in the rope.

44. Upon responding to a call for a cardiac arrest, you discover that the victim has been dead for hours; this appears to be an unattended death. To help preserve a possible crime scene, you should:
    a. leave the body in the position found.
    b. bag the victim's clothing in a brown paper bag for the police.
    c. wait for the police before touching the body to assess for signs of life.
    d. use the telephone at the victim's residence to call his doctor and ask about any advance directives.

45. While caring for the victim of a rape, the EMT can help to preserve evidence by:

    a. waiting for the police to arrive before talking to the patient.
    b. putting all the victim's clothing into one red bag and taking it along to the hospital.
    c. asking the victim not to change clothes or bathe.
    d. waiting for the police to interview the patient before treating any injuries.

46. Which of the following actions would be inappropriate for an EMT who is working at the scene of a call?

    a. assure scene safety
    b. provide patient care
    c. observe and document anything unusual at the scene
    d. document any suspicions based on prior calls to the scene

47. You are treating a 7-year-old girl who was bitten on the arm and hand by her neighbor's dog. The skin is broken and bleeding is controlled. The patient's mother has allowed you to care for the wounds but is refusing transport to the hospital and says that she will follow up with her pediatrician. This type of call is:

    a. reportable because of the animal bite.
    b. most likely to be associated with abuse.
    c. reportable because the patient is a minor.
    d. non-reportable.

48. An EMT is caring for a female who complains of abdominal pain. During the assessment and history taking, the patient reveals that she has been raped, but asks that this information not be disclosed to the police. Which of the following statements is most accurate regarding reporting of the rape?

    a. Failure to report this incident may actually be a crime.
    b. The EMT must keep the patient's information confidential upon her request.
    c. The patient has suffered a traumatic event and is not of sound mind to make such a request.
    d. The EMT can keep the information confidential from the hospital staff if the patient reports the crime on a hotline within 24 hours.

49. After responding to a call for an 80-year-old female who is unconscious, the EMT suspects that the patient may have taken too much of her medication, either accidentally or on purpose. The EMT should:

    a. consider this a crime scene and notify the police immediately.
    b. provide care for the patient, protect potential evidence, and notify the ED staff of his suspicions.
    c. provide care for the patient and wait to report the incident until the hospital can confirm an overdose.
    d. accurately document all suspicions and let the hospital make a report to the police.

50. Which statement is most accurate about avoiding lawsuits while working as an EMT?

    a. Only the EMT in charge of the call can be sued.
    b. Provide the right care and you can never be sued.
    c. Even if you provide the right care to your patient, you can be sued.
    d. Accurate documentation indicates good patient care, which can never result in a lawsuit.

Chapter 3 Answer Form

	A	B	C	D		A	B	C	D
1.	❏	❏	❏	❏	26.	❏	❏	❏	❏
2.	❏	❏	❏	❏	27.	❏	❏	❏	❏
3.	❏	❏	❏	❏	28.	❏	❏	❏	❏
4.	❏	❏	❏	❏	29.	❏	❏	❏	❏
5.	❏	❏	❏	❏	30.	❏	❏	❏	❏
6.	❏	❏	❏	❏	31.	❏	❏	❏	❏
7.	❏	❏	❏	❏	32.	❏	❏	❏	❏
8.	❏	❏	❏	❏	33.	❏	❏	❏	❏
9.	❏	❏	❏	❏	34.	❏	❏	❏	❏
10.	❏	❏	❏	❏	35.	❏	❏	❏	❏
11.	❏	❏	❏	❏	36.	❏	❏	❏	❏
12.	❏	❏	❏	❏	37.	❏	❏	❏	❏
13.	❏	❏	❏	❏	38.	❏	❏	❏	❏
14.	❏	❏	❏	❏	39.	❏	❏	❏	❏
15.	❏	❏	❏	❏	40.	❏	❏	❏	❏
16.	❏	❏	❏	❏	41.	❏	❏	❏	❏
17.	❏	❏	❏	❏	42.	❏	❏	❏	❏
18.	❏	❏	❏	❏	43.	❏	❏	❏	❏
19.	❏	❏	❏	❏	44.	❏	❏	❏	❏
20.	❏	❏	❏	❏	45.	❏	❏	❏	❏
21.	❏	❏	❏	❏	46.	❏	❏	❏	❏
22.	❏	❏	❏	❏	47.	❏	❏	❏	❏
23.	❏	❏	❏	❏	48.	❏	❏	❏	❏
24.	❏	❏	❏	❏	49.	❏	❏	❏	❏
25.	❏	❏	❏	❏	50.	❏	❏	❏	❏

Medical Terminology
and
Anatomy and Physiology

1. The _____ position is the stance of the body when it is erect with the arms and hands to the side, palms facing forward.
   a. prone
   b. supine
   c. anatomical
   d. recumbent

2. Terms related to the surface and depth of body parts include all of the following *except:*
   a. plane.
   b. parietal.
   c. internal.
   d. superficial.

3. Which of the following posterior regions of the spine contains seven vertebrae?
   a. cervical
   b. thoracic
   c. lumbar
   d. sacral

4. When describing the location of an injury to the wrist, which of the following statements is correct?
   a. bilateral to the hand
   b. distal to the forearm
   c. proximal to the elbow
   d. superior to the forearm

5. The _____ position is the body lying in a horizontal position with the face up.
   a. prone
   b. lateral
   c. supine
   d. anatomical

6. The quadrants of the abdomen are named for the:
   a. underlying organs in each.
   b. technique used to assess the abdomen.
   c. position on the body they occupy.
   d. physician who discovered them.

7. Which of the following structures lies mostly in the midline of the body?
   a. stomach
   b. heart
   c. esophagus
   d. large intestine

8. You are caring for an 18-year-old male who fell while skateboarding and broke his forearm in the middle. How would you describe the location of the fracture?
   a. The fracture is proximal to the shoulder.
   b. The fracture is midshaft in the forearm.
   c. The fracture is superior to the elbow.
   d. The fracture is located on the inferior portion of the humerus.

9. The imaginary line that runs vertically from the armpit down to the ankle is the:
   a. midline.
   b. mid-clavicular line.
   c. bilateral line.
   d. mid-axillary line.

10. You have just finished palpating the cervical spine of a victim involved in a motor vehicle collision. This area is referred to as the _____ neck.
    a. lateral
    b. inferior
    c. posterior
    d. transverse

11. The _____ is the cavity connecting the nose and mouth with the esophagus and trachea.
    a. glottis
    b. nares
    c. sinus
    d. pharynx

12. The cavity that contains the vocal cords or "voice box" is the:
    a. larynx.
    b. pharynx.
    c. glottis.
    d. nasal.

13. The _____ prevents food from entering the larynx.
    a. tongue
    b. trachea
    c. glottis
    d. epiglottis

14. Oxygen and carbon dioxide exchange takes place in the:
    a. alveoli.
    b. bronchi.
    c. bronchioles.
    d. alveolar ducts.

15. Lungs are held in an inflated state by:
    a. ligaments.
    b. negative pressure.
    c. positive pressure.
    d. the mediastinum.

16. The primary muscles involved in breathing are the _____ and the _____ muscles.
    a. pleural, pulmonary
    b. diaphragm, glottis
    c. diaphragm, intercostal
    d. intercostal, extracostal

17. The prefix *pneumo* means:
    a. lung.
    b. air.
    c. breath.
    d. gas.

18. To increase the space in the thorax, the diaphragm _____ and pulls _____.
    a. contracts, upward
    b. relaxes, upward
    c. contracts, downward
    d. relaxes, downward

19. The pleural spaces in the thoracic cavity are filled with:
    a. lobes.
    b. alveoli.
    c. bronchus.
    d. serous fluid.

20. The respiratory system supplies oxygen to the cells of the body and:
    a. removes carbon dioxide.
    b. is a branch of the digestive process.
    c. operates in the senses of smell and taste.
    d. activates the constriction and relaxation of blood vessels.

21. Heart sounds are caused by:
    a. blood rushing through the heart.
    b. the oxygenation of the heart muscle.
    c. offloading of deoxygenated blood from the vena cava.
    d. the opening and closing of valves.

22. The reason you can feel a pulse is:
    a. because of the force of blood on the arterial walls.
    b. because of the electrical impulse traveling through the vessels.
    c. because of the force of blood on the venous walls.
    d. because of the components of which the blood is made up.

23. Which of the following structures drains blood from the lower parts of the body?
    a. aorta
    b. inferior vena cava
    c. superior vena cava
    d. pulmonary artery

24. The _____ valve is the valve on the right side of the heart between the atrium and ventricle.
    a. aortic
    b. tricuspid
    c. bicuspid
    d. pulmonic

25. Which structure carries deoxygenated blood to the lungs?
    a. mitral valve
    b. pulmonary vein
    c. pulmonary artery
    d. superior vena cava

26. Plasma contains which of the following components?
    a. platelets
    b. red blood cells
    c. white blood cells
    d. minerals, salts, and proteins

27. As a baby matures into a child and then an adult, which structure of the heart enlarges to become the most muscular and strongest part of the heart?
    a. left atrium
    b. right atrium
    c. left ventricle
    d. right ventricle

28. Although the heart constantly has blood flowing through it, the heart receives its own blood supply from which vessel(s)?
    a. carotid artery
    b. coronary arteries
    c. pulmonary arteries
    d. superior vena cava

29. Blood is supplied to the extremities by _____ circulation.
    a. portal
    b. hepatic
    c. peripheral
    d. coronary

30. Necrosis, or death, of heart muscle is referred to as:
    a. myocardial infarction.
    b. cardiac tamponade.
    c. myocardial ischemia.
    d. coronary occlusion.

31. Which of the one-way valves of the heart is not working properly when there is a backflow of blood in the right ventricle?
    a. aortic
    b. bicuspid
    c. tricuspid
    d. pulmonary

32. When you are searching for a pulse on the posterior aspect of the medial malleolus, you are palpating the posterior _____ artery.
    a. tibial
    b. femoral
    c. dorsalis pedis
    d. brachial

33. Blood is carried back to the heart by way of:
    a. veins.
    b. arteries.
    c. osmosis.
    d. dialysis.

34. A clot of blood, bubble of air, or other substance that creates an obstruction in a blood vessel is a/an:
    a. edema.
    b. embolism.
    c. varicose.
    d. palpation.

35. The term *conduction* refers to an action in which there is a transmission of _____ through the heart.
    a. pulses
    b. platelets
    c. epinephrine
    d. electrical impulses

36. _____ are a form of connective tissue that are hardened by calcium.
    a. Bones
    b. Tendons
    c. Ligaments
    d. Cartilage

37. _____ is/are a form of connective tissue covering the epiphysis that act(s) as a smooth surface for articulation.
    a. Bones
    b. Cartilage
    c. Tendons
    d. Ligaments

38. While assessing for a radial pulse on an 18-month-old toddler, you palpate the:
    a. medial side of the forearm.
    b. proximal lateral side of the arm.
    c. distal lateral (thumb) side of the forearm.
    d. proximal lateral (thumb) side of the forearm.

39. _____ is a term for the sensation of labored breathing that may be characterized by noisy respirations or increased work of breathing.
    a. Apnea
    b. Dyspnea
    c. Tachypnea
    d. Tachycardia

40. Tenting of the skin is a condition associated with:
    a. alcoholism.
    b. dehydration.
    c. congestive heart failure.
    d. a communicable disease.

41. The 11th and 12th pairs of ribs are commonly referred to as "floating" ribs because:
    a. they are located below the lungs.
    b. they do not connect directly to the sternum.
    c. these two pairs are covered (floating) in synovial fluid.
    d. when fractured, they tend to cause major bleeding.

42. _____ is the term for fractured bone ends that are grinding together.
    a. Crunch
    b. Masticate
    c. Machete
    d. Crepitus

43. _____ is the type of muscle found in the walls of arteries and veins.
    a. Cardiac
    b. Skeletal
    c. Voluntary
    d. Smooth

44. The _____ is the socket of the hip joint where the head or end of the proximal femur fits.
    a. ilium
    b. pubis
    c. ischium
    d. acetabulum

45. The sternum or breastbone is divided into _____ sections.
    a. 2
    b. 3
    c. 4
    d. 5

46. During the secondary assessment, you discover pain and swelling on the humerus, which is located in the:
    a. lower arm.
    b. upper arm.
    c. pelvic girdle.
    d. lower extremity.

47. The central nervous system (CNS) is comprised of the:
    a. cranial nerves and skin.
    b. nerves, skin, and electrons.
    c. muscle receptors and glands.
    d. brain, brain stem, and spinal cord.

48. HEENT is a mnemonic used to help remember the items to examine on the:
    a. back.
    b. extremeties.
    c. head and face.
    d. hips and pelvis.

49. The involuntary nervous system is known as the:
    a. meninges.
    b. control center.
    c. vegetative organism.
    d. autonomic nervous system.

50. While plugging a vacuum cleaner plug into a wall socket, you receive a shock and instinctively pull your hand away. Which structures are responsible for sending the message of pain to your brain?
    a. motor nerves
    b. sensory nerves
    c. sympathetic response
    d. parasympathetic response

51. While you are driving your car, another vehicle unexpectedly pulls into your path. You quickly step on the brake and avoid a collision; simultaneously, you take a deep breath and your heart races. What part of your nervous system has speeded up your heart rate in response to this situation?
    a. autonomic
    b. motor nerves
    c. voluntary
    d. sensory nerves

52. The largest organ of the human body is the:
    a. skin.
    b. intestines.
    c. stomach.
    d. nervous system.

53. Sweat glands are located in which layer(s) of the skin?
    a. dermis
    b. epidermis
    c. subcutaneous
    d. dermis and epidermis

54. The _____ releases hormones that regulate metabolism and growth.
    a. thyroid
    b. kidney
    c. pancreas
    d. mammary gland

55. Except for the palms of the hands and the soles of the feet, the epidermis contains _____ layers.
    a. 2
    b. 3
    c. 4
    d. 5

56. The endocrine system is made up of _____ that produce _____, which help to regulate many body activities and functions.
    a. nerves, impulses
    b. vessels, platelets
    c. glands, hormones
    d. chemicals, plasma

57. The _____ produces insulin, a hormone that is critical in helping the body use glucose for fuel.
    a. thyroid
    b. pancreas
    c. adrenal glands
    d. gonads

58. The endocrine system includes which of the following reproductive organ(s)?
    a. ovaries and testes
    b. uterus
    c. mammary glands
    d. penis

59. The most common type of endocrine emergency that EMTs respond to is:
    a. a seizure.
    b. a diabetic emergency.
    c. a thyroid emergency.
    d. an allergic reaction.

60. Which of the following organs is *not* part of the endocrine system?
    a. kidneys
    b. pituitary gland
    c. thymus gland
    d. adrenal glands

61. The _____ is/are a strong, dome-shaped muscle(s) required for normal respirations.
    a. lungs
    b. tongue
    c. epiglottis
    d. diaphragm

62. The _____ is the pipe-shaped structure through which air moves from the larynx to the lungs.
    a. bronchi
    b. trachea
    c. epiglottis
    d. cricoid cartilage

63. The lower airways are comprised of _____ muscles.
    a. skeletal
    b. cardiac
    c. smooth
    d. voluntary

64. Respiratory exchange between the lung and blood vessels occurs in the:
    a. alveoli.
    b. bronchi.
    c. bronchioles.
    d. coronary vessels.

65. The _____ closes during swallowing to prevent food or liquids from entering the lower airways.
    a. larynx
    b. mouth
    c. trachea
    d. epiglottis

66. The primary respiratory center, which controls the stimulus to breathe, is located in the:
    a. brain.
    b. lungs.
    c. heart.
    d. diaphragm.

67. During exhalation, carbon dioxide is:
    a. converted to energy.
    b. eliminated from the body.
    c. dissolved into the bloodstream.
    d. retained as needed in asthmatics.

68. Hypoxia is defined as a:
    a. total absence of oxygen.
    b. lack of oxygen in the blood.
    c. deficit of red blood cells in the blood.
    d. lack of oxygen in the tissues of the body.

69. One of the major functions of the skin is:
    a. production of fat tissue.
    b. temperature regulation.
    c. the formation of white blood cells.
    d. the release of glucose into the blood.

70. The skin is part of the largest organ system of the body and is the:
    a. first line of defense against infection.
    b. juncture for the formation of red blood cells.
    c. structure that provides nourishment for the cells.
    d. structure that helps stimulates hormone production.

71. The intercostal muscles of the chest are classified as _____ muscle.
    a. skeletal
    b. smooth
    c. cardiac
    d. tensile-strength

72. When muscles contract, the normal result is:
    a. pain.
    b. strain.
    c. pressure.
    d. body movement.

73. A metabolic function of support provided by the skeletal system is the:
    a. production of blood cells.
    b. destruction of blood cells.
    c. regulation of blood glucose.
    d. stimulation of hair and nail growth.

74. The thorax (rib cage), spinal column, and skull are bones that:
    a. stimulate muscle growth.
    b. protect organs of the body.
    c. aid in movement of the body.
    d. contain storage sites for hormones.

75. A fracture that occurs through a process of weakening from disease is called a/an _____ fracture.
    a. epiphyseal
    b. pathological
    c. osteoporotic
    d. nondisplaced

Chapter 4 Answer Form

	A	B	C	D			A	B	C	D
1.	❏	❏	❏	❏		33.	❏	❏	❏	❏
2.	❏	❏	❏	❏		34.	❏	❏	❏	❏
3.	❏	❏	❏	❏		35.	❏	❏	❏	❏
4.	❏	❏	❏	❏		36.	❏	❏	❏	❏
5.	❏	❏	❏	❏		37.	❏	❏	❏	❏
6.	❏	❏	❏	❏		38.	❏	❏	❏	❏
7.	❏	❏	❏	❏		39.	❏	❏	❏	❏
8.	❏	❏	❏	❏		40.	❏	❏	❏	❏
9.	❏	❏	❏	❏		41.	❏	❏	❏	❏
10.	❏	❏	❏	❏		42.	❏	❏	❏	❏
11.	❏	❏	❏	❏		43.	❏	❏	❏	❏
12.	❏	❏	❏	❏		44.	❏	❏	❏	❏
13.	❏	❏	❏	❏		45.	❏	❏	❏	❏
14.	❏	❏	❏	❏		46.	❏	❏	❏	❏
15.	❏	❏	❏	❏		47.	❏	❏	❏	❏
16.	❏	❏	❏	❏		48.	❏	❏	❏	❏
17.	❏	❏	❏	❏		49.	❏	❏	❏	❏
18.	❏	❏	❏	❏		50.	❏	❏	❏	❏
19.	❏	❏	❏	❏		51.	❏	❏	❏	❏
20.	❏	❏	❏	❏		52.	❏	❏	❏	❏
21.	❏	❏	❏	❏		53.	❏	❏	❏	❏
22.	❏	❏	❏	❏		54.	❏	❏	❏	❏
23.	❏	❏	❏	❏		55.	❏	❏	❏	❏
24.	❏	❏	❏	❏		56.	❏	❏	❏	❏
25.	❏	❏	❏	❏		57.	❏	❏	❏	❏
26.	❏	❏	❏	❏		58.	❏	❏	❏	❏
27.	❏	❏	❏	❏		59.	❏	❏	❏	❏
28.	❏	❏	❏	❏		60.	❏	❏	❏	❏
29.	❏	❏	❏	❏		61.	❏	❏	❏	❏
30.	❏	❏	❏	❏		62.	❏	❏	❏	❏
31.	❏	❏	❏	❏		63.	❏	❏	❏	❏
32.	❏	❏	❏	❏		64.	❏	❏	❏	❏

	A	B	C	D		A	B	C	D
65.	❏	❏	❏	❏	71.	❏	❏	❏	❏
66.	❏	❏	❏	❏	72.	❏	❏	❏	❏
67.	❏	❏	❏	❏	73.	❏	❏	❏	❏
68.	❏	❏	❏	❏	74.	❏	❏	❏	❏
69.	❏	❏	❏	❏	75.	❏	❏	❏	❏
70.	❏	❏	❏	❏					

CHAPTER

5

Principles of Pathophysiology

1. In an adult, a fracture of which of the following bones can potentially result in a 1000 mL blood loss?
   a. tibia
   b. fibula
   c. femur
   d. humerus

2. A _____ is an injury to the ligaments around a joint.
   a. strain
   b. sprain
   c. fracture
   d. dislocation

3. Which of the following is not considered a neurological event?
   a. stroke
   b. seizure
   c. heart attack
   d. spinal cord injury

4. Of the following areas for possible dislocations, select the two most potentially serious due to the possibility of complete disruption of blood supply to the distal body part.
   a. knee and elbow
   b. hip and knee
   c. elbow and wrist
   d. shoulder and knee

5. _____ is swelling in the upper airways caused by an infection and is marked by a mild or severe seal-like bark; it usually occurs in children in the 3-month to 3-year age group.
   a. Croup
   b. Asthma
   c. Epiglottitis
   d. Bronchiolitis

6. _____ is an infection that results in a swelling of the lower airways and typically occurs in children less than 2 years of age during the winter and spring seasons.
   a. Croup
   b. Epiglottitis
   c. Bronchiolitis
   d. Emphysema

7. _____ is a whistling sound caused by constriction of the lower airways and is most often heard at the end of exhalation.
   a. Stridor
   b. Croup
   c. Grunting
   d. Wheezing

8. _____ is an abnormal condition that results in a collection of air in the pleural space of the chest; it can cause one or both lungs to collapse.
   a. Pleurisy
   b. Pneumonia
   c. Pneumothorax
   d. Tension pneumothorax

9. A pulmonary embolism is a respiratory abnormality that will affect perfusion by:
   a. causing bronchoconstriction.
   b. filling the lungs with fluid.
   c. blocking a pulmonary artery.
   d. suddenly filling the chest cavity with air.

10. When the heart fails to pump adequately because it has become injured, cardiac output decreases and:
    a. blood backs up in the venous system.
    b. blood backs up in the arterial system.
    c. the kidneys increase urine producing.
    d. the patient will develop ventricular fibrillation.

11. Chronic hypertension (high blood pressure) increases the workload of the heart and:
    a. dilates the coronary arteries.
    b. constricts the pulmonary arteries.
    c. enlarges the left ventricle of the heart.
    d. enlarges the right ventricle of the heart.

12. When an artery to the brain is temporarily occluded by a blood clot, the condition is a:
    a. closed head injury.
    b. non-life-threatening emergency.
    c. life-threatening emergency called a stroke.
    d. life-threatening emergency called a mini-stroke.

13. When a group of neurons in the brain produce excessive electrical discharge, the patient will be experiencing a:
    a. stroke.
    b. seizure.
    c. dementia.
    d. hypertensive crisis.

14. You are treating a patient who is bleeding from an ulcer. She is pale, is breathing rapidly, has a heart rate of 120, and a blood pressure of 128/80. What type of shock is the patient experiencing?
    a. neurogenic
    b. irreversible
    c. compensated
    d. decompensated

15. A patient with signs and symptoms of shock including low blood pressure and a slow heart rate and is not taking any medications is most likely experiencing _____ shock.
    a. cardiogenic
    b. obstructive
    c. anaphylactic
    d. septic

16. Which of the following formulas is correct? CO = cardiac output, BP = blood pressure, and SVR = systemic vascular resistance.
    a. $BP = CO \times SVR$
    b. $CO = BP \times SVR$
    c. $SVR = CO \times BP$
    d. They are all correct.

17. People with diabetes have a _____ that may cause the blood sugar level to become too high or too low.
    a. tumor
    b. cellular injury
    c. hormonal imbalance
    d. hypersensitivity syndrome

18. Which hormone moves sugar molecules from the blood into the cells, where they are stored?
    a. insulin
    b. glucagon
    c. epinephrine
    d. norepinephrine

19. A baseball player was struck in the head and was stunned for several minutes, but never lost consciousness. He now complains of a headache. What type of traumatic brain injury did he most likely experience?
    a. TIA
    b. stroke
    c. contusion
    d. concussion

20. Some diabetic patients develop neuropathy as a complication of the disease. As a result, a patient with neuropathy might not be able to feel:
    a. ulcers on their feet.
    b. trauma from poor fitting shoes.
    c. chest pain from a heart attack.
    d. all of the above.

21. A patient with symptoms of nausea and diarrhea describes his most recent stool as dark and loose. This is an indication of possible:
    a. appendicitis.
    b. food poisoning.
    c. lower gastrointestinal bleeding.
    d. upper gastrointestinal bleeding.

22. A trauma patient has signs of shock but has no external bleeding. What is the most likely source of blood loss?
    a. abdominal injury
    b. closed head injury
    c. myocardial infarction
    d. spinal cord injury

23. _____ is the major cause of a progressive and irreversible disease of the airway called COPD.
    a. Asthma
    b. Smoking
    c. Heredity
    d. An environmental allergy

24. A condition that produced constriction of the bronchi, wheezing, and dyspnea and is the leading cause of chronic illness in children is:
    a. COPD.
    b. croup.
    c. asthma.
    d. bronchitis.

25. _____ is an abnormal accumulation of fluid in the abdominal cavity.
    a. Rales
    b. Rabies
    c. Ascites
    d. Peripheral edema

Chapter 5 Answer Form

	A	B	C	D
1.	❏	❏	❏	❏
2.	❏	❏	❏	❏
3.	❏	❏	❏	❏
4.	❏	❏	❏	❏
5.	❏	❏	❏	❏
6.	❏	❏	❏	❏
7.	❏	❏	❏	❏
8.	❏	❏	❏	❏
9.	❏	❏	❏	❏
10.	❏	❏	❏	❏
11.	❏	❏	❏	❏
12.	❏	❏	❏	❏
13.	❏	❏	❏	❏

	A	B	C	D
14.	❏	❏	❏	❏
15.	❏	❏	❏	❏
16.	❏	❏	❏	❏
17.	❏	❏	❏	❏
18.	❏	❏	❏	❏
19.	❏	❏	❏	❏
20.	❏	❏	❏	❏
21.	❏	❏	❏	❏
22.	❏	❏	❏	❏
23.	❏	❏	❏	❏
24.	❏	❏	❏	❏
25.	❏	❏	❏	❏

CHAPTER

Life Span Development

1. A respiratory rate of 20 to 30 breaths per minute is normal in each of the following age groups, except:
   a. toddlers.
   b. preschool.
   c. school-age.
   d. adolescents.

2. The basics of language are normally mastered by:
   a. infancy.
   b. 36 months.
   c. school-age.
   d. preschool age.

3. During the first year of life, the heart rate of an infant slows to an average of _____ beats per minute.
   a. 120
   b. 140
   c. 160
   d. 180

4. The normal respiratory rate for adolescents is _____ breaths per minute.
   a. 12 to 20
   b. 20 to 30
   c. 25 to 35
   d. 30 to 40

5. In which developmental age group do children lose their primary teeth?
   a. toddler
   b. preschool
   c. school-age
   d. adolescent

6. Which developmental age group has the highest metabolic and oxygen consumption rates?
   a. infants
   b. children
   c. adolescents
   d. adults

7. Proportionate to each age group, which has the most prevalent normal weight gain?
   a. infants
   b. children
   c. adults
   d. the elderly

8. Which of the following vital signs remains the same from adolescence through late adulthood?
   a. temperature
   b. heart rate
   c. respiratory rate
   d. blood pressure

9. Most adolescent girls complete their growth by age:
   a. 13.
   b. 16.
   c. 18.
   d. 20.

10. Separation anxiety or fear and crying when separated from parents or caregivers begins at which age?
    a. 18 months
    b. 2 years
    c. 30 months
    d. 3 years

11. In the _____ age group most primary teeth are lost and replaced with permanent teeth.
    a. toddler
    b. preschool
    c. school
    d. adolescence

12. During adolescence _____ develop(s), producing specific patterns of body hair, fat distribution, and growth of external genitalia.
    a. muscle mass
    b. bone growth
    c. primary sexual characteristics
    d. secondary sexual characteristics

13. Typically, persons reach a peak in physical conditioning between _____ years of age.
    a. 16 and 20
    b. 20 and 25
    c. 25 and 30
    d. 30 and 35

14. The leading cause of death among early adults is:
    a. obesity.
    b. cancer.
    c. accidents.
    d. heart attacks.

15. In which age group does near vision (reading) begin to become more difficult without reading glasses?
    a. adolescence
    b. early adult
    c. middle adult
    d. late adult

16. As a person ages, changes in the _____ have a major effect on the metabolism of many drugs.
    a. respiratory system
    b. gastrointestinal system
    c. endocrine system
    d. renal function

17. In late adulthood, the bone marrow produces fewer red blood cells and may cause which of the following conditions?
    a. anemia
    b. anoxia
    c. arteriosclerosis
    d. atherosclerosis

18. In late adulthood, the heart muscle is less able to respond to exercise because:
    a. the muscle is less elastic.
    b. there is calcium deficiency.
    c. cortisol production increases.
    d. metabolism slows down.

19. Blood vessel walls _____ as adults mature in late adulthood.
    a. thicken
    b. thin out
    c. stretch
    d. become more sensitive

20. Weight control, menopause, and cancer are common and important considerations in the _____ group.
    a. female adolescent
    b. female early adult
    c. female middle adult
    d. female late adult

21. In the late adult group, _____ may result in development of a serious disease with very few signs or symptoms.
    a. hearing loss
    b. decreased reaction times
    c. decreased pain perception
    d. decreased appetite with weight loss

22. People in late adulthood typically go to sleep early and rise early in the morning. The most likely system that contributes to this sleep–wake cycle is:
    a. cardiac.
    b. nervous.
    c. sensory.
    d. endocrine.

23. _____ is/are a major problem associated with diminished visual acuity in the late adult group.
    a. Falls
    b. Alcoholism
    c. Suicide
    d. Loss of appetite

24. Decreased muscle mass in the chest associated with aging results in:
    a. chest wall weakness.
    b. decreased elasticity of the diaphragm.
    c. loss of normal mucous membrane lining.
    d. decreased pain perception in the chest.

25. Major psychosocial challenges of late adulthood include decreased self-worth, declining well-being, and:
    a. financial burdens.
    b. increased peer pressure.
    c. increased self-consciousness.
    d. increased interest in the opposite sex.

Chapter 6 Answer Form

	A	B	C	D		A	B	C	D
1.	❑	❑	❑	❑	14.	❑	❑	❑	❑
2.	❑	❑	❑	❑	15.	❑	❑	❑	❑
3.	❑	❑	❑	❑	16.	❑	❑	❑	❑
4.	❑	❑	❑	❑	17.	❑	❑	❑	❑
5.	❑	❑	❑	❑	18.	❑	❑	❑	❑
6.	❑	❑	❑	❑	19.	❑	❑	❑	❑
7.	❑	❑	❑	❑	20.	❑	❑	❑	❑
8.	❑	❑	❑	❑	21.	❑	❑	❑	❑
9.	❑	❑	❑	❑	22.	❑	❑	❑	❑
10.	❑	❑	❑	❑	23.	❑	❑	❑	❑
11.	❑	❑	❑	❑	24.	❑	❑	❑	❑
12.	❑	❑	❑	❑	25.	❑	❑	❑	❑
13.	❑	❑	❑	❑					

CHAPTER 7

Lifting and Moving Patients

1. The number one injury suffered by prehospital care providers is:
   a. needle stick.
   b. back injury.
   c. airborne infection.
   d. bloodborne infection.

2. _____ refers to safe lifting and moving techniques that help prevent personal injury.
   a. Supination
   b. Body mechanics
   c. Proprioception
   d. Hydraulics

3. To help avoid a back injury when lifting any patient, the EMT should:
   a. keep her back straight and locked.
   b. call the fire department and wait for assistance.
   c. never lift a patient who weighs more than 200 pounds.
   d. only lift with another EMT of the same size and weight.

4. Which of the following is not considered proper form for the EMT who is about to lift and carry a patient who weighs more than 150 pounds?
   a. Lift with the legs, not the back.
   b. Avoid keeping the weight close to one's body.
   c. Avoid lifting on uneven surfaces whenever possible.
   d. Avoid leaning to the left or right to compensate for the weight.

5. To keep a stretcher from becoming unbalanced and possibly tipping, the EMT should:
   a. keep the center of gravity close to the ground.
   b. always use four people to lift the stretcher while moving on stairs.
   c. only raise and lower from the ends of the stretcher, not the sides.
   d. never place a patient weighing more than 250 pounds in the sitting position.

6. The _____ is(are) most commonly utilized by EMTs during safe lifting of a stretcher.
   a. four-person method
   b. power lift and power grip
   c. method with one EMT on each side
   d. none of the above

7. Of the following, the most critical factor in selecting the type of patient-carrying device is:
   a. the age of the patient.
   b. the gender of the patient.
   c. the weight of the patient.
   d. a suspected spinal injury.

8. The extremity lift, direct ground lift, and firefighter's carry are all moving techniques that would be appropriate for moving patients:
   a. who are apneic and pulseless.
   b. with a suspected spinal injury.
   c. with no suspected spinal injury.
   d. who are contaminated with hazardous materials.

9. To avoid injury while carrying a single piece of equipment with only the right hand, it is necessary to:
   a. carry the object in front of the body.
   b. avoid leaning to the left.
   c. lean to the loaded side of the body.
   d. carry another item of equal weight in the other hand to balance the load.

10. You are treating and need to transport a patient who is considerably overweight, but your stretcher will not fit the patient. Now you notify dispatch to:
    a. call the fire department and request transport by fire engine.
    b. request a bariatric stretcher from a mutual aide EMS service.
    c. request a special needs transport bus from the city bus garage.
    d. encourage the patient to go by private vehicle with a family member.

11. Which of the following carrying methods or devices is the least safe for getting a patient down a flight of stairs?

    a. stair chair
    b. long backboard
    c. extremity carry
    d. scoop stretcher

12. The _____ is an ideal lifting device for getting a conscious non ambulatory patient safely out of a basement.

    a. Reeves
    b. stretcher
    c. stair chair
    d. long backboard

13. The only moving technique in which twisting is helpful and not potentially harmful to the EMT is:

    a. lifting.
    b. lowering.
    c. when reaching.
    d. none of the above.

14. Reaching for a piece of equipment or for a patient increases the risk of injury for the EMT and can be avoided by:

    a. moving closer to the object.
    b. leaning forward from the waist.
    c. keeping the knees locked.
    d. extending and locking the elbows.

15. To avoid back injury, the EMT should _____ to keep the back straight while lifting.

    a. exhale while lifting
    b. place both feet together
    c. take a deep breath and hold it
    d. keep the chin tucked to the chest

16. When performing a logroll to get a patient onto a long spine board, the proper reaching technique includes:

    a. reaching with the low back arched.
    b. keeping your head as low as possible.
    c. leaning from the hips with your back locked.
    d. extending and locking the elbows.

17. While pushing and pulling a stretcher from the ambulance, the guidelines recommend:

    a. always push and never pull.
    b. tucking your chin into your chest and locking your back.
    c. keeping your elbows bent and your arms close to your torso.
    d. asking the patient her weight so you can make the proper adjustment.

18. Pushing or pulling equipment and other objects is routine for the EMT. To significantly help decrease the risk of injury, she should avoid pushing or pulling:

    a. overhead.
    b. backward.
    c. a wheeled stair chair.
    d. anything that has wheels.

19. You are treating the victim of a motor vehicle collision (MVC) who has an altered mental status and suspected cervical injury. Her condition is deteriorating rapidly. Which of the following moves is most appropriate for this patient?

    a. direct
    b. urgent
    c. emergency
    d. nonurgent

20. For moving a patient with no suspected spinal injury, which of the following considerations is most commonly utilized by the EMT?

    a. the age of the patient
    b. ease of lifting for the EMT
    c. distance to the hospital
    d. position of comfort for the patient

21. After responding to a call for a respiratory arrest, you find the patient lying on the floor between her bed and the wall. You and your partner move her out into the middle of the room where there is space to work. This move is considered:

    a. an urgent move.
    b. a nonurgent move.
    c. inappropriate without the use of a cervical collar and backboard.
    d. foolish because of the potential for a back injury to the EMTs.

22. In which of the following situations would it be appropriate to use an urgent move?

    a. 43-year-old driver complaining of neck pain entrapped in the driver's side of a stable vehicle
    b. a female in her thirties who is having a seizure while lying on the floor in a department store
    c. a 50-year-old female who collapsed while working outside on a very hot day
    d. a crying 18-month-old infant who is in a car seat at the scene of a minor MVC

23. The _____ stretcher is typically made of canvas and has wooden slats for stability and carrying handles on the sides.

    a. scoop
    b. wheeled
    c. basket
    d. flexible or Reeves

24. A _____ is a carrying device consisting of an aluminum frame and a rectangular tube with shovel-type side flaps for sliding underneath the patient.

a. stair chair
b. scoop stretcher
c. basket stretcher
d. Stokes® basket

25. When moving a patient who has a suspected spinal injury, which of the following methods or devices would not be appropriate?

a. logroll
b. extremity lift
c. basket stretcher
d. short spine board

Chapter 7 Answer Form

	A	B	C	D
1.	❏	❏	❏	❏
2.	❏	❏	❏	❏
3.	❏	❏	❏	❏
4.	❏	❏	❏	❏
5.	❏	❏	❏	❏
6.	❏	❏	❏	❏
7.	❏	❏	❏	❏
8.	❏	❏	❏	❏
9.	❏	❏	❏	❏
10.	❏	❏	❏	❏
11.	❏	❏	❏	❏
12.	❏	❏	❏	❏
13.	❏	❏	❏	❏

	A	B	C	D
14.	❏	❏	❏	❏
15.	❏	❏	❏	❏
16.	❏	❏	❏	❏
17.	❏	❏	❏	❏
18.	❏	❏	❏	❏
19.	❏	❏	❏	❏
20.	❏	❏	❏	❏
21.	❏	❏	❏	❏
22.	❏	❏	❏	❏
23.	❏	❏	❏	❏
24.	❏	❏	❏	❏
25.	❏	❏	❏	❏

SECTION

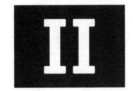

II

AIRWAY

CHAPTER

8

Airway

1. The upper airway consists of the:
   a. mouth, uvula, and carina.
   b. nose, mouth, and bronchioles.
   c. mouth, nasopharynx, and oropharynx.
   d. oropharynx, nasopharynx, and bronchi.

2. The potential space between the visceral and parietal pleura is known as the:
   a. epiglottis.
   b. alveoli sac.
   c. diaphragm.
   d. pleural space.

3. The lower airway begins at which of the following structures?
   a. carina
   b. bronchi
   c. larynx
   d. diaphragm

4. The right and left lungs are separated in the chest by the:
   a. vallecula.
   b. mediastinum.
   c. glottic opening.
   d. mainstem bronchi.

5. _____ reflex is a reliable indication that a patient is unable to protect her own airway.
   a. A positive gag
   b. Loss of the gag
   c. A positive cough
   d. Loss of the sneezing

6. You are managing an unresponsive patient and attempt to establish a patent airway by performing a head-tilt, chin-lift maneuver. There is no need to suction, so the next step is to:
   a. insert an oral airway.
   b. obtain an SpO_2 reading.
   c. hyperventilate the patient.
   d. intubate with a large ET tube.

7. Managing a patient's airway with simple or advanced techniques is a messy skill and always requires:
   a. suction.
   b. body substance isolation.
   c. the use of sterile procedures.
   d. the use of endotracheal tubes.

8. An unresponsive patient who is seizing has clenched teeth and abnormal respirations. Which of the following airway adjuncts would be appropriate for this patient?
   a. oral intubation
   b. French catheter
   c. oropharyngeal airway
   d. nasopharyngeal airway

9. One of the easiest and least invasive methods of correcting airway obstruction caused by the tongue is:
   a. the head-tilt chin-lift maneuver.
   b. to suction the oropharynx as needed.
   c. to awaken the patient as soon as possible.
   d. to insert a nasopharyngeal airway into one or both nostrils.

10. When performing the head-tilt chin-lift maneuver, the EMT should begin by:
    a. moving the patient onto a long backboard.
    b. placing the patient in a supine position.
    c. moving the patient into the recovery position.
    d. turning the patient over into the prone position.

11. The head-tilt chin-lift maneuver is helpful in all of the following situations, except for a/an:
    a. unresponsive diabetic who is drooling.
    b. postictal seizure patient who is alert to painful stimuli.
    c. 75-year-old male found in cardiac arrest on the floor at home.
    d. basketball player who was knocked unconscious and has not awakened.

12. A 2-year-old child was reported to have been choking on a foreign body while in his high chair, and became unresponsive just prior to your arrival. The first step you take to open and maintain his airway is to:

    a. use a jaw-thrust maneuver.
    b. measure and insert an oral airway.
    c. perform a head-tilt chin-lift maneuver.
    d. roll him into the recovery position and perform back blows.

13. You have been called to care for a patient with an altered mental status, whom you suspect has a head injury as a result of a traumatic injury. While you are immobilizing the patient, he becomes unresponsive. Which method is the recommended procedure to open and maintain this patient's airway?

    a. Place the patient supine and use a jaw-thrust maneuver.
    b. Place the patient supine and use a head-tilt chin-lift maneuver.
    c. Roll the patient into the recovery position, allowing secretions to drain from the mouth.
    d. Finish immobilizing the patient on a long board and hold the mouth open with your thumb and forefinger.

14. Your patient is the driver of a vehicle that was hit head on. He is still belted into the driver's seat, and there is evidence that his neck struck the steering wheel. He is having difficulty breathing and is becoming unresponsive. The first step you take to open and maintain his airway is to:

    a. suction the mouth and nose, then insert an oral airway.
    b. hold cervical stabilization while your partner applies a non-rebreather mask with high flow.
    c. quickly place a cervical collar on the patient and perform a rapid extrication.
    d. hold cervical stabilization while you sit him up and open his airway using the jaw-thrust maneuver.

15. When performing the jaw-thrust maneuver, the EMT places his fingers on:

    a. the patient's chin and bridge of the nose.
    b. each side of the patient's head just above the ears.
    c. the patient's chin and upper jaw just below the nose.
    d. each side of the patient's lower jaw just below the ears.

16. The primary objective of the jaw-thrust maneuver is to:

    a. not stimulate a gag reflex.
    b. open the airway as soon as possible.
    c. open the airway without moving the head or neck.
    d. clear any obstructions or secretions as soon as possible.

17. The optimal position for the EMT while performing a jaw-thrust maneuver is:

    a. over the patient's torso with one hand on each side of the patient's lower jaw.
    b. beside the patient's head with one hand on each side of the patient's upper jaw.
    c. beside the patient's torso with one hand on each side of the patient's head.
    d. at the top of the patient's head with elbows resting on the same surface as the patient's head.

18. Suction units with rigid-tip catheters are designed for removal of:

    a. big chunks of food.
    b. blood and broken teeth.
    c. blood, fluid, and secretions.
    d. foreign body airway obstructions (FBAOs).

19. The danger of aspirating vomitus is that:

    a. stomach acids can easily destroy lung tissue.
    b. it can paralyze the vocal cords.
    c. it increases the ability to ventilate.
    d. it can cause the tongue to swell creating an airway obstruction.

20. When suctioning the oropharynx of an adult, the _____ device is preferred because you can direct where the tip is going.

    a. rigid-tip
    b. soft-tip
    c. semi-rigid
    d. French catheter

21. As a general rule for suctioning the upper airway of a patient, the suction is applied:

    a. before, during, and on the way out of the oropharynx.
    b. while guiding the catheter around the airway adjunct.
    c. after insertion of the catheter tip into the oropharynx and on the way out.
    d. after measuring the catheter and during insertion of the catheter into the oropharynx.

22. Suctioning a patient carries a high risk of exposure for the EMT. The recommended PPE includes:

    a. mask, gloves, and gown.
    b. eye protection and gloves.
    c. gloves, gown, and eye protection.
    d. gloves, eye protection, and mask.

23. While suctioning a patient with a soft or flexible catheter, oxygen delivery is:

    a. discontinued only while suctioning.
    b. reduced until suction is completed.
    c. discontinued only during insertion of the catheter.
    d. never discontinued, as oxygen delivery is very important.

24. Pocket face masks are made of clear plastic so that the EMT can:

    a. protect himself from exposure to vomitus.

    b. see if the mask is properly placed on the face.

    c. recognize when the patient needs to be suctioned.

    d. observe the mouth and nose for signs of spontaneous breathing.

25. When measuring an oropharyngeal airway for insertion into a patient, the EMT measures:

    a. from the tip of the nose to the angle of the jaw.

    b. from the center of the chin to the earlobe.

    c. the length of the patient's pinky (fifth digit or little) finger.

    d. the distance from the center of the lips to the angle of the jaw.

26. Oropharyngeal airways (OPAs) are made of hard plastic and are designed to:

    a. prevent the tongue from obstructing the glottis.

    b. keep the patient from choking on secretions.

    c. prevent the patient from aspirating vomit.

    d. prevent the patient from gagging.

27. The use of an OPA is indicated when a patient:

    a. is experiencing a seizure.

    b. is unconscious without a gag reflex.

    c. has an altered mental status and is choking.

    d. has broken teeth as a result of trauma to the face.

28. Before inserting a nasopharyngeal airway (NPA) into a patient, the EMT must:

    a. lubricate the tube with petroleum jelly.

    b. perform a head-tilt chin-lift maneuver.

    c. lubricate the tube with a water-soluble jelly.

    d. hyperventilate the patient using high-flow oxygen.

29. Dispatch has sent your unit to a fast-food restaurant for a choking victim. Arrival time was very short since you were returning from another call. When you arrive, bystanders summon you to a 16-year-old male who is in the men's room. The patient is responsive, cyanotic, and working hard to breathe. When you get closer, you hear faint stridor when he tries to breathe in. What do these findings indicate?

    a. complete airway obstruction

    b. partial airway obstruction with poor air exchange

    c. partial airway obstruction with adequate air exchange

    d. partial airway obstruction requiring immediate suctioning

30. (Continuing with the previous question) What immediate intervention is appropriate?

    a. Perform abdominal thrusts.

    b. Suction the patient's oropharynx.

    c. Administer high-flow oxygen and transport him.

    d. Assist ventilations with a bag mask device and high-flow oxygen.

Chapter 8 Answer Form

	A	B	C	D			A	B	C	D
1.	❏	❏	❏	❏		16.	❏	❏	❏	❏
2.	❏	❏	❏	❏		17.	❏	❏	❏	❏
3.	❏	❏	❏	❏		18.	❏	❏	❏	❏
4.	❏	❏	❏	❏		19.	❏	❏	❏	❏
5.	❏	❏	❏	❏		20.	❏	❏	❏	❏
6.	❏	❏	❏	❏		21.	❏	❏	❏	❏
7.	❏	❏	❏	❏		22.	❏	❏	❏	❏
8.	❏	❏	❏	❏		23.	❏	❏	❏	❏
9.	❏	❏	❏	❏		24.	❏	❏	❏	❏
10.	❏	❏	❏	❏		25.	❏	❏	❏	❏
11.	❏	❏	❏	❏		26.	❏	❏	❏	❏
12.	❏	❏	❏	❏		27.	❏	❏	❏	❏
13.	❏	❏	❏	❏		28.	❏	❏	❏	❏
14.	❏	❏	❏	❏		29.	❏	❏	❏	❏
15.	❏	❏	❏	❏		30.	❏	❏	❏	❏

CHAPTER

Respiration and Artificial Respiration

1. Oxygenated blood from the lungs enters the _____ of the heart and is pumped to the tissues of the body.
   a. left atrium
   b. left ventricle
   c. right atrium
   d. right ventricle

2. Which of the following is a sign of inadequate breathing?
   a. skin color that is pink or flushed
   b. air movement out of the mouth and nose
   c. equal and prolonged exhalations with grunting
   d. equal expansion of both sides of the chest during inhalation

3. To properly assess a pediatric patient for adequate breathing, the EMT will need to:
   a. position the patient upright.
   b. expose the torso to perform a complete exam.
   c. reposition the patient in semi-Fowler's position.
   d. assess by looking, listening, and feeling for signs of adequate breathing.

4. Which of the following is most likely an indication of inadequate breathing?
   a. a pulse oximetry reading of 90 percent
   b. slow and deep respirations while sleeping
   c. snoring respirations while sleeping
   d. wheezing sounds that can be heard without a stethoscope

5. When a patient is showing signs of inadequate breathing, the first step the EMT should take is:
   a. apply high-flow oxygen.
   b. assure that the airway is open and will remain open.
   c. expose the chest and stabilize any holes or fractures.
   d. insert an airway adjunct and suction as necessary.

6. _____ is a condition characterized by blue or gray skin color as a result of hypoxia.
   a. COPD
   b. Cyanosis
   c. Epistaxis
   d. Diaphoresis

7. Ventilating a patient with a pocket mask requires that the EMT be able to do all of the following, *except*:
   a. maintain a good mask seal over the patient's mouth only.
   b. maintain a good mask seal over the patient's mouth and nose.
   c. suction and properly insert an airway adjunct prior to ventilating.
   d. hold the mask firmly in place while maintaining the proper head tilt.

8. Which of the following statements is most correct about ventilations provided with a pocket face mask?
   a. Pocket face masks are one-size-fits-all patients.
   b. When used properly, the face mask will deliver higher volumes of air than a bag mask device.
   c. All pocket face masks protect the rescuer from exposure to patient secretions.
   d. When used with supplemental oxygen, the face mask will deliver an oxygen concentration of 90 percent.

9. You need to ventilate a child patient with a bag mask device while using the jaw-thrust maneuver. Ventilations will be delivered:
   a. over 1 to 1½ seconds.
   b. over 1½ to 2 seconds.
   c. before securing the pop-off valve.
   d. after you have confirmed that there is no suspected spinal injury.

10. Ventilating a patient with a bag mask device while using the jaw-thrust maneuver requires a minimum of _____ rescuer(s).
    a. one
    b. two
    c. three
    d. four

11. When ventilating an unresponsive apneic patient with a bag mask device, the EMT should squeeze in _____ cc without oxygen connected and squeeze in _____ cc with oxygen connected.
    a. 600; 800
    b. 800; 600
    c. 1,000; 800
    d. 1,200; 1,000

12. When a patient's chest does not appear to be rising and falling adequately, it is appropriate to use which of the following oxygen delivery devices first?
    a. nasal cannula at 6 lpm
    b. positive pressure ventilation
    c. automatic transport ventilator
    d. high-flow oxygen by non-rebreather mask

13. Using the jaw-thrust maneuver while ventilating with a bag mask device is indicated:
    a. on a patient with a suspected neck, spine, or head injury.
    b. on an adult patient who is experiencing status epilepticus.
    c. for the patient who is entrapped and awaiting extrication.
    d. when the head-tilt chin-lift maneuver is not adequate for opening the airway.

14. One of the primary advantages of a bag mask device is that the:
    a. bag mask device can be used with one hand.
    b. EMT can easily decontaminate the device for reuse on another patient.
    c. bag mask device provides an infection control barrier between the EMT and the patient.
    d. EMT can deliver higher volumes of air than ventilations with a pocket face mask.

15. Bag mask device systems are available in _____ sizes.
    a. one-size-fits-all
    b. adult and child
    c. adult, child, and infant
    d. obese adult, adult, and child

16. Which of the following items is not a part of a bag mask device system?
    a. nasal prongs
    b. oxygen tubing
    c. reservoir bag
    d. clear face mask

17. The greatest disadvantage for one rescuer ventilating a patient with a bag mask device is:
    a. not squeezing the bag fast enough.
    b. not squeezing the bag hard enough.
    c. obtaining a proper mask seal on the face.
    d. there is no disadvantage for one rescuer ventilating with a bag mask device.

18. When two EMTs are ventilating an adult patient using a bag mask device, one EMT will squeeze the bag:
    a. once every 6 seconds.
    b. enough to assure that the patient is hyperventilated.
    c. to produce a minimum ventilation of 1,500 mL.
    d. to produce a minimum ventilation of 1,000 mL.

19. Before beginning two-rescuer ventilations with a bag mask device, one EMT should:
    a. call for backup assistance.
    b. immobilize the patient's head and neck.
    c. check the patient's wallet for identification.
    d. suction as needed and insert an airway adjunct.

20. Several minutes after you use a bag mask device to ventilate a patient who is in respiratory distress, you reassess the patient and find that your ventilations are adequate. Which of the following signs have you found?
    a. improved skin color
    b. rapid spontaneous breathing
    c. resistance to your ventilations
    d. air is moving out of the mouth and nose

21. Which of the following is an indication that your ventilations with a bag mask device are adequate?
    a. equal chest expansion and rise
    b. a heart rate that decreases from 60 to 40 beats per minute
    c. it takes more strength to squeeze the bag
    d. the abdomen rises with each squeeze of the bag

22. Which of the following methods is most reliable for assessing the adequacy of ventilations with a bag mask device?
    a. getting a pulse oximetry reading over 95 percent
    b. noting good compliance while squeezing the bag
    c. auscultating both sides of the chest with a stethoscope
    d. noting that the reservoir bag is filling completely between ventilations

23. Using a bag mask device, you are ventilating an unresponsive patient who initially was breathing too slowly. Squeezing the bag is difficult and after a couple of minutes you see no improvement. Which of the following is most likely the problem?
    a. No airway adjunct is in place.
    b. The patient is having a heart attack.
    c. You are not squeezing the bag fast enough.
    d. You are not allowing the bag enough time to refill with oxygen.

24. Which of the following conditions will most likely be the cause of inadequate ventilation with the use of a bag mask device?
    a. poor mask seal
    b. ventilating with one rescuer
    c. no oxygen supply to the reservoir
    d. squeezing the bag with two hands

25. No chest rise, difficulty squeezing the bag, and decreased breath sounds are all:
    a. signs that the patient requires suction.
    b. indications that the patient is in shock.
    c. signs of inadequate ventilation using a bag mask device.
    d. indications that oxygen is not attached to the bag mask device.

26. You have just arrived on the scene where an elderly female is unresponsive. The family suspects she may have taken too much of her pain medication by accident. Her respirations are slow and shallow; pulse rate is 60, strong and regular; you have not obtained a BP yet. You begin to assist her ventilations with a bag mask device and find that you are unable to make a good mask seal because her dentures are out. What can you do to improve ventilations?
    a. Squeeze the bag faster.
    b. Squeeze the bag harder.
    c. Use two hands to make the mask seal.
    d. Reinsert the dentures and try to ventilate again.

27. When the relief valve is activated on a flow-restricted, oxygen-powered ventilation device (FROPVD), it will cause:
    a. an audible alarm.
    b. a pneumothorax.
    c. gastric distention.
    d. the device to shut off.

28. A primary advantage of using a FROPVD is that:
    a. it never has to be decontaminated.
    b. the trigger is an inexpensive, disposable item.
    c. this device does not need a lot of oxygen as a power source.
    d. one rescuer can use both hands to maintain a seal while triggering the device.

29. A major disadvantage of using a FROPVD is that:
    a. it can be used only on adult patients.
    b. there is no disadvantage with the use of this device.
    c. it cannot be used on a patient with a suspected spinal injury.
    d. gastric distention is a common problem when using this device.

30. When providing mouth-to-mask ventilations with no oxygen source, each ventilation should be delivered over:
    a. 1½ to 2 seconds in children.
    b. 1½ to 2 seconds in adults.
    c. 1½ to 2 seconds in infants.
    d. 1½ to 2 seconds in all patients.

31. To obtain to good seal while ventilating a patient with a partial stoma, the EMT must:
    a. use a water-soluble jelly.
    b. cover the mouth and nose.
    c. ventilate with a minimum of 800 mL.
    d. insert an oropharyngeal airway prior to ventilating.

32. A very common problem associated with ventilation through a stoma is:
    a. using the wrong size bag mask device.
    b. not squeezing the bag hard enough.
    c. not being able to properly attach a bag mask device.
    d. that mucus and secretions create an obstruction.

33. Which of the following components of an oxygen delivery system must be hydrostatically tested on a regular schedule?
    a. oxygen cylinder
    b. pressure regulator
    c. the cascade system
    d. positive pressure ventilator

34. When a patient is not breathing adequately, which of the following devices cannot be used to ventilate oxygen into the lungs?
    a. bag mask device
    b. pocket face mask
    c. oxygen cylinder
    d. positive pressure regulator

35. The basic components of an oxygen delivery system used in the prehospital setting by EMTs include a/an:
    a. pocket mask, suction, and humidifier.
    b. bag mask device, airway adjunct, and non-rebreather mask.
    c. suction, airway adjunct, and pressure regulator.
    d. oxygen cylinder, pressure regulator, and delivery device.

36. When a patient who is wearing a non-rebreather mask inhales, he receives oxygen-enriched gas from the:
    a. reservoir bag.
    b. partial-rebreather bag.
    c. two-way valve on a supplied line.
    d. one-way valve on a supplied line.

37. A non-rebreather mask is indicated whenever a patient needs oxygen and:
    a. is apneic.
    b. is in respiratory arrest.
    c. is in cardiac arrest.
    d. can maintain the airway.

38. Of the following devices, the _____ is the oxygen delivery device that can provide the highest oxygen concentration enrichment.
    a. humidifier
    b. nasal cannula
    c. non-rebreather mask
    d. pocket mask with an oxygen port

39. To enrich the oxygen of a stoma patient with mild respiratory distress, the preferred oxygen delivery device is a:
    a. nasal cannula.
    b. bag-valve mask.
    c. non-rebreather mask.
    d. flow-restricted, oxygen-powered ventilation device.

40. The use of a nasal cannula for a hypoxic patient is preferred over a non-rebreather mask in which of the following cases?
    a. facial injury
    b. infants and children
    c. a patient who refuses to wear a mask
    d. foreign body airway obstruction

41. In which of the following cases would an NRB be indicated rather than a nasal cannula?
    a. a preschool child with a croupy cough who is crying
    b. a newly born infant with poor respiratory effort after 1 minute
    c. a patient in the second stage of active labor who feels nauseated
    d. a COPD patient who fainted, but is now awake with no respiratory distress

42. In the prehospital setting, the EMT occasionally responds to a patient who is wearing a cannula and is not in respiratory distress. When transporting this patient, the EMT should:
    a. change the cannula to an NRB on 10 liters.
    b. leave the cannula in place, but adjust the liter flow to 6.
    c. leave the cannula in place using the same liter flow as found.
    d. begin transport without the cannula and request advice from Medical Control while en route.

43. Which of the following is an indication for use of a nasal cannula?
    a. severe hypoxia
    b. mouth breathing
    c. poor respiratory effort
    d. moderate oxygen enrichment for long periods

44. A common problem associated with the use of a nasal cannula is:
    a. that prolonged use causes nausea.
    b. drying of the nasal mucous membranes.
    c. that the device is difficult to use and uncomfortable to adjust.
    d. that the patient has to be weaned off after long periods of use.

45. Your unit was the first to arrive at a residence for a difficulty-breathing call; ALS is also en route. You discover an elderly male in bed, unresponsive and gasping for breath. His airway is open and clear. With auscultation, you find that there is no air movement, the distal pulse is weak and fast, and his skin CTC is pale, warm, and dry. You begin assisting ventilations with a bag mask device. Your partner attempts to insert an OPA and the patient gags, but does not vomit. ALS notifies you on the radio that they are 5 minutes away. What steps do you take next?
    a. Insert an NPA and place a non-rebreather mask on the patient.
    b. Insert an NPA and continue ventilations with the bag mask device once every 6 seconds.
    c. Continue ventilations with the bag mask device and hyperventilate the patient in preparation for intubation.
    d. Attempt to reinsert the OPA again and be prepared to suction if the patient vomits.

46. (Continuing with the preceding question) Five minutes later, a paramedic arrives and you give report. The paramedic rapidly assesses the patient, asks you to continue with your interventions, and decides to intubate the patient. The paramedic quickly assembles the necessary equipment and is ready to intubate. Now she asks you to stop what you are doing and prepare to assist her to visualize the vocal cords by:
    a. lifting the patient's tongue.
    b. turning on every light in the room.
    c. placing cricoid pressure on the patient.
    d. holding the patient's head in a neutral position.

47. A local nursing home has called EMS this morning for an elderly patient who fell out of bed during the night. Staff reports that the patient denied any injury at the time of the fall, so they put her back to bed. This morning the patient has a decreased mental status and the following vital signs: respiratory rate 12 and shallow, with decreased lung sounds on both sides; pulse 58 and regular; BP 100/60; skin CTC is cyanotic, warm, and dry. The patient opens her eyes when touched and spoken to. She denies any neck or back pain, but points to her chest. You discover a bruise and tenderness on her left chest. What do you suspect is the patient's immediate problem?

a. inadequate ventilations due to injured ribs
b. decompensated shock due to tension pneumothorax
c. compensated hypovolemic shock due to intraabdominal bleeding
d. inadequate breathing due to an acute myocardial infarction (AMI)

48. (Continuing with the preceding question) You begin treatment by administering high-flow oxygen and observe that the patient has pain in the left lateral chest with movement. Based on your assessment of the patient's immediate problem, what is your initial management plan for this patient?

a. Lay the patient on her back, elevate her legs, provide warmth, and provide rapid transport to the ED.
b. Splint the left arm to the chest using a sling and swathe and coach the patient to take deeper breaths.
c. Assist the patient with the administration of nitroglycerin for chest pain and call for an ALS intercept.
d. Treat the patient for shock and call for an ALS intercept for a possible chest decompression due to tension pneumothorax.

49. Early in the evening, you are dispatched to a call for a sick patient. After arriving at a residence, you discover that a 30-year-old female, her husband, and their two sons are experiencing flu-like symptoms. You suspect carbon monoxide poisoning, request the fire department to the scene, and evacuate the family out to your ambulance. The female's symptoms are the worst, with headache, nausea, and vomiting. While you administer oxygen to each family member and obtain vital signs, your partner talks to the firefighters and confirms that there is an elevated CO reading in the home. In addition to obtaining vital signs, you obtain pulse oximetry readings while the patients are on oxygen. What would you expect for an SPO_2 reading for the female in this case?

a. The SpO_2 reading will be low, but inaccurate.
b. The SpO_2 reading will be low and accurate.
c. The SpO_2 reading will be high, but inaccurate.
d. The SpO_2 reading will be high and accurate.

50. (Continuing with the previous question) What is the most likely reason for the female to be experiencing more severe symptoms than other members of the household?

a. The female had the longest exposure to CO.
b. All females are more susceptible to CO poisoning.
c. Females do not recover from hypoxic states as easily as males.
d. The affinity for hemoglobin to bind to CO is greater in females of childbearing age.

Chapter 9 Answer Form

	A	B	C	D		A	B	C	D
1.	❑	❑	❑	❑	26.	❑	❑	❑	❑
2.	❑	❑	❑	❑	27.	❑	❑	❑	❑
3.	❑	❑	❑	❑	28.	❑	❑	❑	❑
4.	❑	❑	❑	❑	29.	❑	❑	❑	❑
5.	❑	❑	❑	❑	30.	❑	❑	❑	❑
6.	❑	❑	❑	❑	31.	❑	❑	❑	❑
7.	❑	❑	❑	❑	32.	❑	❑	❑	❑
8.	❑	❑	❑	❑	33.	❑	❑	❑	❑
9.	❑	❑	❑	❑	34.	❑	❑	❑	❑
10.	❑	❑	❑	❑	35.	❑	❑	❑	❑
11.	❑	❑	❑	❑	36.	❑	❑	❑	❑
12.	❑	❑	❑	❑	37.	❑	❑	❑	❑
13.	❑	❑	❑	❑	38.	❑	❑	❑	❑
14.	❑	❑	❑	❑	39.	❑	❑	❑	❑
15.	❑	❑	❑	❑	40.	❑	❑	❑	❑
16.	❑	❑	❑	❑	41.	❑	❑	❑	❑
17.	❑	❑	❑	❑	42.	❑	❑	❑	❑
18.	❑	❑	❑	❑	43.	❑	❑	❑	❑
19.	❑	❑	❑	❑	44.	❑	❑	❑	❑
20.	❑	❑	❑	❑	45.	❑	❑	❑	❑
21.	❑	❑	❑	❑	46.	❑	❑	❑	❑
22.	❑	❑	❑	❑	47.	❑	❑	❑	❑
23.	❑	❑	❑	❑	48.	❑	❑	❑	❑
24.	❑	❑	❑	❑	49.	❑	❑	❑	❑
25.	❑	❑	❑	❑	50.	❑	❑	❑	❑

SECTION

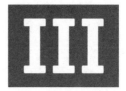

PATIENT ASSESSMENT

Scene Size-Up and Primary Assessment

1. The EMT performs a scene size-up to obtain valuable information about the:
   a. need for standard precautions.
   b. safety issues at the scene.
   c. mechanism of injury (MOI) or nature of illness (NOI).
   d. all of the above.

2. It is late at night and you have responded to a residence that appears to have no lights on. What should you do next?
   a. Put on your BSI equipment.
   b. Suspect a potentially threatening environment.
   c. Bring your flashlight, because the power might be out.
   d. Begin forming your general impression of the patient.

3. After responding to a private residence for a 42-year-old female with a severe headache and nausea, you discover that other family members in the house have the same symptoms, but not as severe. What action should you take first?
   a. Transport the entire family because of flu-like symptoms.
   b. Put a face mask on the patient and each family member.
   c. Put on a face mask and have your crew members do the same.
   d. Evacuate the house and call the fire department to have the residence checked for a carbon monoxide gas leak.

4. While sizing up the scene of a two-car motor vehicle collision, which of the following hazards would be more dangerous for you than for any of the vehicle occupants?
   a. undeployed airbags
   b. downed power lines
   c. a vehicle occupant using a cell phone
   d. broken glass on the vehicle and ground

5. When you are dispatched to a scene for a traumatic injury with hemorrhage, what is the minimum personal protective equipment (PPE) you will need?
   a. gloves
   b. gown
   c. turnout gear
   d. HEPA mask

6. You are entering a single-family residence for an elderly woman who lives alone. Her chief complaint is chest pain. Which of the following could present as a hazard for you and your crew, but probably not the patient?
   a. pet poodle
   b. small doorways
   c. family member
   d. expired nitroglycerin prescription

7. The term "secure scene" is a police term that means:
   a. EMS must remain in a staging area near the scene.
   b. a perpetrator at a crime scene is the injured patient.
   c. police have attempted to make a potentially violent scene as safe as possible.
   d. there are hazardous materials on the scene, but do not present an immediate danger.

8. Before entering a motor vehicle that was involved in a collision, to care for an injured passenger, which of the following actions should the EMT take *first* to quickly stabilize the vehicle?
   a. Let the air out of two of the tires.
   b. Turn off the engine and set the parking brake.
   c. Instruct the occupants to keep their seat belts on.
   d. Check to see if the doors are unlocked before breaking any glass.

9. How can the EMT stabilize a vehicle that has been turned on its side in order to gain access to a patient?
   a. Do not do anything until the fire department arrives.
   b. With help from your crew, push the vehicle right side up.
   c. Place cribbing around the vehicle to keep it from tipping.
   d. With help from your crew, push the vehicle onto its roof.

10. Which of the following conditions is considered a traumatic injury?
    a. seizure
    b. thermal burn
    c. asthma attack
    d. hypoglycemia

11. During the scene size-up of a motor vehicle collision, it becomes obvious to you that the driver of the vehicle involved was unrestrained and went up and over the steering column. In which of the following areas would you expect to find *primary* injuries?
    a. head, face, and neck
    b. head, chest, and knees
    c. face, chest, and femurs
    d. neck, back, and abdomen

12. A common injury pattern seen when a/an _____ pedestrian is struck by a vehicle is called *Waddell's triad*. This pattern consists of injuries to the torso, legs, and then head.
    a. infant
    b. child
    c. adult
    d. pregnant woman

13. The police are on the scene of a domestic violence call. A husband and wife were fighting and both were injured during the altercation. One has minor injuries and the other is potentially unstable. How many ambulances will be needed?
    a. One ambulance for each patient.
    b. Both can go in one ambulance, because neither is a high-priority patient.
    c. None; both have been charged with assault and can be transported by the police to the hospital after processing at the police station.
    d. Two; one for the couple and one for their children, as the children cannot be left unattended.

14. Upon arrival at a scene where a vehicle is off the road in the woods, you find that the windshield is broken out and is lying on the hood. The driver is behind the wheel and appears to be unrestrained and unconscious. While you begin your approach to the vehicle, your partner does a perimeter sweep for:
    a. snakes.
    b. signs of any hunters in the area.
    c. other occupants who may have been ejected.
    d. any personal items that may have been tossed from the vehicle.

15. Your ambulance is the second to arrive at the scene of a potentially large multiple casualty incident (MCI). You are directed to make a quick count of all the patients. You have been asked to do this because the:
    a. transport officer has to make room for incoming fire apparatus.
    b. incident commander needs to assess for appropriate resources.
    c. triage officer needs to know how many triage tags will be needed.
    d. incident commander does not trust the triage officer to make the count.

16. The last component of scene size-up is determining:
    a. which level of PPE to don.
    b. the need for additional resources.
    c. when it is safe for your crew members to proceed onto the scene.
    d. none of the above.

17. During your assessment of an elderly patient, whom you are going to transport to the hospital for evaluation of a minor laceration that requires sutures, it becomes apparent that the patient's disabled spouse cannot be left alone. What action would you take?
    a. Take the spouse along to the hospital.
    b. Call a friend or relative to come over after you leave.
    c. Notify adult protective services before leaving the scene.
    d. Ask dispatch to send a police unit over to handle the matter.

18. You are the incident commander at the scene of an MCI. There are two critical and two stable patients. With adequate resources and a two-person crew for each ambulance, what is the minimum number of ambulances you need to effectively transport all the patients?
    a. one
    b. two
    c. three
    d. four

19. While walking up to a residence where dispatch sent you for a medical emergency, your partner states that he forgot a piece of equipment; he returns to the ambulance to retrieve it. Which of the following actions is most appropriate for you and your partner now?
    a. You wait until your partner returns and enter the residence together.
    b. Your partner conducts a scene size-up as he enters the residence.
    c. You enter the residence and conduct a scene size-up and advise your partner when he enters.
    d. You wait for your partner to return and allow him to perform the scene size-up, as he is the senior crew member.

20. Which of the following statements is most correct about the scene size-up?
    a. The scene size-up is completed only one time for each EMS call.
    b. The scene size-up is the responsibility of the most senior EMT on the call.
    c. The most junior EMT on the call is never responsible for completing the scene size-up.
    d. The elements of the scene size-up should be reconsidered throughout the entire time on the scene.

21. The police have advised you that the scene is safe to enter at the residence of a patient who is experiencing a behavioral emergency. The patient is agitated after failing to complete a suicide attempt. You approach the patient to begin your primary assessment and ask your partner to _____ as an additional safety measure.
    a. call another ambulance to assist
    b. have the police handcuff the patient
    c. keep the exit accessible at all times
    d. tie the patient's wrists with a cravat

22. While sizing up the scene of an accidental injury to a child, you get the impression that the MOI does not fit the injuries you discover. Your plan of action now includes:
    a. confronting the caregiver with your suspicions.
    b. transporting the child, but not telling anyone of your suspicions.
    c. immediately calling for the police while you wait on scene.
    d. not confronting the caregiver or calling the police, but notifying the ED staff.

23. After being dispatched to a residence for an elderly gentleman who is unable to get out of bed, it quickly becomes obvious to you that his living conditions are unhealthy and possibly dangerous. This information is:
    a. necessary to report to the ED staff.
    b. irrelevant to your care of the patient.
    c. reportable to the health department once you notify the police.
    d. reportable to the health department once you notify your supervisor.

24. Your crew has just loaded the only patient involved in a MVC into the ambulance and you are ready to transport him. The EMS supervisor who was on scene hands you a Polaroid snapshot of the patient's vehicle to take with you. The photograph was taken so that:
    a. you can add it to your EMS photo collection.
    b. the patient can use it later for the insurance claim.
    c. the ED staff may appreciate the MOI better when they have a photograph for reference.
    d. your crew will be protected in litigation, because the patient mentioned getting a lawyer.

25. Which of the following hazards poses the highest risk for EMTs working at the scene of an auto accident?
    a. traffic
    b. broken glass
    c. loaded bumper
    d. undeployed airbag

26. Your general or first impression of a patient helps you to:
    a. ensure that the scene is safe.
    b. rapidly identify all threats to life.
    c. fully appreciate the mechanism of injury or illness.
    d. get a sense of how serious the patient's condition is.

27. When forming a general impression of a patient, which of the following components is usually not a factor?
    a. allergies
    b. the environment
    c. patient's age
    d. patient's level of distress

28. When using the mnemonic AVPU to assess a patient's mental status, a rating of "V" relates to:
    a. how well the patient speaks.
    b. the inability of the patient to speak.
    c. the tone of the patient's voice.
    d. how the patient responds to your voice.

29. After physically stimulating a patient who initially appeared unresponsive, the patient moaned loudly and pushed your hand away. Using the mnemonic AVPU, rate this patient's mental status.

a. alert
b. verbal
c. painful
d. unresponsive

30. You are assessing an elderly patient who is not answering your questions appropriately. How can you determine if this is normal for the patient or a new onset?

a. Obtain a Glasgow Coma Score (GCS).
b. Test the patient's blood sugar level.
c. Wait to check the patient's medical records at the hospital.
d. Discuss your findings with the patient's spouse or caregiver.

31. A reliable way of determining the mental status of a child or infant is to:

a. ask the caregiver if the patient has ingested any poisons.
b. keep the patient with the caregiver when you perform your examination.
c. use a favorite toy to distract the patient while you assess reflexes.
d. ask the caregiver if the patient is acting different today and if so, how.

32. Which of the following conditions would lead you to suspect that a conscious patient has a potentially serious airway problem?

a. epistaxis
b. broken jaw and nose
c. patient with active tuberculosis
d. drooling as a result of a dental procedure

33. The primary method for assessing the airway in a patient of any age is:

a. palpation.
b. auscultation.
c. visual inspection.
d. talking to the patient.

34. On the scene of a construction site accident, witnesses state that the patient fell to the ground from a height of 25 feet. The patient is alert, oriented, and denies any pain or injury. Which of the following statements is least accurate?

a. If the patient has no pain, there is no cervical injury.
b. The MOI is reason enough to take cervical precautions.
c. It is possible to have a broken neck without having any pain.
d. Anyone who falls from a height of 25 feet is likely to have a cervical injury.

35. In most cases, the _____ is(are) the most reliable evidence that a patient experienced a significant MOI.

a. environment
b. patient's report
c. witnesses on scene
d. police on scene

36. _____ is(are) a reliable indication that an adult patient's breathing is not adequate.

a. Retractions
b. Slow speech
c. Delayed capillary refill
d. A low pulse oximeter reading

37. In the unresponsive patient, the EMT initially assesses _____ by looking for rise and fall of the chest.

a. breathing
b. oxygenation
c. airway patency
d. perfusion status

38. An 18-month-old infant is postictal after experiencing febrile seizure. She is sleepy; her airway is clear; her respiratory rate is 28; and her skin is pink, warm, and moist. How would you characterize her breathing and state the initial care to be given?

a. Breathing is adequate; do nothing at this point.
b. Breathing is inadequate; assist with positive pressure ventilations.
c. Breathing is adequate; administer high-flow oxygen with a non-rebreather mask.
d. Breathing is inadequate; administer high-flow oxygen with a non-rebreather mask.

39. You have completed a primary assessment on an unresponsive medical patient and have determined that the airway is clear and breathing and circulation are adequate. Your initial care would now include:

a. suction the airway and apply a nasal cannula at 4 to 6 liters per minute.
b. attempt to insert an airway adjunct and begin ventilations with a bag mask device.
c. insert an oral airway and administer high-flow oxygen with a non-rebreather mask.
d. position the patient on his side and administer high-flow oxygen with a non-rebreather mask.

40. You are called to care for a 2-year-old male who is wheezing and has been sick for 3 days. The patient's mental status is alert to his mother's presence; respiratory rate of 36 with nasal flaring; and the skin is pale, warm, and dry. What would you do next?

a. Keep the child calm, reassess, and transport.
b. Keep the child calm and administer blow-by oxygen.
c. Administer high-flow oxygen with a non-rebreather mask.
d. Ask the child's mother to help you assist ventilations with positive pressure.

41. A 30-year-old male fell approximately 20 feet off a ladder and landed on his side. His chief complaint is left-side rib pain. His respirations are shallow and he has guarding over his rib cage. No deformities or external bleeding are apparent. Initial interventions for this patient are cervical stabilization and:
   a. rapid packaging and transport.
   b. assisting the patient with positive pressure ventilations.
   c. keeping the patient calm and administering oxygen by nasal cannula.
   d. encouraging the patient to take deeper breaths and administering high-flow oxygen by non-rebreather mask.

42. Which skin finding distinctly indicates decreased oxygenation associated with inadequate breathing?
   a. pale
   b. moist
   c. yellow
   d. cyanosis

43. In which age group is the impact of a stuffy nose from a cold the most significant?
   a. ages 2 to 4
   b. first 4 weeks of life
   c. last 4 months of life
   d. under 5 years of age

44. _____ and nasal flaring are indications that an infant is having difficulty breathing.
   a. Coughing
   b. Flushed skin
   c. Grunting
   d. An elevated temperature

45. You are assisting a small child with positive pressure ventilations. You know the ventilations are adequate when:
   a. there are equal breath sounds.
   b. the skin color improves.
   c. there is a good mask seal and the chest rises.
   d. all of the above.

46. The lower airways are softer and more flexible than in any other age group in:
   a. infants up to 1 year old.
   b. adolescents.
   c. elderly patients older than 75 years.
   d. elderly patients older than 90 years.

47. In infants, the pulse is assessed in the brachial artery in the:
   a. medial aspect of the upper arm.
   b. medial aspect of the lower arm.
   c. thumb side of the lower arm near the wrist.
   d. left side of the chest near the sternal margin.

48. As part of the primary assessment of an unresponsive 8-year-old child, the EMT performs the American Heart Association's "quick check" by assessing the _____ pulse.
   a. apical
   b. carotid
   c. radial
   d. brachial

49. During the primary assessment of a patient with a deep laceration of the forearm, you recognize that the bleeding is arterial. Your next step is to:
   a. call for ALS.
   b. prioritize the patient as critical.
   c. prioritize the patient as unstable.
   d. manage the bleeding immediately.

50. When a patient has life-threatening external bleeding, the EMT should _____ during the initial assessment.
   a. attempt to control the bleeding
   b. estimate the rate of blood loss
   c. report to the emergency department
   d. classify the stage of shock as grade I, II, or III

51. A patient suffering from acute hepatitis or renal failure may exhibit skin color that is:
   a. blue.
   b. yellow.
   c. anemic.
   d. dark around the eyes.

52. Skin color is best assessed by looking at the:
   a. eyes, ears, and nose.
   b. eyes, lips, and nail beds.
   c. palms and soles of the feet.
   d. tongue and mucous membranes.

53. An ill patient who has been lying in bed all day in a room with a comfortable ambient temperature has skin that appears flushed, hot, and moist. This patient is most likely experiencing:
   a. a high fever.
   b. dehydration.
   c. a medication overdose.
   d. a mild allergic reaction.

54. Goose pimples, chattering teeth, and pale skin suggest that the patient has:
   a. been exposed to cold temperatures.
   b. an infection.
   c. pain or fever.
   d. all of the above.

55. A capillary refill time of less than _____ seconds is considered normal in a healthy 3-year-old child.
   a. 2
   b. 3
   c. 4
   d. 5

56. A delayed capillary refill time in an infant is:

a. a finding that suggests a circulation problem.

b. not a problem unless it exceeds five seconds.

c. a finding that suggests there are no peripheral pulses.

d. normal in children with dark skin.

57. As the team leader on a crew, you may be the provider who will prioritize a patient as part of the primary assessment. Completing this task:

a. sets the tone for a management plan.

b. lets the crew know you are clearly in charge of the call.

c. allows you to gain permission to treat the patient.

d. is reassuring to the patient and the patient's family.

58. The primary reason for prioritizing a patient for treatment and transport is:

a. to know when to stabilize a patient on the scene or call for ALS.

b. to determine the need for rapid transport for definitive care.

c. that no other task is as important in the first phase of patient contact.

d. to be able to locate and manage life-threatening conditions affecting the airway, breathing, and circulation.

59. You have arrived at the side of an unconscious adult patient who is breathing. You are unable to locate a radial pulse, and find the carotid pulse to be present and weak. What does this finding suggest about the patient's blood pressure?

a. The patient will have a low blood pressure.

b. The diastolic can be estimated as at least 70 mm Hg.

c. The patient will have a systolic but no diastolic pressure.

d. This finding is not associated with the patient's blood pressure.

60. A construction worker has fallen from a height of 10 feet. When you arrive, he is conscious, but confused about how the fall occurred. He tells you that he is having difficulty breathing and cannot feel his legs. What is the first priority in the initial assessment of this patient?

a. Open the airway.

b. Take spinal precautions.

c. Obtain a blood pressure.

d. Check for distal pulses, motor function, and sensation.

61. Your ambulance is dispatched to an office building for a 24-year-old male who is having difficulty breathing. As you approach the patient, he appears anxious and is talking fast and in long sentences. He looks well and skin color is good, yet he tells you that he is having trouble catching his breath. What is your priority consideration for this patient?

a. Provide high-flow oxygen.

b. Do nothing and observe for a while.

c. Consider that he is faking being sick to get out of work.

d. Have him breathe into a paper bag for one minute, then reevaluate.

62. A patient tells you "I feel bloated and my stomach hurts." This is referred to as the:

a. field diagnosis.

b. chief complaint.

c. objective finding.

d. general impression.

63. The family of an elderly patient tells you that they have been unable to wake her up this morning. You approach and shake her arm gently; as you speak to her, she awakens and is able to tell you her name, day of the week, and where she is. She cannot tell you the date. You classify her mental status as:

a. alert.

b. verbal.

c. painful.

d. unresponsive.

64. Which of the following statements is most correct with regard to making a priority decision about a patient's condition?

a. Every patient will need definitive care within the "Golden Hour."

b. When a presenting problem could be either more or less serious, consider it to be more serious.

c. When a presenting problem could be either more or less serious, consider it to be less serious.

d. When a presenting problem could be either more or less serious, let the crew chief make the priority decision.

65. The Glasgow Coma Scale is useful for assessing mental status and for making a priority decision about a patient. It does not, however, provide you with information about the best _____ response.

a. verbal

b. motor

c. sensation

d. eye-opening

Chapter 10 Answer Form

	A	B	C	D			A	B	C	D
1.	❏	❏	❏	❏		34.	❏	❏	❏	❏
2.	❏	❏	❏	❏		35.	❏	❏	❏	❏
3.	❏	❏	❏	❏		36.	❏	❏	❏	❏
4.	❏	❏	❏	❏		37.	❏	❏	❏	❏
5.	❏	❏	❏	❏		38.	❏	❏	❏	❏
6.	❏	❏	❏	❏		39.	❏	❏	❏	❏
7.	❏	❏	❏	❏		40.	❏	❏	❏	❏
8.	❏	❏	❏	❏		41.	❏	❏	❏	❏
9.	❏	❏	❏	❏		42.	❏	❏	❏	❏
10.	❏	❏	❏	❏		43.	❏	❏	❏	❏
11.	❏	❏	❏	❏		44.	❏	❏	❏	❏
12.	❏	❏	❏	❏		45.	❏	❏	❏	❏
13.	❏	❏	❏	❏		46.	❏	❏	❏	❏
14.	❏	❏	❏	❏		47.	❏	❏	❏	❏
15.	❏	❏	❏	❏		48.	❏	❏	❏	❏
16.	❏	❏	❏	❏		49.	❏	❏	❏	❏
17.	❏	❏	❏	❏		50.	❏	❏	❏	❏
18.	❏	❏	❏	❏		51.	❏	❏	❏	❏
19.	❏	❏	❏	❏		52.	❏	❏	❏	❏
20.	❏	❏	❏	❏		53.	❏	❏	❏	❏
21.	❏	❏	❏	❏		54.	❏	❏	❏	❏
22.	❏	❏	❏	❏		55.	❏	❏	❏	❏
23.	❏	❏	❏	❏		56.	❏	❏	❏	❏
24.	❏	❏	❏	❏		57.	❏	❏	❏	❏
25.	❏	❏	❏	❏		58.	❏	❏	❏	❏
26.	❏	❏	❏	❏		59.	❏	❏	❏	❏
27.	❏	❏	❏	❏		60.	❏	❏	❏	❏
28.	❏	❏	❏	❏		61.	❏	❏	❏	❏
29.	❏	❏	❏	❏		62.	❏	❏	❏	❏
30.	❏	❏	❏	❏		63.	❏	❏	❏	❏
31.	❏	❏	❏	❏		64.	❏	❏	❏	❏
32.	❏	❏	❏	❏		65.	❏	❏	❏	❏
33.	❏	❏	❏	❏						

27. Capillary refill in infants is considered a very reliable indicator of the:
    a. perfusion status.
    b. distal sensory status.
    c. neurological status.
    d. accurate pulse rate.

28. When the ambient light is so bright that your patient's pupils are fully constricted, you can stimulate a pupillary response by:
    a. shining a really large flashlight into both eyes.
    b. asking the patient to hold his breath for 30 seconds.
    c. shading both eyes for 30 seconds, while watching for dilation.
    d. there is no way to stimulate a pupillary response under these conditions.

29. Examination of the head includes assessment of the pupils. Which of the following includes an accurate measurement of the pupil?
    a. diameter in millimeters
    b. diameter in centimeters
    c. circumference in centimeters
    d. circumference in millimeters

30. When a light is shined into the right pupil in an effort to get it to constrict, which of the following would be considered a normal response?
    a. Both pupils react equally.
    b. The left pupil gets large.
    c. The right pupil gets large.
    d. Only the right pupil constricts.

31. The normal blood glucose range is _____ mg/dl.
    a. 60–80
    b. 60–100
    c. 100–120
    d. 80–120

32. During an initial assessment of an 18-year-old female with an isolated cut on her arm from a utility knife, you notice that her pupils are unequal. She denies any loss of consciousness or any other injury. What is the appropriate action to take regarding your abnormal finding?
    a. Ask her if this is normal for her.
    b. Consider the possibility of a head injury and immobilize her.
    c. Consider the possibility of a stroke and perform a stroke exam.
    d. Just ignore the finding, because the present problem is totally unrelated.

33. While assessing a 62-year-old male who had fallen and injured his hip, you note that he has unequal pupils. His wife tells you that this is not normal for him, so one of the first things you consider as the cause for the abnormal finding is:
    a. shock.
    b. stroke.
    c. hypotension.
    d. hypoglycemia.

34. You are assessing an alert, 40-year-old male who struck his head after falling from a standing position. He did not lose consciousness and denies any significant pain or injury. When you assess his pupils, you find that his right pupil is nonreactive to light. You consider _____ to be the possible cause for the abnormal finding.
    a. fright
    b. pink eye
    c. a concussion
    d. an artificial eye

35. Taking a blood pressure by palpation would be most reasonable in which situation?
    a. when the patient has no distal pulse
    b. when auscultation is taking too long
    c. when the BP cuff gauge is not calibrated
    d. when the sirens are turned on en route to the hospital

36. You are obtaining a blood pressure on a patient by auscultation. As you release the pressure in the cuff, the first sound you hear indicates the:
    a. systolic reading.
    b. diastolic reading.
    c. cardiac output.
    d. stroke volume.

37. The systolic blood pressure relates to the:
    a. contraction of the ventricles.
    b. relaxation of the ventricles.
    c. contraction of the atria.
    d. none of the above.

38. During the normal heart cycle, the pressure created within the arteries is known as the _____ blood pressure.
    a. atrial
    b. systolic
    c. diastolic
    d. ventricular

39. The diastolic blood pressure relates to the:
    a. contraction of the heart.
    b. atria refilling with blood.
    c. relaxation phase of the heart cycle.
    d. conduction phase of the heart cycle.

40. The unit of measure "mm Hg" refers to the:
    a. ancient Greek formula of liquid measure.
    b. Latin measure of liquid under hydrostatic pressure.
    c. apothecary unit of measure for liquid mercury hydraulic pressure.
    d. height of mercury in millimeters to which the blood pressure elevates a column of liquid mercury in a glass tube.

41. _____ is an assessment of the level of carbon dioxide exhaled by the patient.
    a. Oximetry
    b. Spirometry
    c. Capnography
    d. Tracheostomy

42. Which of the following statements about blood pressure readings is most accurate?
    a. The method of obtaining a BP by auscultation is more accurate than by palpation.
    b. Obtaining a BP by palpation is more accurate than by auscultation.
    c. It is easier to obtain a BP by palpation than by auscultation.
    d. Both auscultation and palpation are equally accurate.

43. The "E" in the mnemonic SAMPLE represents:
    a. episodes of a similar nature.
    b. evidence of the mechanism of injury.
    c. events that have been previously diagnosed for the patient.
    d. events that led up to what the patient was doing when the current episode began.

44. When a patient is unconscious or has an altered mental status, obtaining the SAMPLE history:
    a. is not going to matter.
    b. can be completed by the police.
    c. can wait until the patient becomes alert.
    d. may be attempted with family or a caretaker.

45. Which of the following is considered a symptom rather than a sign?
    a. edema
    b. dizziness
    c. fainting
    d. wheezing

46. Which of the following is considered a sign rather than a symptom?
    a. headache
    b. crepitus
    c. numbness
    d. blurred vision

47. Recording the baseline set of vital signs, followed by a reassessment of vital signs during the reassessment, is:
    a. helpful to find all life-threatening injuries.
    b. referred to as *trending*.
    c. only necessary with critical patients.
    d. only necessary with trauma patients.

48. Ideally, vital signs should be taken and recorded every _____ minutes on a stable patient.
    a. 5
    b. 10
    c. 15
    d. 20

49. Some patients keep a written record of their medical information and place it in a container called a Vial of Life®. This container is typically stored:
    a. by the telephone.
    b. in the refrigerator.
    c. with the closest relative.
    d. with the next-door neighbor.

50. An example of critical but nonemergent medical information the EMT should record and relay to the next health care provider receiving the patient is:
    a. the name and address of the patient's closest relative.
    b. any evidence of neglected yard work and a sloppy garage.
    c. the number and type of pets found in the patient's residence.
    d. any evidence of the patient's inability to perform activities of daily living.

Chapter 11 Answer Form

	A	B	C	D			A	B	C	D
1.	❑	❑	❑	❑		26.	❑	❑	❑	❑
2.	❑	❑	❑	❑		27.	❑	❑	❑	❑
3.	❑	❑	❑	❑		28.	❑	❑	❑	❑
4.	❑	❑	❑	❑		29.	❑	❑	❑	❑
5.	❑	❑	❑	❑		30.	❑	❑	❑	❑
6.	❑	❑	❑	❑		31.	❑	❑	❑	❑
7.	❑	❑	❑	❑		32.	❑	❑	❑	❑
8.	❑	❑	❑	❑		33.	❑	❑	❑	❑
9.	❑	❑	❑	❑		34.	❑	❑	❑	❑
10.	❑	❑	❑	❑		35.	❑	❑	❑	❑
11.	❑	❑	❑	❑		36.	❑	❑	❑	❑
12.	❑	❑	❑	❑		37.	❑	❑	❑	❑
13.	❑	❑	❑	❑		38.	❑	❑	❑	❑
14.	❑	❑	❑	❑		39.	❑	❑	❑	❑
15.	❑	❑	❑	❑		40.	❑	❑	❑	❑
16.	❑	❑	❑	❑		41.	❑	❑	❑	❑
17.	❑	❑	❑	❑		42.	❑	❑	❑	❑
18.	❑	❑	❑	❑		43.	❑	❑	❑	❑
19.	❑	❑	❑	❑		44.	❑	❑	❑	❑
20.	❑	❑	❑	❑		45.	❑	❑	❑	❑
21.	❑	❑	❑	❑		46.	❑	❑	❑	❑
22.	❑	❑	❑	❑		47.	❑	❑	❑	❑
23.	❑	❑	❑	❑		48.	❑	❑	❑	❑
24.	❑	❑	❑	❑		49.	❑	❑	❑	❑
25.	❑	❑	❑	❑		50.	❑	❑	❑	❑

CHAPTER

12

Assessment of the Trauma Patient

1. While sizing up the scene at a trauma incident, you determine that the mechanism of injury (MOI) is potentially life-threatening. However, the patient appears to be in stable condition. You should now:

   a. get the patient's SAMPLE history.

   b. provide care appropriate for the stable condition.

   c. begin treatment and transport based on the MOI.

   d. treat the patient only if she begins to become unstable.

2. When determining the severity of the MOI, the EMT will:

   a. recognize all potential injuries.

   b. identify when a patient is in shock.

   c. relate the forces of energy to the pathology of injury.

   d. recognize which patients will make it through to hospital discharge.

3. When assessing the trauma patient, the EMT must consider what the patient needs and:

   a. what treatment he can provide.

   b. what type of insurance the patient has.

   c. when was the patient's last medical exam.

   d. whether the patient can tolerate lying on a long back board.

4. A 12-year-old male rode through a stop sign at the bottom of a hill and hit a passing vehicle, breaking the side view mirror and denting the passenger side door. He is lying on the street crying, and there is a first responder holding c-spine stabilization. A witness reports the patient was not wearing a helmet and did not lose consciousness, but did not get up. What is the first action to take?

   a. talk to the patient

   b. take over c-spine stabilization

   c. obtain a pulse rate and blood pressure

   d. apply oxygen with a non-rebreather mask

5. (Continuing with the previous questions) You examine the patient and find his airway is open, his lung sounds are clear with a good respiratory effort, and his distal pulse is strong and regular. His injuries include a large bump (hematoma) on the side of his head and scrapes on his hands and legs. He continues to cry and is asking for his mother. How would you classify the patient at this point?

   a. critical with a significant mechanism of injury

   b. critical without a significant mechanism of injury

   c. noncritical with a significant mechanism of injury

   d. noncritical without a significant mechanism of injury

6. While performing the secondary assessment on a trauma patient, the EMT:

   a. will not discover injuries that could become life-threatening later.

   b. may discover life-threatening injuries not found in the primary assessment.

   c. will obtain the past medical history and history of present illness.

   d. will obtain pulse oximetry, blood glucose reading, and an EKG.

7. After performing a secondary assessment on a patient who was involved in a serious motor vehicle collision, your partner obtains a second set of vital signs. You find that the patient's rapid heart rate is persisting despite having no apparent injuries. Your next step is to:

   a. repeat the primary assessment.

   b. calm her down, and the heart rate will slow.

   c. treat her as a high-priority patient with possible internal bleeding.

   d. repeat the rapid trauma assessment, as you have probably missed an injury.

8. While assessing the chest of a trauma patient with a significant mechanism of injury, which of the following findings suggests the most serious injury?
   a. chest symmetry
   b. paradoxical motion
   c. tenderness on the sternum
   d. abrasions on the upper left side

9. The findings obtained from a rapid trauma exam:
   a. will help you identify all life-threatening conditions.
   b. can help you determine the patient's final outcome.
   c. will help you determine what care to provide on the way to the hospital.
   d. will help you stabilize the patient on the scene prior to beginning transport.

10. Crepitus is an abnormal finding of the _____ and will typically be discovered during the rapid trauma assessment.
    a. flank
    b. hips
    c. scalp
    d. abdomen

11. _____ is a mnemonic that is helpful in remembering what should be evaluated about the patient in the secondary assessment.
    a. MOI
    b. SAMPLE
    c. OPQRST
    d. D-CAP-BTLS

12. Paradoxical motion is an abnormal finding of the _____, which may be discovered in a secondary assessment.
    a. neck
    b. eyes
    c. chest
    d. abdomen

13. While conducting an assessment on an unconscious patient, you discover a medical alert device that identifies the patient as a diabetic. What action should you take next?
    a. Administer oral glucose.
    b. Finish conducting the secondary assessment.
    c. Look for the patient's glucometer and obtain a reading.
    d. Attach AED electrodes and turn on the device.

14. You are performing a secondary assessment of a conscious patient who had a witnessed seizure. During your assessment of the head and neck, the patient begins to seize again. Your next action is to:
    a. suction the airway.
    b. administer high-flow oxygen.
    c. gently lay the patient supine, protecting the head.
    d. pry open the airway with an OPA.

15. The secondary assessment is generally performed in a head-to-toe manner, except when:
    a. the patient is unconscious.
    b. there are multiple patients.
    c. there is a suspected spinal injury.
    d. a life-threatening injury is discovered.

16. You and your partner respond to a call for a fall from a ladder. When you arrive, you find an elderly male lying on the ground next to an eighteen-foot broken ladder outside of his home. He is conscious, confused, bleeding from the scalp, and smells of tobacco and alcohol. From the scene size-up information, which of the following is most concerning initially?
    a. the broken ladder
    b. the patient is confused
    c. probable alcohol use
    d. bleeding from the scalp

17. (Continuing with the previous question) Your partner takes hold of cervical stabilization and you begin the patient interview. The patient knows his name but is unsure of his age or what is happening. He confirms having pain at the site of the wound on his scalp and denies difficulty breathing. What should be assessed next?
    a. lung sounds
    b. blood sugar
    c. neck, back, and spine
    d. the amount of blood lost from the scalp wound

18. (Continuing with the previous two questions) The first set of vital signs are respiratory rate 22 non labored, pulse rate 66 and regular, and blood pressure 180/120. His scalp wound is oozing blood and he has blood draining from the right ear. What is the appropriate transport decision for this patient?
    a. Request ALS to the scene and wait to transport.
    b. Request helicopter transport to the trauma center.
    c. Begin immediate transport to the nearest hospital (10 minutes).
    d. Begin immediate transport to the trauma center (20 minutes).

19. The driver involved in a serious MVC is uncooperative and quarrelsome. There is no evidence of intoxication, and you consider _____ to be a possible reason for his behavior.
    a. hypoxia
    b. hypertension
    c. that he has something to hide
    d. that this is his normal character

20. During the physical exam of a trauma patient, in which of the following areas or regions would you be least likely to find crepitus?
    a. back
    b. face
    c. sternum
    d. abdomen

21. You are caring for a victim who has a gunshot wound (GSW) through the leg. In the primary assessment, the patient is alert, is breathing adequately, has a strong distal pulse, and has minimal external bleeding from a wound in his upper thigh. After completing a secondary assessment, you find no other holes and you bandage his leg wound. What should you do next?
    a. Obtain vital signs.
    b. Transport immediately.
    c. Repeat the secondary assessment.
    d. Repeat the initial assessment.

22. For the patient in the previous question, which of the following factors can best help you determine if the wound is an entry or exit GSW?
    a. the amount of blood lost
    b. the gender of the shooter
    c. the shell type of ammunition used
    d. presence of powder residue at the injury site

23. Asymmetry, crepitus, and paradoxical motion are abnormal findings consistent with traumatic injury to the:
    a. pelvis.
    b. skull.
    c. chest.
    d. abdomen.

24. You have discovered signs and symptoms of a pelvic injury during a secondary assessment of a patient who was involved in a motorcycle collision. Your next step should be to:
    a. stabilize the pelvis.
    b. obtain a blood pressure.
    c. not move the patient until ALS arrives.
    d. finish the remainder of the secondary assessment.

25. The Glasgow Coma Scale (GCS) is an objective measure of _____,verbal response, and motor response, with a numerical score from 3 to 15 that is used to establish priority care for head-injured patients.
    a. skin color
    b. temperature
    c. capillary refill
    d. eye opening response

26. You have responded to a residence for a 34-year-old woman complaining of neck pain. She appears to be guarding her neck muscles as she tells you that she was involved in a minor motor vehicle collision yesterday. She was evaluated at an emergency department and the x-rays were clear. The pain and guarding are most likely associated with:
    a. arthritis.
    b. muscle strain.
    c. osteoporosis.
    d. a new case of meningitis.

27. The driver of a snowmobile struck a tree and was thrown from the sled. A witness confirms that there was a brief loss of consciousness; that was why he called 9-1-1. The patient is awake when you reach him. Which of the following is the most significant finding concerning the MOI?
    a. the condition of the rider's helmet
    b. the amount of damage to the snowmobile
    c. the number of years experience riding a snowmobile
    d. the amount of time the patient has been out in the cold

28. Injury patterns associated with specific MOIs, from which the EMT can anticipate the potential for shock or other problems, are referred to as:
    a. nature of illness.
    b. predictable shock.
    c. index of suspicion.
    d. history of traumatic impression.

29. The police have called you to evaluate 11-year-old twins who were seat-belted into the back seat of a minivan that was involved in a moderate-speed collision. The children deny any injury, but after 15 minutes on the scene, one has a rapid heart rate and appears pale. Which of the following is the likely cause of the persistent rapid heart rate?
    a. anxiety
    b. head injury
    c. hypoglycemia
    d. internal bleeding

30. While you were obtaining equipment from the ambulance, your partner performed a primary assessment on an unconscious male who had been struck by a car. You help conduct the secondary assessment and discover a life-threatening injury that was missed in the primary assessment. What should you do?
    a. Immediately manage the life threat.
    b. Have a discussion with your partner.
    c. Call the EMS supervisor to the scene.
    d. Complete the rapid trauma exam and begin the secondary assessment.

Chapter 12 Answer Form

	A	B	C	D		A	B	C	D
1.	❑	❑	❑	❑	16.	❑	❑	❑	❑
2.	❑	❑	❑	❑	17.	❑	❑	❑	❑
3.	❑	❑	❑	❑	18.	❑	❑	❑	❑
4.	❑	❑	❑	❑	19.	❑	❑	❑	❑
5.	❑	❑	❑	❑	20.	❑	❑	❑	❑
6.	❑	❑	❑	❑	21.	❑	❑	❑	❑
7.	❑	❑	❑	❑	22.	❑	❑	❑	❑
8.	❑	❑	❑	❑	23.	❑	❑	❑	❑
9.	❑	❑	❑	❑	24.	❑	❑	❑	❑
10.	❑	❑	❑	❑	25.	❑	❑	❑	❑
11.	❑	❑	❑	❑	26.	❑	❑	❑	❑
12.	❑	❑	❑	❑	27.	❑	❑	❑	❑
13.	❑	❑	❑	❑	28.	❑	❑	❑	❑
14.	❑	❑	❑	❑	29.	❑	❑	❑	❑
15.	❑	❑	❑	❑	30.	❑	❑	❑	❑

CHAPTER 13

Assessment of the Medical Patient

1. You arrive at the residence of a 23-year-old male, who called because he had a sudden onset of severe chest pain "like no other pain he has ever had before." Now he states that the pain is completely gone and is refusing transportation for evaluation. With no prior history and the quick resolution of pain, what should you do now?
   a. Let the patient refuse.
   b. Convince the patient to get evaluated at the hospital.
   c. Ask the patient to call his own physician and follow up.
   d. Convince the patient to drive to the hospital if the pain comes back.

2. You are about to interview a patient about her chief complaint of "nausea and vomiting." Which mnemonic can you use to remember which questions to ask about the chief complaint?
   a. AVPU
   b. OPQRST
   c. SAMPLE
   d. D-CAP-BTLS

3. While obtaining a focused history from an elderly patient, it becomes obvious that he is having trouble remembering certain things. Except for your crew, the patient is alone in his residence. What can you use at the residence to help discover the patient's past medical history?
   a. Call the patient's pharmacy.
   b. Locate any medications prescribed for the patient.
   c. Ask your dispatcher who called 9-1-1 for this patient.
   d. Look in the patient's closet.

4. Which of the following patient complaints would make you suspect that the patient is most likely experiencing a new onset of diabetes?
   a. fainting twice in a month
   b. increased frequency of thirst and urination
   c. feeling sweaty for no apparent reason
   d. feeling short of breath with exertion

5. Which of the following clues may indicate that a patient has a cardiac history?
   a. a midline scar on the chest
   b. aspirin in the medicine cabinet
   c. a bottle of medication in the refrigerator
   d. a prescribed inhaler on the bedside table

6. When assessing a patient with an unprotected airway and the patient begins to vomit, _____ is the immediate potential complication for the patient.
   a. aspiration
   b. dehydration
   c. infectious exposure
   d. gastrointestinal bleeding

7. You have been called to care for a diabetic patient who was found unresponsive, on the floor, by strangers. She is breathing, but remains unresponsive upon scene size-up. Your next action is to:
   a. assess the SpO_2.
   b. check for a pulse.
   c. ensure cervical stabilization.
   d. back off and wait for the police.

8. After performing a primary assessment of an unresponsive patient, you determine that the ABCs are adequate. What do you do next?
   a. Obtain a set of vital signs.
   b. Connect AED electrodes and turn the unit on.
   c. Connect AED electrodes and do not turn the unit on.
   d. Look for a diabetic Medic Alert tag.

9. Your primary concern for the unresponsive medical patient is:
   a. airway patency.
   b. administering oxygen.
   c. completing a physical exam.
   d. getting a history of the present illness.

10. A 23-year-old female shows you a rash on both arms and tells you that this rash is new and is occurring for the first time. She has no other symptoms, but is very upset about the rash. You suspect that she is:
    a. poisoned.
    b. contagious.
    c. trying to get attention.
    d. going into anaphylaxis.

11. For the medical patient complaining of dizziness, getting a history and performing a secondary assessment are performed:
    a. en route to the hospital.
    b. after placing the patient on the stretcher.
    c. after the primary assessment.
    d. before the primary assessment.

12. The SAMPLE history for a medical patient does not include the patient's:
    a. age.
    b. primary symptom.
    c. history of smoking.
    d. history of the last trip to the hospital.

13. The police have requested transport for a male in his twenties who appears to be intoxicated. The patient does not appear to be injured, but is not very alert. Your approach to this patient is to:
    a. let him sleep it off during the transport.
    b. assume there is a head injury until proven otherwise.
    c. complete an examination and keep an open mind about the intoxication.
    d. restrain him so he does not become violent or a threat to you and your crew.

14. When caring for a medical patient, whether the patient is conscious or unconscious, the highest priority is:
    a. airway maintenance.
    b. positioning the patient.
    c. getting a SAMPLE history.
    d. making a transportation decision.

15. After being dispatched for a cardiac arrest, you arrive to find that the patient is unconscious, is breathing, and has a pulse. Once the primary assessment is completed, you obtain a baseline set of vital signs and:
    a. contact medical control.
    b. complete a secondary assessment.
    c. call the dispatcher and cancel the police.
    d. obtain a SAMPLE history from the patient's physician.

16. The adult patient you are caring for is experiencing an asthma attack, with severe difficulty breathing and speaking. How would you proceed with the focused history?
    a. Call medical control for advice.
    b. Phrase your questions for yes or no answers.
    c. Wait to ask any questions until the patient is stable.
    d. Wait to ask questions until after you have assisted the patient with her inhaler.

17. During your interview, a patient complains of chest pain. Which of the following pieces of information is least helpful for the presenting problem?
    a. There is a family history of cardiac disease.
    b. The spouse and children are currently out of town.
    c. The patient has no known allergies to medications.
    d. The patient took his own nitroglycerin with no relief of pain.

18. While assessing an unresponsive medical patient, you discover a transdermal patch on the upper left chest. You do not recognize the name of the product on the patch but suspect the medication from the patch is the cause of the patient's unresponsiveness. Which action is most appropriate regarding the transdermal patch?
    a. Leave the patch in place.
    b. Treat the patient for shock.
    c. Contact medical control for directions.
    d. With gloves on, immediately remove the patch.

19. When your general impression is that a patient appears to have an altered mental status, the first person from whom you try to get patient information is:
    a. the patient.
    b. a friend or neighbor.
    c. the caretaker or parent.
    d. the patient's physician.

20. The _____ is(are) the information obtained from the patient or bystanders about the current event and what led up to it.
    a. baseline data
    b. demographics
    c. focused history
    d. chief complaint

21. A baseline set of vital signs taken during a patient assessment is:
    a. the most important set of vital signs.
    b. the first set of vital signs used to establish a trend.
    c. completed on scene only if a life-threatening condition exists.
    d. the responsibility of the most senior EMS provider on scene.

22. When your patient says that she is having multiple symptoms, which one do you consider to be the chief complaint?
    a. the symptom that worries her the most
    b. the first symptom the patient describes
    c. the last symptom the patient describes
    d. all of the symptoms are considered part of the chief complaint

23. You have been dispatched to a medical call for chest pain. As you assess and interview the patient, she tells you the chest pain began 15 minutes ago and is very intense. She vomited and now feels nauseous and is having difficulty taking a breath. She appears pale and sweaty. From the information above, which is(are) the associated symptom(s)?
    a. acute onset of chest pain
    b. nausea and dyspnea
    c. pale and sweaty skin
    d. all of the above

24. After assisting a patient who was complaining of chest pain to take his prescribed nitroglycerin, the patient tells you that the pain is gone. What do you do now?
    a. Transport the patient to the hospital.
    b. Wait 15 minutes before releasing the patient.
    c. Transport the patient to his doctor's office for follow-up.
    d. Release the patient and tell him to call 9-1-1 if the pain returns.

25. While transporting a patient who has generalized weakness, your patient's eyes roll back and he begins to have a seizure. Which of the following actions should you take first?
    a. Prepare for vomiting.
    b. Call for ALS to meet you en route.
    c. Tell the driver to turn on the lights and siren.
    d. Make sure the patient is securely strapped in.

26. During your interview of a 61-year-old patient, you learn that she has a pacemaker. Where would you expect to see the scar associated with the implantation of such a device?
    a. in the upper-left thigh area
    b. in the midline of the chest
    c. in the upper-right or upper-left chest
    d. below the left armpit (midaxillary line)

27. While assessing a 48-year-old male with a complaint of chest pain, you obtain a history, including SAMPLE and OPQRST questions. Which of the following is considered to be a pertinent negative when managing a patient with chest pain?
    a. The patient confirms having a pacemaker.
    b. The patient has no shortness of breath or difficulty breathing.
    c. The patient feels better after taking nitroglycerin and now refuses transportation for evaluation at the hospital.
    d. The patient has had chest pain in the past.

28. You have arrived at the apartment of an elderly couple with a report of a fainting episode. When you ask for information about the patient, the spouse tells you they have a Vial of Life®. What is this?
    a. a prescription vitality medication
    b. an over-the-counter vitality medication
    c. a subscription service with an 800 number that provides patient information
    d. a small plastic container that holds a rolled piece of paper with patient information

29. You are transporting a cancer patient who complains of generalized weakness. From your first impression, it is obvious that the patient has yellow in the normally white part of the eyes. He tells you that he has had jaundice before, and this is not bad. What precautions do you need to take first with this patient?
    a. None; jaundice is not contagious.
    b. Wear gloves and eyewear and wash your hands.
    c. Place a mask on the patient and yourself.
    d. Notify the hospital that you are bringing in a highly infectious patient.

30. While assessing a patient who has flu symptoms, you quickly notice that the patient has a persistent cough. Now your first priority is to:
    a. provide high-flow oxygen immediately.
    b. be prepared for nausea and vomiting.
    c. ask the patient if she is contagious.
    d. take precautions for yourself and put on a mask.

Chapter 13 Answer Form

	A	B	C	D		A	B	C	D
1.	❏	❏	❏	❏	16.	❏	❏	❏	❏
2.	❏	❏	❏	❏	17.	❏	❏	❏	❏
3.	❏	❏	❏	❏	18.	❏	❏	❏	❏
4.	❏	❏	❏	❏	19.	❏	❏	❏	❏
5.	❏	❏	❏	❏	20.	❏	❏	❏	❏
6.	❏	❏	❏	❏	21.	❏	❏	❏	❏
7.	❏	❏	❏	❏	22.	❏	❏	❏	❏
8.	❏	❏	❏	❏	23.	❏	❏	❏	❏
9.	❏	❏	❏	❏	24.	❏	❏	❏	❏
10.	❏	❏	❏	❏	25.	❏	❏	❏	❏
11.	❏	❏	❏	❏	26.	❏	❏	❏	❏
12.	❏	❏	❏	❏	27.	❏	❏	❏	❏
13.	❏	❏	❏	❏	28.	❏	❏	❏	❏
14.	❏	❏	❏	❏	29.	❏	❏	❏	❏
15.	❏	❏	❏	❏	30.	❏	❏	❏	❏

CHAPTER

14

Reassessment, Critical Thinking, and Decision Making

1. Your primary assessment of a 55-year-old male complaining of abdominal pain revealed that he has tachycardia and that his skin is pale, warm, and moist. In your reassessment, you found that there was increased tachycardia and that he still looks pale and is now hypotensive. These findings indicate:

   a. shock.
   b. anxiety.
   c. hypoglycemia.
   d. intracranial bleeding.

2. Repeating the primary assessment as part of the ongoing assessment en route to the hospital is necessary to:

   a. reevaluate the treatment priorities for the patient.
   b. predict all possible trends before arriving at the ED.
   c. have all information documented before arriving at the ED.
   d. provide any needed definite care prior to arriving at the ED.

3. The primary reason for conducting a reassessment on all patients is to:

   a. correct any life-threatening conditions.
   b. identify changes in a patient's condition.
   c. determine if the patient is competent to give consent.
   d. be able to complete the patient care report accurately.

4. After reassessing your patient, you document your findings. Each of the following components should be documented as part of the reassessment, *except*:

   a. serial vital signs.
   b. response to interventions.
   c. pertinent past medical history.
   d. findings from the repeat focused assessment.

5. Which of the following is most often repeated first in the reassessment?

   a. vital signs
   b. primary assessment
   c. checking interventions
   d. status of chief complaint

6. _____ is the primary focus of the reassessment.

   a. Assessing interventions
   b. Providing definitive care
   c. Reconsidering the MOI or NOI
   d. Early notification of the patient's status to the ED

7. In addition to vital signs, which of the following assessment components is used to establish a trend?

   a. pulse oximetry
   b. compliance with medications
   c. events leading up to the current episode
   d. time of onset of symptoms

8. On the way to the hospital, you take repeated sets of vital signs on a conscious medical patient and compare them to the baseline set of vital signs. This skill is known as:

   a. trending.
   b. reporting.
   c. appraising.
   d. reassuring.

9. You are en route to the hospital with a trauma patient whom you are treating for internal bleeding and head injury. While conducting the reassessment, you find that the systolic blood pressure has decreased from 110 to 100, and is now 92. What is the significance of this finding?

   a. The patient is in irreversible shock.
   b. The patient is in compensated shock.
   c. The patient is in decompensated shock.
   d. The patient has lost approximately 55 percent of his blood volume.

10. You are caring for a 30-year-old male who suspects that he has cracked or fractured a rib after falling. He has had broken ribs before and tells you that it hurts to take a deep breath. During your reassessment, you recognize that the patient is guarding his chest and his breathing seems much shallower. The emergency care for this patient includes:

    a. placing the patient on a pulse oximeter.
    b. providing high-flow oxygen and keeping the patient still.
    c. encouraging the patient to take deeper breaths and providing high-flow oxygen.
    d. encouraging the patient to take deeper breaths despite the increase in pain; no oxygen is necessary.

11. The reassessment of a patient with an isolated extremity injury includes reassessing:

    a. lung sounds and adequacy of the splint.
    b. pulse, blood pressure, and pulse oximetry.
    c. mental status and vital signs every 5 minutes.
    d. distal pulse, motor and sensory functions, and the adequacy of the splint.

12. When providing high-flow oxygen to a patient with a history of COPD, reassessment of this intervention includes assessing the skin color, checking the tank pressure and flow rate, and:

    a. documenting the procedure.
    b. removing nail polish to observe the nail beds.
    c. watching the patient for decreased respiratory effort.
    d. assessing for the development of congestive heart failure.

13. When assisting a patient who has chest pain to take his nitroglycerin, the EMT should reassess the _____ 3 to 5 minutes after the administration and before any additional medication is taken.

    a. pulse rate
    b. mental status
    c. blood pressure
    d. position of comfort

14. The driver of a mid-sized vehicle that was involved in a low-speed collision initially complained of cervical tenderness, with no other injuries. Your crew put on a cervical collar and immobilized her to a long backboard. En route to the hospital, the patient tells you that she is now experiencing low back spasms. This finding:

    a. is a pertinent negative.
    b. is not uncommon for this situation.
    c. indicates that the patient was improperly immobilized.
    d. indicates that the injury was missed during the physical exam.

15. In the primary assessment of a patient with chest trauma, you discovered a flail segment and immediately stabilized it. During the secondary assessment of the patient, you:

    a. reassess the injury for stability.
    b. reassess the injury only if there is significant bleeding.
    c. skip over the stabilized injury, but listen to lung sounds.
    d. reassess the injury only if the patient's breathing becomes worse.

16. En route to the hospital, the reassessment will often guide the EMT to:

    a. provide additional interventions.
    b. revise the plan of care for a patient.
    c. make the patient more comfortable.
    d. determine if the care provided is appropriate.

17. Which of the following statements about reassessment is most correct?

    a. Reassessment of the trauma patient with a significant MOI should be performed only by a paramedic.
    b. The reassessment of critically ill patients should be performed by the most senior EMT on the call.
    c. Anyone who is trained as an EMT may reassess any patient.
    d. The time interval for reassessing an unstable trauma patient is the same as for an unstable medical patient.

18. You are assessing a conscious patient who was reported to have passed out briefly. As you are talking to him and getting ready to move him onto your stretcher, you see his face get very pale and he starts sweating. What should you do next?

    a. Check to see if he has a pacemaker.
    b. Take off the oxygen mask and prepare for him to vomit.
    c. Elevate the patient's legs and reassess the blood pressure.
    d. Increase the flow of oxygen and sit him up in case he vomits.

19. When attempting to establish a trend, the EMT must obtain at least _____ vital sign(s).

    a. one
    b. two
    c. three
    d. four

20. Before documenting any trends observed during the time spent with the patient, the EMT should:

    a. reconsider the MOI.
    b. reassess the need for standard precautions.
    c. reassess the need for ALS.
    d. perform serial assessments.

21. Which of the following is one of the only times during the care of a patient that the EMT may omit the reassessment?
    a. short transport time
    b. treating a life-threatening condition
    c. when the patient is faking the complaint
    d. when a patient is too scared or embarrassed to be touched

22. You are transporting a conscious 34-year-old male who was hit by a car while walking in a parking lot. He has a broken lower leg, which is splinted, and he is fully immobilized to a long backboard. His last set of vital signs was: pulse 94/regular, respirations 26 and adequate, and BP 130/74. During the ride to the hospital, you reassess:
    a. every 5 minutes.
    b. every 15 minutes.
    c. after every intervention.
    d. only if there is a change in his condition.

23. (Continuing with the preceding question) Reassessment of the injured extremity should include:
    a. assessing for loss of range of motion.
    b. alternating cold and heat packs to the injured site.
    c. reassessing the distal pulse, motor and sensory functions.
    d. reassessing the proximal pulse and skin color, temperature, and condition.

24. Which of the following is an example of nondiagnostic information obtained in the patient assessment?
    a. allergies
    b. temperature
    c. blood glucose
    d. pulse oximetry

25. As you perform a detailed physical exam of the neck on a patient who is immobilized to a long backboard, you observe the presence of jugular vein distention (JVD). This finding:
    a. indicates hypertension.
    b. is normal in a supine patient.
    c. is an abnormal finding in a supine patient.
    d. indicates a possible life-threatening condition.

26. How often should a conscious patient be reassessed?
    a. every 5 minutes
    b. every 10 minutes for a high-priority patient
    c. typically once while en route to the hospital
    d. every time there is a change in the patient's condition

27. Which of the following statements about trauma patients with significant MOIs is most correct?
    a. The baseline vital signs appear better than they actually are.
    b. The MOI will help the EMT decide when to obtain baseline vital signs.
    c. Baseline vital signs should be obtained prior to performing the secondary assessment.
    d. The patient's level of consciousness will help to determine when to perform the secondary assessment.

28. The secondary assessment is typically performed in a head-to-toe order because:
    a. this order is the quickest method.
    b. most local protocols mandate this order.
    c. the patient is usually most cooperative with this order of assessment.
    d. using this same order every time helps to minimize missing any pertinent findings.

29. What is the value of a secondary assessment?
    a. Performing a secondary assessment will really impress the ED staff.
    b. The EMT may discover information not obtained in the primary assessment.
    c. Completing a secondary assessment will keep the EMT from becoming involved in a lawsuit.
    d. Completion of a secondary assessment helps to establish a better rapport with the patient.

30. When a patient has a chief complaint of chest pain the EMT must ask several questions to attempt to determine if the pain is cardiac in nature or from another source. The list of possible causes of chest pain the EMT formulates as he interviews the patient is called the:
    a. patient history.
    b. past medical history.
    c. differential diagnosis.
    d. comprehensive assessment.

31. The EMT is assessing a 65-year-old male with a chief complaint of difficulty breathing. One of the early questions she asks the patient is "Are you having any chest pain?" The patient replies "No." This is an example of a/an:
    a. diagnostic information.
    b. pertinent positive reply.
    c. effective communication.
    d. pertinent negative response.

32. During your assessment of your patient's pupils, you note that they both respond to light but are unequal in size. Your next action should be to:

    a. call medical control for advice.
    b. do nothing and reassess in 5 minutes.
    c. ask the patient if this is normal for her.
    d. provide high-flow oxygen and rapid transport.

33. The EMT is caring for patient who is presenting with stroke symptoms. The patient is conscious but unable to speak. No one at the patient's home can speak for the patient. What can the EMT use to obtain information about the patient's medical history?

    a. vital signs
    b. advanced directives
    c. prescription medications
    d. SpO_2 and blood sugar readings

34. Your ambulance was dispatched for a "fainting episode." When you arrive, the patient is awake and complaining of neck and back pain. After the primary assessment, your plan of action should be to:

    a. assess the neck and back pain first.
    b. assess for a medical cause for the fainting first.
    c. call for ALS, as the patient is too unstable for BLS.
    d. obtain vital signs followed by a secondary assessment.

35. You have arrived on scene at a supermarket on a call for an unconscious checkout clerk, who is lying on the floor beneath the register. Who would likely provide the best information about what has just happened to the patient?

    a. the patient
    b. the patient's boss
    c. the customer at the checkout who witnessed the episode
    d. the police officer on the scene

Chapter 14 Answer Form

	A	B	C	D		A	B	C	D
1.	❏	❏	❏	❏	19.	❏	❏	❏	❏
2.	❏	❏	❏	❏	20.	❏	❏	❏	❏
3.	❏	❏	❏	❏	21.	❏	❏	❏	❏
4.	❏	❏	❏	❏	22.	❏	❏	❏	❏
5.	❏	❏	❏	❏	23.	❏	❏	❏	❏
6.	❏	❏	❏	❏	24.	❏	❏	❏	❏
7.	❏	❏	❏	❏	25.	❏	❏	❏	❏
8.	❏	❏	❏	❏	26.	❏	❏	❏	❏
9.	❏	❏	❏	❏	27.	❏	❏	❏	❏
10.	❏	❏	❏	❏	28.	❏	❏	❏	❏
11.	❏	❏	❏	❏	29.	❏	❏	❏	❏
12.	❏	❏	❏	❏	30.	❏	❏	❏	❏
13.	❏	❏	❏	❏	31.	❏	❏	❏	❏
14.	❏	❏	❏	❏	32.	❏	❏	❏	❏
15.	❏	❏	❏	❏	33.	❏	❏	❏	❏
16.	❏	❏	❏	❏	34.	❏	❏	❏	❏
17.	❏	❏	❏	❏	35.	❏	❏	❏	❏
18.	❏	❏	❏	❏					

CHAPTER

15

Communications and Documentation

1. You need to contact medical control for an order to assist a patient with his medication. Ideally, the contact should be made by:
   a. contacting the patient's physician using the patient's phone.
   b. getting dispatch to call the hospital and make the request using any method that is recorded for quality assurance.
   c. cell phone, as it is the quickest way to make contact and obtain an order.
   d. landline from the patient's residence, as it is the clearest form of communication.

2. The proper method of establishing radio contact between two units is to:
   a. push the PTT button and wait to be acknowledged.
   b. speak with your upper lip touching the microphone.
   c. say the name of the unit being called followed by the name of your unit.
   d. say the name of your unit followed by the name of the unit being called.

3. To effectively initiate a radio call, the EMT must first:
   a. learn all the radio codes.
   b. anticipate what the unit being called is going to say next.
   c. monitor the channel for a clear frequency before beginning the transmission.
   d. all of the above.

4. Safety hazards, patient condition, number of patients, and confirmation of the number of ambulances needed are all pieces of information that should be provided:
   a. while at the scene.
   b. en route to the scene.
   c. en route to the hospital.
   d. upon returning to service.

5. The ambulance-to-hospital communication should:
   a. be less than 30 seconds long.
   b. never be more than 90 seconds long.
   c. follow the standard medical case presentation.
   d. begin with the estimated time of arrival at the hospital.

6. A typical medical radio report is presented in which order?
   a. vital signs, chief complaint, allergies, mental status, and ETA
   b. patient's age, sex, chief complaint, severity, treatment, and ETA
   c. ETA, patient's name, chief complaint, and Social Security number
   d. chief complaint, past medical history, date of birth, and health insurance number

7. An EMT's inability to communicate effectively about the patient may lead to:
   a. delayed care and transfer of the patient.
   b. a possible better outcome for the patient.
   c. practice of professional patient advocacy.
   d. a smoother transition of the patient between health care providers.

8. Standard radio operating procedures are created and designed to:
   a. reduce the number of misunderstood messages.
   b. get the units back in service as soon as possible.
   c. allow dispatch to know where all units are at all times.
   d. keep users from using complicated codes in their transmissions.

9. Which of the following factors directly interferes with effective radio communication of patient information to the hospital?
   a. background noise
   b. patient's condition
   c. training level of EMS provider
   d. the EMS provider's years of experience

10. Which of the following is considered an essential component of the verbal report for patient registration?
    a. SAMPLE history
    b. patient's address and telephone number
    c. pertinent positive and negative findings
    d. emergency care provided to the patient

11. Upon arrival at the hospital, the EMT will first provide the staff with a _____ report about the patient.
    a. rapid
    b. verbal
    c. written
    d. controlled

12. The _____ is responsible for giving report of the patient to the hospital staff.
    a. ambulance driver
    b. most senior crew member
    c. EMT in charge of the patient
    d. highest-ranking crew member

13. You are taking a report from a registered nurse (RN) in a nursing home about an elderly patient who has dementia and hearing deficit. What can you do to increase the effectiveness of your communication with this type of patient?
    a. Look into the patient's eyes when you speak.
    b. Shout in a clear tone and at a normal rate.
    c. Make eye contact and shout as you speak.
    d. Whisper into the right ear.

14. Which of the following practices is appropriate when talking to dispatch on an approved radio frequency?
    a. using clear and brief communication
    b. including personal patient information
    c. using "please" and "thank you"
    d. using a tone of voice that implies anger, frustration, or extreme emotion

15. You are caring for a 4-year-old who seems to be frightened of you and your crew. How can you appear less threatening and begin effective communication with the patient?
    a. Let the parent be the liaison for you.
    b. Tell the patient that you are not the police and promise her a toy.
    c. Use an authoritative tone and tell the child you will not give her any shots.
    d. Keep a friendly smile on your face and kneel down to her height as you speak.

16. When two units transmit at the same time:
    a. only one unit will be heard.
    b. both transmissions will be heard.
    c. neither transmission will be heard.
    d. both units can be subject to a fine for improper communication.

17. The _____ is the agency that assigns and licenses radio frequencies.
    a. Homeland Security Agency
    b. Federal Telecommunications Commission
    c. Federal Corrections Commission
    d. Federal Communications Commission

18. Slang terms should be avoided when making transmissions using a:
    a. repeater.
    b. two-way communication device.
    c. mobile or portable radio.
    d. cell phone.

19. Which of the following is an inappropriate form of communication that should be avoided when interacting with a patient?
    a. Use the patient's surname when making an introduction with a patient.
    b. Take off your glove to shake hands when making an introduction with a patient.
    c. Allow the patient to describe his concerns before asking the SAMPLE questions.
    d. Use the patient's first name or nickname to put the patient at ease when making an introduction with a patient.

20. How can the EMT best communicate with an elderly patient who cannot hear without his hearing aids?
    a. Shout into the ear that has the best hearing.
    b. Use sign language to communicate your questions.
    c. Make sure that the patient is wearing his hearing aids and that they are turned on.
    d. Look into the patient's face and exaggerate your lip movement when speaking.

21. You are caring for a patient who speaks a foreign language and does not appear to understand English. Which of the following methods of communications will be most useful in this situation?
    a. Make eye contact and maintain friendly facial expressions.
    b. Avoid talking to the patient; instead, draw pictures to communicate.
    c. Call the hospital and advise them that the patient is in need of an interpreter.
    d. Avoid talking to or touching the patient unless he becomes unresponsive.

22. You have just loaded your patient into the ambulance when a neighbor runs over to you and asks what is going on. You tell the neighbor:
    a. that the patient is going to be fine and not to worry.
    b. that you are taking the patient to the hospital and nothing else.
    c. to call the patient's family if she wants to know what is happening.
    d. everything that has happened on the scene and to meet you at the hospital if she wishes.

23. You are treating a 55-year-old female for symptoms of chest pain and dizziness. As you are getting ready to move the patient to the ambulance, the family asks you how she is doing. You should tell the patient's family:

    a. that the patient is going to be fine and not to worry at this point.
    b. nothing and let the emergency department physician explain.
    c. what you suspect is happening and what you are going to do en route to the hospital.
    d. that the patient has a 50/50 chance of going into cardiac arrest and that you need to get going.

24. Using medical terminology when discussing a patient's present condition or past medical history is not appropriate when:

    a. documenting your patient care report.
    b. presenting your patient in case review.
    c. giving report to the next health care provider.
    d. demonstrating your expertise to the patient's family.

25. You are contacting medical control to obtain an order to assist a patient with a medication. The typical request should be stated by:

    a. describing the patient's condition, requesting the order, and confirming the order.
    b. requesting the order, describing the patient's condition, and asking questions if you do not understand the order.
    c. requesting the order, confirming the order, describing the patient's condition, and never questioning the order.
    d. describing the patient's condition, requesting the order, repeating the order, confirming the order, and never asking questions about the order.

26. In which order does the communication between dispatch and a transporting ambulance occur?

    a. The ambulance notifies dispatch, when leaving the scene, of the destination and when they will arrive; dispatch acknowledges with a time check.
    b. Dispatch assigns the destination hospital; the ambulance acknowledges and calls out upon arrival at that hospital.
    c. The ambulance advises of ETA at the hospital; dispatch acknowledges and approves transport; the ambulance calls out when arriving.
    d. The ambulance calls dispatch after arriving at the hospital, relaying the time it left the scene, time of arrival at the hospital, and time back in service; dispatch acknowledges.

27. When reporting time data on a patient care report (PCR), which of the following are typically included?

    a. date, time the report was written, and time back in service
    b. time of dispatch, arrival at the scene, leaving the scene, and arrival at the hospital
    c. time the initial call for help was received, time of dispatch, time of arrival at the scene and leaving the scene, and time the report was written
    d. time of call received, time of acknowledgment of call received, on-scene time, and time of end of shift when the shift end occurs during a call

28. When tracking the times on a written report, the EMT should use:

    a. the time provided by dispatch.
    b. universal Greenwich Mean Time.
    c. his watch and convert to military time.
    d. the clock in the ambulance and convert to military time.

29. The _____ has standardized a minimum data set to be included in all prehospital care reports.

    a. Surgeon General
    b. American Ambulance Association
    c. National Highway Traffic Safety Administration
    d. Occupational Safety and Health Administration

30. Patient information that includes age, date of birth, gender, address, and telephone number is considered:

    a. universal statistics.
    b. assessment findings.
    c. patient demographics.
    d. past medical history.

31. The _____ portion of the written prehospital care report includes information that is most useful to the next health care provider to care for the patient.

    a. narrative
    b. runtimes
    c. insurance
    d. administrative

32. When completing a written report, the emergency care provided to a patient by the EMT should be documented:

    a. in the narrative.
    b. on the billing form.
    c. in check boxes provided.
    d. on the back of the patient care report.

33. In the EMS profession, times are recorded in military time because:
   a. fire departments and police agencies use it.
   b. it helps to minimize documentation and recording errors.
   c. the government has ultimate oversight over such matters.
   d. compliance is mandated by the American Medical Association.

34. Many prehospital care reports include use of the Glasgow Coma Scale, which provides information about a patient's mental status in the form of a:
   a. trend.
   b. number.
   c. disposition.
   d. brief narrative.

35. During the scene size-up and while forming a general impression of a trauma patient, you discovered that your unconscious patient has no identification. This information should be documented in which portion of the patient care report?
   a. administrative
   b. chief complaint
   c. demographics
   d. statistics and research

36. Which of the following patients should the EMT allow to refuse treatment or transport?
   a. a competent 12-year-old with a minor abrasion from a skateboard accident
   b. a 17-year-old married female with a black eye and multiple new cuts and bruises on her body
   c. a 30-year-old with a possible sprained ankle who admits to having had two beers
   d. a 32-year-old mother of three who is home without transportation and has a child who choked, but appears fine upon your initial assessment

37. When a patient refuses care or transport, the EMT should disclose and document what information to the patient?
   a. billing information
   b. dispatch information
   c. treatment recommendations
   d. transportation considerations

38. You are assessing a patient who was involved in an MVC. He complains of neck pain as a result of the collision. The patient has requested transport to the hospital for evaluation, but is refusing to be immobilized because he fears being confined. You should:
   a. refuse to transport without immobilization.
   b. transport the patient without any immobilization.
   c. request police intervention to get the patient to comply with standard immobilization practices.
   d. document the refusal of care, have the patient sign the refusal, and transport the patient.

39. After completing your written report on a patient, you realize that you forgot to document an important finding from the primary assessment. How should you correct this error?
   a. Verbally report the omitted finding to the patient's nurse.
   b. Make the change on your copy only, then initial and date it.
   c. Make the change on all copies of the written report, then initial and date it.
   d. Make the change on your copy and have your supervisor initial and date it.

40. A written patient care report that is _____ may give rise to a presumption that the proper care was omitted or lacking.
   a. legible
   b. intelligible
   c. incomplete
   d. comprehensible

41. A written report is considered credible when the EMT completes it accurately, objectively, promptly, and:
   a. upholds stereotyping.
   b. preserves judgmental biases.
   c. maintains patient confidentiality.
   d. includes extraneous statements.

42. Reporting suspected abuse of an elderly patient by a family member:
   a. is mandated by AARP.
   b. varies from state to state.
   c. is mandatory in all 50 states.
   d. is optional and not required in all 50 states.

43. While inside the home of a patient, you notice some unusual findings. Which of the following are you mandated to report?
   a. suspected child abuse
   b. calendars with nudity
   c. whips and restraining devices
   d. a couple hundred full and empty liquor bottles

44. _____ are often used as the first form of documentation at a multiple casualty incident (MCI).
   a. Triage tags
   b. Colored tape
   c. Patient care reports
   d. Special incident reports

45. Using medical terminology when completing a written patient care report is appropriate in which of the following cases?
   a. when the term is spelled incorrectly
   b. when the medical terms are used duly
   c. only when the report is one page long
   d. only when the report is two or more pages long

46. Which of the following would be considered a pertinent negative on your written report?
    a. the MOI
    b. trending vital signs
    c. the position in which the patient was found
    d. head injury without a loss of consciousness

47. You have successfully assisted a diabetic who has an altered mental status to take oral glucose. Which of the following should you document on your written report?
    a. time of absorption
    b. time of medication administration
    c. contraindications for oral glucose
    d. date of expiration on the oral glucose

48. Which of the following is an example of something that should be documented on the patient care report?
    a. radio failure
    b. route of transport
    c. exposure to blood
    d. standard operating procedures

49. In a court of law, poor documentation is often characterized as:
    a. forgetfulness.
    b. poor assessment.
    c. improper training.
    d. delegation of authority.

50. After administering oxygen by non-rebreather mask to a patient with respiratory distress, what information should be documented on the patient care report?
    a. the liter flow of oxygen
    b. the steps to apply the mask
    c. the size of the oxygen tank that was utilized
    d. the hydrostatic date on the oxygen cylinder

Chapter 15 Answer Form

	A	B	C	D			A	B	C	D
1.	❏	❏	❏	❏		26.	❏	❏	❏	❏
2.	❏	❏	❏	❏		27.	❏	❏	❏	❏
3.	❏	❏	❏	❏		28.	❏	❏	❏	❏
4.	❏	❏	❏	❏		29.	❏	❏	❏	❏
5.	❏	❏	❏	❏		30.	❏	❏	❏	❏
6.	❏	❏	❏	❏		31.	❏	❏	❏	❏
7.	❏	❏	❏	❏		32.	❏	❏	❏	❏
8.	❏	❏	❏	❏		33.	❏	❏	❏	❏
9.	❏	❏	❏	❏		34.	❏	❏	❏	❏
10.	❏	❏	❏	❏		35.	❏	❏	❏	❏
11.	❏	❏	❏	❏		36.	❏	❏	❏	❏
12.	❏	❏	❏	❏		37.	❏	❏	❏	❏
13.	❏	❏	❏	❏		38.	❏	❏	❏	❏
14.	❏	❏	❏	❏		39.	❏	❏	❏	❏
15.	❏	❏	❏	❏		40.	❏	❏	❏	❏
16.	❏	❏	❏	❏		41.	❏	❏	❏	❏
17.	❏	❏	❏	❏		42.	❏	❏	❏	❏
18.	❏	❏	❏	❏		43.	❏	❏	❏	❏
19.	❏	❏	❏	❏		44.	❏	❏	❏	❏
20.	❏	❏	❏	❏		45.	❏	❏	❏	❏
21.	❏	❏	❏	❏		46.	❏	❏	❏	❏
22.	❏	❏	❏	❏		47.	❏	❏	❏	❏
23.	❏	❏	❏	❏		48.	❏	❏	❏	❏
24.	❏	❏	❏	❏		49.	❏	❏	❏	❏
25.	❏	❏	❏	❏		50.	❏	❏	❏	❏

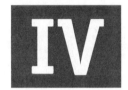

MEDICAL EMERGENCIES

CHAPTER 16

General Pharmacology

1. One of the major functions of the liver is to detoxify and metabolize drugs so the _____ can easily eliminate them.
   a. kidneys
   b. stomach
   c. colon
   d. lungs

2. Which of the following medications does not require a written prescription from a physician?
   a. oxygen
   b. Atrovent
   c. Benadryl
   d. nitroglycerin

3. Which of the following medications requires a prescription and therefore is not typically carried on a BLS ambulance?
   a. oxygen
   b. nitroglycerin
   c. oral glucose
   d. activated charcoal

4. A single drug usually affects:
   a. one organ.
   b. vital signs.
   c. more than one organ.
   d. every organ except the brain.

5. The official name of a drug is the _____ name followed by the initials USP or NF.
   a. brand
   b. product
   c. generic
   d. chemical

6. The EMT is responsible for knowing the generic and _____ names of the medications carried on the unit.
   a. trade
   b. slang
   c. official
   d. chemical

7. You have been dispatched on a seizure call. When you arrive, the patient is unresponsive, breathing, and has a pulse. A family member reports that the patient has diabetes and just finished having a second seizure, with a brief period of alertness between the two seizures. Which medication should you assist the patient with?
   a. oxygen
   b. oral glucose
   c. activated charcoal
   d. prescribed nitroglycerin

8. A 30-year-old female with a history of asthma is complaining of difficulty breathing and chest tightness. She appears anxious and slightly confused, yet you can hear her wheezing. Which of the following medications will you assist her with?
   a. albuterol
   b. oral glucose
   c. nitroglycerin
   d. epinephrine auto-injector

9. The EMT may assist a patient with _____ when the patient is exhibiting signs of wheezing, airway swelling, tachycardia, and hives.
   a. prescribed nitroglycerin
   b. over-the-counter Benadryl
   c. prescribed bronchodilator inhaler
   d. prescribed epinephrine auto-injector

10. _____ is the trade name for a common preparation of oral glucose that EMTs can give as a treatment if authorized by medical control.
    a. Glutose
    b. Orajel™
    c. Fructose
    d. Maltose

11. EpiPen™ is the _____ name for an epinephrine auto-injector.
    a. brand
    b. official
    c. generic
    d. street

12. You are going to be assisting an asthma patient with her medication. Your partner brings you several of her metered dose inhalers. Of the following medication names, which is the generic form?

a. ventolin
b. albuterol
c. proventil
d. combivent

13. Liquids that contain dissolved drugs are called:

a. solutions.
b. suspensions.
c. suppositories.
d. transdermals.

14. A _____ is a single dose of medication that is shaped like a disc and can be chewed or swallowed whole.

a. tablet
b. capsule
c. suppository
d. suspension

15. _____ are a form of medication consisting of liquids with solid particles mixed within them, but not dissolved.

a. Syrups
b. Tinctures
c. Solutions
d. Suspensions

16. For the patient who is experiencing an asthma attack, the EMT should first assist the patient with _____ followed by:

a. oxygen, the patient's inhaler.
b. the patient's inhaler, a position of comfort.
c. a position of comfort, the patient's inhaler.
d. oxygen, an epinephrine auto-injector.

17. Epinephrine works on a patient who is experiencing anaphylaxis by:

a. blocking the release of histamines.
b. dilating coronary vessels and improving oxygenation.
c. dilating peripheral vessels to relieve itching and hives.
d. relaxing airway passages and constricting the blood vessels.

18. Activated charcoal works with poisons that have been:

a. inhaled.
b. injected.
c. ingested.
d. absorbed through the skin.

19. Epinephrine is a powerful vasoconstrictor that causes:

a. increased blood pressure.
b. decreased blood pressure.
c. no change in blood pressure.
d. increased bronchoconstriction.

20. Which of the following is not a "right" of medication administration?

a. right drug
b. right dose
c. right patient
d. right standard precautions

21. Bronchodilators, antihistamines, and antihypertensives are all examples of:

a. forms of medications.
b. routes of medications.
c. classifications of medications.
d. medications the EMT can assist a patient with.

22. A/An _____ warns that something is inappropriate as a treatment.

a. side effect
b. classification
c. adverse effect
d. contraindication

23. _____ is/are derived from both animal and human sources.

a. Benadryl
b. Oral glucose
c. Activated charcoal
d. Epinephrine and insulin

24. _____ is not a route of drug administration.

a. Inhalation
b. Intravenous
c. Immunization
d. Intramuscular

25. Which of the following is a route for administering medication?

a. gas
b. syrup
c. sublingual
d. suspension

26. A/An _____ is a response to a drug that is not the principal intent for giving that drug.

a. defect
b. side effect
c. additive effect
d. contraindication

27. The most significant side effect of epinephrine is:

a. anxiety.
b. increased heart rate.
c. decreased blood pressure.
d. decreased respiratory rate.

28. Nitroglycerin works to decrease chest pain by:
    a. constricting coronary vessels and increasing the blood pressure.
    b. dilating coronary vessels, thus increasing blood supply to the heart.
    c. constricting coronary vessels, thus improving oxygenation to the heart.
    d. dilating coronary vessels, thus decreasing the muscle spasm of the heart.

29. _____ is a side effect of bronchodilators.
    a. Increased heart rate
    b. Decreased heart rate
    c. Altered mental status
    d. Increased respiratory rate

30. In a patient with poisoning (whether intentional or unintentional), activated charcoal works by:
    a. absorbing most of the poison.
    b. inactivating the chemical composite.
    c. causing the patient to vomit the poison.
    d. allowing the poison to be reabsorbed, causing dilution.

31. Your unit has been dispatched to a high school for an allergic reaction to a bee sting. In the school nurse's office, a 16-year-old female is sitting up and appears very ill. She is working hard to breathe and looks pale and moist, one side of her face is swollen, and she has hives on her neck and arms. The nurse reports that the patient's pulse is 130, weak and regular, and that her BP is 78/40. The patient has a history of allergies to bee stings, and used her epinephrine auto-injector shortly after being stung on the face approximately 20 minutes ago. What is the patient's present condition?
    a. She is potentially unstable.
    b. She is in anaphylactic shock.
    c. She is experiencing hypotension as a side effect of the epinephrine.
    d. She has signs and symptoms of a possible reaction to epinephrine as well as the bee sting.

32. (Continuing with the preceding question) You administer high-flow oxygen and confirm that ALS is en route. Further examination findings include wheezing, hives on the front and back torso, and new patient complaints of a swollen tongue, dizziness, and chest tightness. The nurse has additional epinephrine auto-injectors, as well as a few over-the-counter medications, on hand. Which treatment or medication would be the most appropriate for the patient now?
    a. Benadryl™.
    b. Contact medical control for another dose of epinephrine.
    c. Do not administer any more epinephrine, but treat for shock.
    d. Provide only high-flow oxygen and wait for ALS to arrive.

33. The aunt of a 4-year-old male called EMS when the child developed shortness of breath and wheezing while the child was in her care. She tells you that the child does have a history of asthma and that she has his metered dose inhaler (MDI). However, she has never had to give it until today and she is not sure that she did it correctly. You assess the child and find him to be very anxious; he has audible wheezing and his skin is pale, warm, and moist. Respiratory rate is 40 and labored, and his pulse is 120, strong and regular. You verify that the MDI is the patient's and obtain permission from medical control to assist the patient with the MDI. You attempt to assist with the MDI, but cannot be sure that any medication was inhaled. The child begins to exhibit tremors and has a significant decrease in mental status. What do you suspect is the cause of the sudden change in the patient's condition?
    a. The medication is beginning to work.
    b. The patient has received a lethal dose of medication.
    c. The tremors and decreased mental status indicate that the patient may have received too much medication.
    d. Tremors are a side effect of the medication and the child's decreased mental status is a sign of inadequate breathing.

34. (Continuing with the preceding question) What is the appropriate action to take next?
    a. Rapidly administer an additional dose.
    b. Stop giving the medication and assist ventilations with a bag mask device.
    c. Request ALS for a possible overdose of medication from the MDI.
    d. Stop giving the medication and administer high-flow oxygen by non-rebreather mask.

35. An elderly male is experiencing respiratory distress from recently diagnosed pneumonia. The patient has a history of COPD, specifically emphysema, and for most of the day and night uses a nasal cannula. Since being discharged from the hospital two days ago for pneumonia, the patient has had progressively worsening dyspnea. He is cyanotic, warm, and dry; lung sounds are diminished on the right; respiratory rate is 28 and labored, pulse is 110 and irregular, and BP is 144/90. You administer high-flow oxygen by non-rebreather mask and prepare the patient for transport. En route to the ED, you see the patient become sleepy, and his respiratory rate and effort decrease. What action is appropriate for this patient now?
    a. Assist the patient's ventilations using a bag mask device.
    b. Gently wake the patient and encourage him to stay awake.
    c. Replace the non-rebreather mask with a nasal cannula turned on at 2 lpm.
    d. Remove the oxygen and observe the patient for the duration of the transport.

Chapter 16 Answer Form

	A	B	C	D		A	B	C	D
1.	❏	❏	❏	❏	19.	❏	❏	❏	❏
2.	❏	❏	❏	❏	20.	❏	❏	❏	❏
3.	❏	❏	❏	❏	21.	❏	❏	❏	❏
4.	❏	❏	❏	❏	22.	❏	❏	❏	❏
5.	❏	❏	❏	❏	23.	❏	❏	❏	❏
6.	❏	❏	❏	❏	24.	❏	❏	❏	❏
7.	❏	❏	❏	❏	25.	❏	❏	❏	❏
8.	❏	❏	❏	❏	26.	❏	❏	❏	❏
9.	❏	❏	❏	❏	27.	❏	❏	❏	❏
10.	❏	❏	❏	❏	28.	❏	❏	❏	❏
11.	❏	❏	❏	❏	29.	❏	❏	❏	❏
12.	❏	❏	❏	❏	30.	❏	❏	❏	❏
13.	❏	❏	❏	❏	31.	❏	❏	❏	❏
14.	❏	❏	❏	❏	32.	❏	❏	❏	❏
15.	❏	❏	❏	❏	33.	❏	❏	❏	❏
16.	❏	❏	❏	❏	34.	❏	❏	❏	❏
17.	❏	❏	❏	❏	35.	❏	❏	❏	❏
18.	❏	❏	❏	❏					

CHAPTER

17

Respiratory Emergencies

1. A 45-year-old male is complaining of difficulty breathing that began 15 minutes ago, right after returning home from a walk. The EMT should assess breathing *first* by:
   a. using pulse oximetry (SpO_2).
   b. listening to lung sounds in the apecies.
   c. listening to lung sounds in the back.
   d. feeling for equal chest wall expansion.

2. For patients who are significantly overweight, the ideal place to listening for lung sounds is the:
   a. back.
   b. upper chest.
   c. lower chest.
   d. middle of the chest.

3. _____ is an abnormal breathing sound caused by an upper airway obstruction.
   a. Croup
   b. Stridor
   c. Wheezing
   d. Coughing

4. A 26-year-old female with a history of asthma is wheezing and complaining of breathing difficulty and chest tightness. She also complains of dizziness and tingling in her hands. You should:
   a. provide high-flow oxygen and assist her with her inhaler.
   b. lay her down to relieve the dizziness and assist her with her inhaler.
   c. provide high-flow oxygen for the breathing difficulty and assist her with nitroglycerin for the chest tightness.
   d. get her to slow her breathing to relieve the dizziness and tingling; then, after those symptoms are relieved, administer high-flow oxygen.

5. Which of the following is a symptom rather than a sign of breathing difficulty?
   a. The patient is coughing.
   b. The patient has an altered mental status.
   c. The patient has a sustained increased heart rate.
   d. The patient tells you that it is hard to take a deep breath.

6. You are assessing a patient who is complaining of difficulty breathing. She is speaking in full sentences with no trouble, her skin signs are good, and her lung sounds are clear in all fields. You should:
   a. consider that she may be faking the complaint.
   b. believe her complaint and provide her with high-flow oxygen.
   c. tell her that she is okay for now and have her go to her own doctor.
   d. believe her complaint, but withhold oxygen until signs of respiratory distress are present.

7. During a routine return transport of an elderly nursing home resident, from his dental appointment back to the nursing home, you notice that he has fallen asleep. Suddenly the patient has snoring and gurgling respirations. The first action you should take is to:
   a. check for a pulse.
   b. assess responsiveness.
   c. lay the patient supine and suction his airway.
   d. do nothing, as the snoring will stop without intervention.

8. For a patient who is having breathing difficulty, a _____ is indicated whenever the patient needs oxygen, has a good respiratory effort, and is not apneic.
   a. nasal cannula
   b. bag mask device
   c. simple face mask
   d. non-rebreather mask

9. Oxygen delivery by nasal cannula is usually tolerated well by most patients, but is contraindicated when a:
   a. patient is a mouth breather.
   b. hypoxic patient will not tolerate a mask.
   c. child with respiratory distress pushes away a non-rebreather mask.
   d. patient with no distress is receiving low to moderate oxygen enrichment for long periods.

10. All of the following patients are having breathing difficulty. For which one would you need medical direction to assist in emergency medical care?

   a. a 14-year-old female with asthma, who is wheezing after gym class
   b. a 30-year-old female with a respiratory rate of 30 after a near-fainting event
   c. an 18-month-old infant who choked on a hot dog and is breathing without distress
   d. a postictal seizure patient who is awake but confused, with a respiratory rate of 16 breaths per minute

11. A 65-year-old female who is having difficulty breathing tells you that she has a history of COPD, hypertension, and diabetes. You listen to her breath sounds and hear faint wheezing. Vital signs are: respiratory rate 26; pulse 78, regular; BP 150/100. Her skin signs are good. Which of the following would you consider assisting her with?

   a. her home nebulizer
   b. her metered dose inhaler
   c. the scheduled insulin dose she is late with
   d. increasing the flow rate on her home oxygen unit

12. Your ambulance has been dispatched for a 16-year-old male who is having difficulty breathing. In the primary assessment, you find that he is alert; gasping for air; and has hives on his neck, arms, and chest. Your partner quickly administers high-flow oxygen and you:

   a. look for a possible poisoning agent.
   b. look into the airway for a possible foreign body airway obstruction.
   c. contact medical control for an order to assist with a bronchodilator inhaler.
   d. assist the patient with an epinephrine auto-injector, after obtaining permission from medical control.

13. An elderly man with a history of chronic bronchitis wears a nasal cannula delivering 2 to 4 lpm of oxygen most of the time. He appears distressed and complains of having had increased difficulty breathing since he was recently discharged from the hospital with pneumonia. Initial management of this patient will include:

   a. gentle handling, position of comfort, warmth, and high-flow oxygen by NRB mask if tolerated.
   b. high-flow oxygen by non-rebreather mask and being prepared to assist with bag mask ventilations.
   c. sitting the patient upright, giving high-flow oxygen by non-rebreather mask, and assisting with a bronchodilator inhaler.
   d. keeping the patient calm, turning up the oxygen flow on the cannula to 8 lpm, and providing warmth and gentle transport.

14. After responding to a call for a cardiac arrest, you find an unresponsive elderly male who is breathing at a rate of 6 breaths per minute and has a pulse of 60. You attempt to place an OPA, but the patient gags. Now you should:

   a. suction the patient and provide blow-by oxygen.
   b. administer high-flow oxygen via non-rebreather mask.
   c. insert an NPA and provide bag mask ventilations once every 6 seconds.
   d. insert an NPA and provide bag mask ventilations once every 3 seconds.

15. You are attempting to coach an asthmatic patient, who is in respiratory distress, to use her inhaler. You tell her to:

   a. exhale, then inhale while spraying, and then hold her breath.
   b. take a deep breath while spraying and hold her breath; then repeat.
   c. slow her breathing, lean forward, spray, inhale, exhale deeply, and repeat.
   d. put her head back, exhale, inhale while spraying, swallow, and hold her breath.

16. You have decided to assist ventilations with a bag mask device for a patient with severe breathing difficulty. You know you are providing effective ventilations when:

   a. the chest rises with each ventilation.
   b. the pulse oximetry reading is above 95 percent.
   c. the patient begins to fight or pushes you away.
   d. there is little or no resistance squeezing the bag.

17. You are assessing and treating a patient who is in respiratory distress. Which of the following signs would give you the indication to assist the patient with bag mask ventilations?

   a. decreased wheezing respirations and increased retractions
   b. a fast pulse rate and a change in mental status
   c. respiratory rate of 30 and change in pulse rate from 48 to 88 bpm
   d. hyperventilation with flushed skin

18. In which of the following patients would a nasal pharyngeal airway be most appropriate?

   a. an 80-year-old male in cardiac arrest
   b. a 2-year-old with stridor and drooling
   c. an 18-year-old male who is experiencing a seizure
   d. an alert 24-year-old female who is having an asthma attack

19. In forming a general impression of the patient, the EMT can rapidly assess for adequate air exchange by:
    a. noting the skin color.
    b. getting a pulse oximetry reading.
    c. assuring an open and patent airway.
    d. observing movement of the diaphragm.

20. When a patient is receiving ventilations with a bag mask device, the EMT should assess for adequate ventilations by:
    a. assuring a tight mask seal.
    b. assessing pupillary reactions.
    c. relying on pulse oximeter readings.
    d. assuring that the oxygen flow rate is high.

21. The three signs of adequate air exchange are:
    a. regular rhythm, inability to speak, and warm and pink skin.
    b. alert mental state, equal breath sounds, and a regular rhythm.
    c. high pulse oximetry reading, unilateral breath sounds, and no wheezing.
    d. a rate of 12 to 20 breaths per minute in an adult, pink and dry skin, and unequal chest rise and fall.

22. Before assisting a patient who has respiratory difficulty to administer a dose of his prescribed inhaler, the EMT must assure all of the following "rights," except right:
    a. dose.
    b. vital signs.
    c. medication.
    d. prescription for the patient.

23. Which of the following conditions is not an indication for the EMT to assist a patient with difficult breathing to use her own prescribed inhaler?
    a. The patient has two different prescribed inhalers.
    b. The patient is experiencing anxiety and a fast pulse rate.
    c. Vital signs and a focused history have yet to be obtained.
    d. An asthma patient has severe breathing difficulty, but no wheezing.

24. A prescribed inhaler containing albuterol causes which of the following actions?
    a. dilates coronary vessels
    b. reduces airway constriction
    c. increases mucus production
    d. decreases mucus production

25. You are using a bag mask device to assist ventilations for a 7-year-old child who has severe breathing distress. You squeeze the bag once every _____ seconds.
    a. 3
    b. 4
    c. 5
    d. 6

26. For a child who is experiencing respiratory distress due to asthma or bronchiolitis, _____ is the most important treatment the EMT can provide.
    a. oxygen
    b. rapid transport
    c. a bronchodilator
    d. a prescribed inhaler

27. A 12-month-old infant is suspected of having swallowed a marble and is now unresponsive. The correct sequence for treating a foreign body airway obstruction (FBAO) when no foreign body is visible in the airway is to:
    a. open the airway, do a finger sweep, and give a breath and back blows.
    b. open the airway, give a breath, administer abdominal thrusts, and repeat.
    c. open the airway and give a breath, back blows, and chest thrusts. Repeat as needed.
    d. perform back blows, chest thrusts, and a finger sweep, and give a breath.

28. Signs and symptoms of _____ include pain and difficulty swallowing, profound drooling, a sore throat, and difficulty breathing.
    a. croup
    b. epiglottitis
    c. bronchitis
    d. pneumonia

29. A 9-month-old child appears sick. Her mother tells you that the child has had an ear infection and her temperature is 100.5 degrees F. She is not eating or drinking well today. When you listen to lung sounds, the child begins coughing. The sound is a distinct seal-like bark. Which condition do you suspect?
    a. croup
    b. asthma
    c. foreign body obstruction
    d. pneumonia

30. (Continuing with the previous question) You listen to lung sounds and find clear sounds, but an increased respiratory rate. What should be assessed next?
    a. the throat
    b. circulation
    c. ears, nose, and throat
    d. chest, back, and belly

31. _____ causes an excessive intake of oxygen and an excessive elimination of carbon dioxide.
    a. Snoring
    b. Sedation
    c. Hypoventilation
    d. Hyperventilation

32. You and your crew have responded to a call for difficulty breathing. When you arrive, a woman lets you in and directs you to her husband who is sitting up leaning forward in his chair. He is working hard to breathe and is wearing a nasal cannula. His skin color is pale and gray and he is unable to speak more than two words without gasping for air. What position is the patient presenting?
    a. tripod
    b. Fowler's
    c. Semi-Fowler's
    d. recumbent

33. (Continuing with the previous question) You approach the patient and listen to lung sounds with your stethoscope and notice that his neck veins are greatly distended. His lung sounds are diminished and sound wet in the lower lobes. He has peripheral edema and his stomach is distended. What do these findings indicate?
    a. COPD
    b. asthma attack
    c. left-sided heart failure
    d. right-sided heart failure

34. (Continuing with the two previous questions) The patient's wife tells you that he has had increased difficulty breathing for several days and was up early this morning looking worse. He is taking an antibiotic for a respiratory infection. You smell and see cigarette butts in a tray near his chair. Your partner is obtaining vital signs and you begin treatment by:
    a. putting on a non-rebreather mask.
    b. turning up the lifer flow on his cannula.
    c. assisting him with his own nitroglycerin.
    d. laying him down so he does not fall out of his chair.

35. EMS was called for an unresponsive male at a bus stop. Police are on the scene and wave you onto the scene reporting "the male appears to be intoxicated." He does not have any signs of injury, but has slow, shallow snoring respirations. Vomit is present on his face and clothing. Using standard precautions, your first action is to:
    a. open his airway.
    b. suction his airway.
    c. turn him on his side.
    d. obtain a pulse rate and blood pressure.

36. (Continuing with the previous question) The patient has no reaction as you assess and begin to care for him. His skin color and condition is pale, warm, and dry. He smells of vomit, alcohol, and urine. Your partner obtains vital signs, which are respiratory rate 6 and shallow, pulse rate 48 and regular, and blood pressure 130/100. Which action do you perform next?
    a. Obtain a blood sugar reading and look for a head injury.
    b. Apply a cervical collar and immobilize on a long back board.
    c. Insert an airway adjunct and ventilate with a bag mask device.
    d. Insert an airway adjunct and apply a non-rebreather mask.

37. A person with breathing distress may be found in a tripod position because this position:
    a. prevents air trapping in the upper airways.
    b. reduces pressure in the pulmonary vessels.
    c. allows more expansion of the rib cage and lungs.
    d. helps to prevent excessive use of accessory muscles to breathe.

38. _____ occurs with exhalation against a partially opened epiglottis and is an abnormal sound heard primarily in infants and small toddlers. It is usually a sign of breathing distress.
    a. Stridor
    b. Grunting
    c. Gasping
    d. Whooping cough

39. An irregular breathing pattern associated with diabetic acidosis is referred to as:
    a. hyperventilation.
    b. agonal respirations.
    c. Kussmaul's respirations.
    d. Cheyne-Stokes respirations.

40. When a patient with breathing distress tells you that she has been coughing up green sputum, this is a sign of:
    a. hypoxia.
    b. a respiratory infection.
    c. a chronic breathing disorder.
    d. impending respiratory failure.

41. For a patient with breathing difficulty, what is the significance of a history of cigarette smoking?
    a. Smoking may cause a drop in blood pressure.
    b. Smoking may exacerbate a recent respiratory infection.
    c. Smoking may have caused liver disease or worsened it.
    d. Smoking only becomes a problem after 20 years of continuous use.

42. When listening to breath sounds with a stethoscope, the _____ sounds are louder and clearer than the _____ sounds.
    a. posterior, anterior
    b. anterior, posterior
    c. wheezing, stridorous
    d. rales, wheezing

43. When connecting a bag mask device to an oxygen source, which piece attaches to the regulator?
    a. the bag
    b. the reservoir
    c. the pop-off valve
    d. the oxygen tubing

44. _____ is used to measure the percentage of hemoglobin saturated with oxygen.
    a. Capnography
    b. Capillary refill
    c. Hypoxic drive
    d. Pulse oximetry

45. When a patient with COPD has an acute exacerbation of this condition, it means that the patient:
    a. is compensating.
    b. is rapidly decompensating.
    c. is maintaining a certain baseline.
    d. has a loss of elastic recoil of the lungs.

46. COPD is a progressive and irreversible lung disease that is prevalent in which age group?
    a. the elderly
    b. young adults
    c. the middle-aged
    d. persons more than 90 years of age

47. A person experiencing an asthma attack may also be described as having:
    a. COPD.
    b. bronchospasm.
    c. Kussmaul's respirations.
    d. foreign body airway obstruction.

48. Hyperventilation results in too much intake of _____ and an excessive elimination of _____.
    a. oxygen, glucose
    b. oxygen, carbon dioxide
    c. carbon dioxide, oxygen
    d. oxygen, carbon monoxide

49. Which of the following traumatic injuries is associated with breathing distress?
    a. broken rib
    b. lower lumbar injury
    c. bruised pelvis
    d. neck pain

50. During the physical examination of a child who has severe breathing distress, where would you expect to see retractions?
    a. nares
    b. mouth
    c. neck and chest
    d. chest and back

Chapter 17 Answer Form

	A	B	C	D		A	B	C	D
1.	❑	❑	❑	❑	26.	❑	❑	❑	❑
2.	❑	❑	❑	❑	27.	❑	❑	❑	❑
3.	❑	❑	❑	❑	28.	❑	❑	❑	❑
4.	❑	❑	❑	❑	29.	❑	❑	❑	❑
5.	❑	❑	❑	❑	30.	❑	❑	❑	❑
6.	❑	❑	❑	❑	31.	❑	❑	❑	❑
7.	❑	❑	❑	❑	32.	❑	❑	❑	❑
8.	❑	❑	❑	❑	33.	❑	❑	❑	❑
9.	❑	❑	❑	❑	34.	❑	❑	❑	❑
10.	❑	❑	❑	❑	35.	❑	❑	❑	❑
11.	❑	❑	❑	❑	36.	❑	❑	❑	❑
12.	❑	❑	❑	❑	37.	❑	❑	❑	❑
13.	❑	❑	❑	❑	38.	❑	❑	❑	❑
14.	❑	❑	❑	❑	39.	❑	❑	❑	❑
15.	❑	❑	❑	❑	40.	❑	❑	❑	❑
16.	❑	❑	❑	❑	41.	❑	❑	❑	❑
17.	❑	❑	❑	❑	42.	❑	❑	❑	❑
18.	❑	❑	❑	❑	43.	❑	❑	❑	❑
19.	❑	❑	❑	❑	44.	❑	❑	❑	❑
20.	❑	❑	❑	❑	45.	❑	❑	❑	❑
21.	❑	❑	❑	❑	46.	❑	❑	❑	❑
22.	❑	❑	❑	❑	47.	❑	❑	❑	❑
23.	❑	❑	❑	❑	48.	❑	❑	❑	❑
24.	❑	❑	❑	❑	49.	❑	❑	❑	❑
25.	❑	❑	❑	❑	50.	❑	❑	❑	❑

CHAPTER

18

Cardiac Emergencies

1. The _____ is the largest artery in the cardiovascular system.
   a. aorta
   b. superior vena cava
   c. left pulmonary artery
   d. right pulmonary artery

2. The _____ pump(s) blood into the pulmonary circulation.
   a. left ventricle of the heart
   b. right ventricle of the heart
   c. diaphragm
   d. coronary arteries

3. Which of the following statements is most correct regarding the function of the heart?
   a. Contraction and relaxation of the heart normally occur simultaneously.
   b. The four valves of the heart normally open and close at the same time.
   c. Heart sounds are generated by the sound of contracting coronary blood vessels.
   d. The four valves of the heart normally open and close to carry the flow of blood forward.

4. When a patient is experiencing chest pain or discomfort, place the patient:
   a. in a position of comfort.
   b. lying down with legs elevated, after assisting with nitroglycerin.
   c. supine, because this is the best position if CPR becomes necessary.
   d. on the side, because nausea and vomiting are common with chest pain.

5. When the EMT is assessing a patient who is experiencing acute chest discomfort, she should:
   a. assess for a possible pneumothorax.
   b. call medical control before transporting the patient.
   c. look for signs of trauma before starting any treatment.
   d. treat the patient as if he is having a life-threatening event.

6. When treating a patient who has chest pain, the goal for the EMT is to:
   a. help increase the workload on the heart.
   b. relax skeletal muscle with nitroglycerin if possible.
   c. reduce the patient's blood pressure with nitroglycerin.
   d. provide high-flow oxygen and transport quickly without increasing the patient's anxiety.

7. The EMT should attach an AED to a patient who is unresponsive(,):
   a. with no signs of circulation, and is apneic.
   b. and is under the supervision of hospice care.
   c. seizing, and is breathing at a rate of 6 breaths per minute.
   d. and was witnessed to be choking prior to becoming unresponsive.

8. Which of the following situations indicates a need to use an AED?
   a. a 60-year-old cancer patient who is unresponsive, is not breathing, and has no pulse
   b. an 8-year-old who is unresponsive after being hit in the chest with a soccer ball, but has a pulse
   c. a 54-year-old male who is complaining of severe chest pain, and has profuse sweating and no distal pulse
   d. an unresponsive elderly patient in a nursing home who was found in bed and who is not breathing, but has a pulse

9. You are treating a patient whom you suspect is having a heart attack. For which of the following reasons would you attach an AED?
   a. You witness an arrest en route to the hospital.
   b. The patient has taken his nitroglycerin three times with no relief.
   c. The patient tells you he has had two heart attacks in the last 10 years.
   d. The patient is responsive but has an implanted defibrillator that is firing.

10. You are treating a patient with a complaint of substernal chest pain. Your local protocol allows you to assist a patient with nitroglycerin, administer aspirin, oxygen, and call for ALS. In which order is the protocol most appropriate for a patient with vital signs of respiratory rate of 28 labored, pulse rate of 88 irregular, and blood pressure of 160/60?
    a. oxygen, aspirin, nitroglycerin, and call for ALS
    b. call for ALS, oxygen, aspirin, and nitroglycerin
    c. call for ALS nitroglycerin, oxygen, and aspirin
    d. call for ALS aspirin, oxygen, and nitroglycerin

11. You are alone in the back of the ambulance treating and transporting a patient for chest pain when suddenly she becomes unresponsive, pulseless, and stops breathing. Now you should:
    a. attach and turn on the AED.
    b. start CPR and attach the AED.
    c. advise the driver to turn on the siren and lights.
    d. attach the AED, start CPR, and ventilate the patient.

12. The role of the EMT in the Chain of Survival is early:
    a. access and CPR.
    b. advanced life support.
    c. CPR and defibrillation.
    d. defibrillation and advanced care.

13. For the morbidly obese patient, defibrillation:
    a. has a better response to high-energy doses.
    b. is less successful than in patients of normal weight.
    c. is more successful than in patients of normal weight.
    d. is administered in energy doses that are the same as for any other patient.

14. A patient with a history of angina has which of the following conditions?
    a. a history of having a heart attack
    b. a history of having two or more heart attacks
    c. a history of carotid artery disease
    d. Narrowing of one or more cardiac arteries

15. A patient with crushing chest pain and no difficulty breathing also complains of weakness and dizziness when he tries to walk. The most likely position of comfort for this patient will be _____ position.
    a. semi-Fowler's
    b. high Fowler's
    c. Trendelenburg
    d. left lateral recumbent

16. For the patient with acute breathing difficulty, crackles in the lungs, and a history of congestive heart failure, the most likely position of comfort will be:
    a. lying down.
    b. sitting upright.
    c. lying on the side.
    d. Trendelenburg position.

17. You are treating an 85-year-old female who woke up in the middle of the night with difficulty breathing and severe chest pain. While you are taking her vital signs, her mental status decreases significantly and you lay her down. At this point you:
    a. suction her airway and insert an OPA.
    b. do nothing, as she is still breathing on her own.
    c. attempt to insert an OPA and begin to ventilate with a bag mask device.
    d. make sure the non-rebreather mask fits properly and then turn up the flow rate.

18. The primary goal of airway management for the patient who is in cardiac arrest is to:
    a. suction for no longer than 15 seconds.
    b. insert an OPA and maintain cervical stabilization.
    c. hyperventilate the patient until her color improves.
    d. maintain a good mask seal and assure chest rise.

19. You are working with a paramedic when a call comes in for a cardiac arrest. The paramedic asks you to provide basic life support while he prepares his equipment. You begin by:
    a. checking vital signs, suctioning, and ventilating with a bag mask device.
    b. verifying pulselessness and starting CPR.
    c. hyperventilating the patient so that the paramedic can intubate.
    d. directing bystanders to assist with CPR so you can set up the IV bag.

20. You have successfully converted a witnessed cardiac arrest with one shock from the AED. The patient now has a pulse, is breathing, and is awakening. At this point you should:
    a. cancel ALS and transport.
    b. be prepared for the patient to arrest again.
    c. take the AED off the patient and transport.
    d. be prepared to give the patient nitroglycerin if chest pain returns.

21. An AED is being utilized in an unwitnessed cardiac arrest. When should the Analyze button be pressed?
    a. after 1 minute of CPR
    b. after 2 minutes of CPR
    c. after 5 minutes of CPR
    d. immediately after the electrodes are applied

22. When the heart is unable to produce effective contractions because of disorganized electrical conduction, the AED will rapidly:
    a. indicate "No shock advised."
    b. reanalyze after 60 seconds.
    c. recognize V-fib as a shockable rhythm.
    d. recognize slow V-tach as a shockable rhythm.

23. A 32-year-old female is complaining of chest pain in the left lower side of her chest. She denies shortness of breath, but states that it hurts to take a deep breath. You find an antibiotic, which she is taking for a respiratory infection. She is also a smoker with a new productive cough. Your treatment should include:
    a. oxygen, attachment of the AED, and nitroglycerin.
    b. oxygen, position of comfort, and nitroglycerin.
    c. position of comfort, routine transport, and reassessment.
    d. oxygen, position of comfort, and routine transport.

24. You have assisted a 56-year-old male to take his nitroglycerin. His chest pain came on suddenly as he was shoveling snow, and was totally relieved with oxygen and nitroglycerin. Now you should:
    a. let the patient sign a refusal and refer him to his cardiologist.
    b. attach the AED, monitor him, and transport the patient to the hospital.
    c. attach the AED and give another nitroglycerin if his blood pressure is adequate.
    d. continue oxygen therapy and perform ongoing assessments en route to the hospital.

25. When Advanced Cardiac Life Support (ACLS) is available in the prehospital setting to patients with a cardiac emergency:
    a. the AED will never be needed.
    b. the patient will always have a better outcome.
    c. defibrillation is secondary to the medications the patient can receive.
    d. advanced airway management and emergency medications may improve survival.

26. For the victim of cardiac arrest, the chance of survival is:
    a. highest when ACLS is available in the prehospital setting.
    b. higher when ACLS is available upon arrival at the hospital.
    c. highest if ACLS is not available in the prehospital setting.
    d. best when ACLS is available immediately following early defibrillation.

27. Upon completing an assessment of a 74-year-old female with severe chest pain, you determine that her blood pressure is quite low, making it a contraindication for assisting with nitroglycerin. You should now:
    a. not move her, call for ALS, and wait for them to provide IV fluids before transporting.
    b. call medical control and ask for an order for nitroglycerin, because the pain is getting worse.
    c. gently lay her supine on your stretcher, treat her for shock, and rapidly transport her to the hospital.
    d. administer high-flow oxygen, place her in Trendelenburg position, and make a routine transport.

28. The patient you are caring for has chest pain and shortness of breath, and appears to be in severe distress. The ALS unit you called for is 15 minutes away and your patient is in the ambulance ready for transport. Because the hospital is 10 minutes away, you decide to:
    a. begin rapid transport to the hospital.
    b. assist the patient with nitroglycerin and meet the ALS unit en route.
    c. get an order to assist with nitroglycerin while you wait for the ALS unit to arrive.
    d. begin routine transport to the hospital and attempt to meet the ALS unit en route.

29. A/An _____ AED delivers approximately 200 joules for the initial shock to an adult in cardiac arrest.
    a. biphasic
    b. implanted
    c. monophasic
    d. investigational

30. A _____ AED supplies nonescalating defibrillation energy doses for patients 25 kg (55 lbs) and larger.
    a. 12-lead
    b. limb-lead
    c. biphasic
    d. monophasic

31. The difference between a fully automated and a semi-automated defibrillator is that the:
    a. automated defibrillator uses less power.
    b. automated defibrillator requires no training.
    c. semi-automated defibrillator requires someone to interpret the rhythm.
    d. semi-automated defibrillator indicates when it is time to press the shock button.

32. The EMT may find a/an _____ AED, prescribed by a physician, in the home of a cardiac patient who is at high risk for V-fib or V-tach.
    a. implanted
    b. experimental
    c. investigational
    d. fully automated

33. While traveling through the airport, you observe a crowd of excited people at the next gate and hear someone yelling "Call 9-1-1." You go over and see an elderly male unresponsive on the floor and an airline employee attaching AED pads to his chest. The employee stops what he is doing when he discovers that the patient's internal defibrillator is firing. What should you do now?
    a. Stand by and watch, as the employee is doing a good job so far.
    b. Offer to do CPR while you wait for the internal defibrillator to stop firing.
    c. Quickly identify yourself as an EMT and push the "Analyze" button on the AED.
    d. Identify yourself as an EMT, offer to help, and quickly encourage the employee to begin the AED sequence.

34. You have responded to the local high school track for a man who has collapsed on the oval track. It is raining; the patient is soaked; and he is unresponsive, is not breathing, and has no pulse. What must be done before utilizing an AED?
   a. Move the patient into the ambulance.
   b. Remove all the wet clothes from the patient.
   c. Check to see if the patient has an implanted defibrillator.
   d. Dry off the patient's chest before applying the electrode.

35. The patient you have been treating for respiratory distress has progressively worsened and now is apneic. Which of the following actions should you take?
   a. Begin CPR, attach the AED pads, turn on the AED, and press "Analyze."
   b. Perform CPR for 1 minute and then assess breathing and pulse.
   c. Move the patient to a long backboard and assess for pulselessness.
   d. Insert an OPA, begin ventilations with a bag mask device, and check for a pulse.

36. Many EMS agencies have a policy stating that the AED should not be used when a patient is found to be breathing or has a pulse. The reason for this is:
   a. to prevent accidental or inappropriate defibrillation.
   b. that the AED will determine if the patient has a pulse.
   c. that AEDs work only for cardiac arrest victims.
   d. that AED electrodes are for a single patient use and expensive to replace.

37. Which of the following conditions may result in inappropriate defibrillation of a patient?
   a. The patient is not lying flat on her back.
   b. The patient is in respiratory arrest and is attached to an AED.
   c. The patient is too obese for the AED to monitor adequately.
   d. The patient is too small for the AED to monitor adequately.

38. Which of the following reasons is rarely the cause of inappropriate shocks?
   a. The user has not been trained in the use of AED.
   b. The AED was giving the prompt "Shock advised."
   c. The AED is one month past due for routine maintenance.
   d. The patient was being moved at the time of rhythm analysis.

39. CPR was started immediately on a 56-year-old woman who collapsed while out running. You arrive and deliver one shock with an AED and take over doing CPR. After 2 minutes, the patient has a pulse. What action should be taken next?
   a. Stop CPR and press Analyze.
   b. Assist ventilations and wait for ALS.
   c. Assess breathing and obtain a blood pressure.
   d. Place the patient on a long backboard and begin transport.

40. After attaching AED pads to a patient, at which point during two-person CPR is it appropriate to interrupt CPR to analyze the patient?
   a. immediately
   b. after the next ventilation is complete
   c. after the patient has been placed on a long backboard
   d. after completing the current cycle of compressions and ventilations

41. AEDs have the capability of recording each event for review after the call and are used for quality assurance purposes by the medical director of an agency. This feature is considered to be a/an:
   a. disadvantage for the user.
   b. advantage of the AED device.
   c. disadvantage in the event of a lawsuit.
   d. nuisance for the record keeper of an EMS agency.

42. _____ is(are) a disadvantage of using AEDs.
   a. Ongoing training and routine maintenance
   b. The minimal steps needed to complete the shock sequence
   c. The time it takes to verify apnea and pulselessness
   d. The amount of time it takes to determine if a rhythm is shockable

43. The amount of time it takes to apply the pads of an AED to a patient, turn on the device, and initiate the analyzing mode:
   a. is a disadvantage of the device.
   b. is easy for most individuals to work within.
   c. impedes the time for delivering the first shock.
   d. takes more than 2 minutes for a trained rescuer.

44. When ventilating a patient in cardiac arrest with a bag mask device, the ventilations should be provided:
   a. once every 6 seconds.
   b. once every 30 seconds.
   c. twice every 30 seconds.
   d. twice between 30 compressions.

45. Defibrillating a patient with an AED is considered to be _____ because the energy is delivered to the patient through remote adhesive pads.
    a. hands-on
    b. hands-off
    c. dangerous
    d. spontaneous

46. The possibility of the user being shocked by an AED is very low because:
    a. of the infrequent use of the device.
    b. the amount of electricity is too weak to reach the user.
    c. of the use of remote defibrillation through adhesive pads.
    d. of the amount of training required for proficiency with the device.

47. After administering several shocks over a period of 15 minutes to a patient who is in cardiac arrest, with no successful conversion, the AED should remain attached and turned on during transport because:
    a. the pads are too difficult to remove.
    b. the hospital will need to check if pad placement is correct.
    c. all patients in cardiac arrest must be monitored for no less than 30 minutes.
    d. the AED will continue to monitor the patient and advise if a shockable rhythm is detected.

48. Which statement about AED rhythm monitoring is most correct?
    a. An AED will never advise you to shock a conscious patient.
    b. The AED will monitor a patient only when in the analyze mode.
    c. All patients at risk for cardiac arrest should be monitored with an AED.
    d. Some AEDs will advise you to shock a patient who is in a fast V-tach rhythm even if the patient has a pulse.

49. Before the AED is used on a patient who is in cardiac arrest, the EMT should:
    a. establish an airway, begin CPR, and call for ALS.
    b. check with the family for a do not resuscitate (DNR) order.
    c. search the patient for a medical identification tag or bracelet.
    d. have checked the batteries and run a test at the start of his shift.

50. While working out in a public gym, a male in his fifties collapsed. You are there and assess him and determine that he has agonal respirations and no detectable pulse. What action do you take next?
    a. Call 9-1-1 and observe the patient.
    b. Direct the staff to bring the AED and call 9-1-1.
    c. Look for an AED and direct a bystander to start CPR.
    d. Begin rescue breathing and direct someone to call 9-1-1.

51. After being on the scene of a cardiac arrest for 10 minutes, you have begun transport to the nearest hospital, which will take 20 minutes. When you are 5 minutes away from the hospital, the AED continues to advise you to shock the patient. You should now:
    a. continue CPR only.
    b. change the batteries in the AED.
    c. continue to shock the patient as advised.
    d. run a test to be sure the AED is working properly.

52. You resume CPR after administering a shock to an apneic and pulseless patient. Now you should:
    a. continue CPR and wait for ALS to arrive.
    b. stop CPR and reanalyze every 10 minutes.
    c. search for a do not resuscitate directive.
    d. continue CPR and place the patient on a long backboard.

53. Shortly after giving a shock and resuming CPR, the AED does an analysis and reads "No shock advised." You prepare the patient for transport and reanalyze the patient, but this time the AED advises you to deliver a shock. At this point, you:
    a. clear the patient and shock as advised.
    b. disregard the "Shock advised" message because of the prior reading.
    c. assume that the AED read the patient's movement as V-fib and reanalyze.
    d. disregard the "Shock advised" message because the patient has been down too long.

54. Two bystanders in an airport successfully converted a pulseless patient with an AED that was hanging on the wall nearby. The patient awoke after being defibrillated twice. While you are getting the patient on the stretcher, he becomes unresponsive, stops breathing, and loses his pulse. What should you do first?
    a. Start CPR.
    b. Check for a blood pressure.
    c. Reanalyze and shock if indicated.
    d. Immobilize the patient's neck and back.

55. When two EMTs with an AED arrive at the side of a patient who is not breathing and has no pulse, they should first:
    a. perform CPR for 2 minutes, call for more help, and attach the AED.
    b. apply the AED as quickly as possible and check for a shockable rhythm.
    c. place the patient on a long backboard, then check for a shockable rhythm.
    d. perform CPR for 3 minutes, then attach the AED and assess for a shockable rhythm.

56. When a single rescuer with an AED arrives at the side of a patient who is not breathing and has no pulse, the steps to take, in order, are:
    a. call for help, turn on and attach the AED, and shock if advised.
    b. attach and turn on the AED, call for help, and shock if advised.
    c. perform CPR for 1 minute, call for help, attach and turn on the AED.
    d. call for help, perform CPR for 2 minutes, attach and turn on the AED.

57. You are about to deliver the first shock with an AED to a pulseless patient. The next pulse check should be taken after:
    a. the first shock.
    b. 2 minutes of CPR.
    c. switching positions with your partner.
    d. the third shock, or when no shock is advised.

58. In an emergency, aspirin is recommended for patients experiencing symptoms of acute coronary syndrome (ACS) because it:
    a. thins the blood.
    b. prevents hypotension.
    c. quickly reduces chest pain.
    d. prevents ventricular fibrillation.

59. Nitroglycerin relaxes vascular smooth muscle which in turn:
    a. increases chest pain.
    b. increases oxygen demand.
    c. decreases the workload of the heart.
    d. increases the workload of the heart.

60. For the last link in the Chain of Survival to be effective, there has to be:
    a. prehospital ACLS available in every community.
    b. rapid transport of the cardiac arrest patient to the emergency department.
    c. an emergency department within a 10-minute transport for each cardiac arrest victim.
    d. practical coordination between ACLS-trained providers and the personnel using the AED.

61. After shocking the victim of an electrocution twice with the AED, you find that the patient has a return of pulses, and no further shocks are advised. What should be done next?
    a. Immobilize the patient to a long backboard.
    b. Quickly search for entrance and exit wounds.
    c. Assist ventilations and obtain a blood pressure.
    d. Administer high-flow oxygen with a non-rebreather mask.

62. Which of the following should the EMT include in the postresuscitation care of a patient resuscitated from V-fib?
    a. Leave the AED attached and turned on.
    b. Leave the AED attached, but turn it off.
    c. Remove the AED pads from the patient.
    d. Allow the patient to assume a position of comfort.

63. For the victim of cardiac arrest with a return of pulses and respirations, _____ is a critical factor in postresuscitation care.
    a. warmth
    b. rapid transport
    c. airway management
    d. C-spine stabilization

64. The victim of a near-drowning, who was initially pulseless, is now breathing and has a pulse after CPR and one shock from the AED. Which of the following complications can you expect with this type of patient?
    a. vomiting
    b. hypoxia
    c. hypothermia
    d. all of the above

65. Which of the following is not an appropriate step in the postresuscitation care of a patient revived from a cardiac arrest?
    a. telling the family that the patient is going to be all right
    b. assisting an ALS provider with ventilation and intubation
    c. obtaining the patient's past medical history from a family member
    d. explaining to the family what is happening and what they can expect at the hospital

66. Postresuscitation care for every victim of cardiac arrest includes:
    a. obtaining one set of vital signs.
    b. endotracheal intubation.
    c. advanced cardiac life support.
    d. rapid transport to the nearest trauma center.

67. You are working with a partner who has been out of work for several months. He asks you to help him get comfortable using the AED again. How can you best help him?
    a. Give him a testing form and let him practice with a simulator.
    b. Have him practice alone with a mannequin and a training video.
    c. Give him a testing form to review and let him watch a training video.
    d. Using a mannequin, practice with him, and provide him with feedback.

68. One of the best ways for an EMT to stay proficient at the use of AEDs is to:
    a. rehearse with a simulator monthly.
    b. watch a training videotape monthly.
    c. complete the operator's checklist each shift.
    d. complete a recertification course once every two years.

69. The AED operator's shift checklist should be completed by:
    a. the supervisor.
    b. the most junior crew member.
    c. the most senior crew member.
    d. anyone on the crew trained to use the AED.

70. One of the most common reasons for failure of an AED to work properly when needed is:
    a. dead batteries.
    b. operator error from lack of practice.
    c. aging of the internal components of the AED.
    d. failure to complete a checklist on a regular basis.

71. For citizens in a community to have the best chance of surviving a cardiac event, which of the following elements has to be in place?
    a. every citizen must be trained in CPR
    b. an EMS system with ACLS-trained personnel
    c. every citizen is trained to use an AED
    d. an AED located in every home and public area

72. In the American Heart Association's "Chain of Survival," early _____ is the first link where the possible use of an AED is set in motion.
    a. CPR
    b. access
    c. defibrillation
    d. advanced life support

73. Before the EMT who works within an EMS agency may use an AED, she must:
    a. meet the medical director.
    b. directly observe its use on a patient.
    c. be trained and certified in its use for at least 30 days.
    d. meet the training requirements of the medical director.

74. The role of the medical director regarding the use of an AED is to:
    a. oversee training and recordkeeping.
    b. provide guidance in the selection and purchase of AEDs.
    c. follow up with the family of every patient on whom an AED was used.
    d. be involved directly or through a designee with each aspect relating to the AED.

75. A case review should be completed following the use of the AED because:
    a. it is a state and federal health care mandate.
    b. if you make a mistake, your partner will not be faulted.
    c. it is an effective tool for improving future skills performance.
    d. if your paperwork gets lost, the AED will have a record of the events.

76. When the victim of a cardiac arrest does not survive, how can the EMT be assured that his skill performance on the call was appropriate?
    a. Talk to the patient's family.
    b. Obtain a copy of the autopsy report.
    c. Ask the supervisor to evaluate the patient care report.
    d. Obtain feedback on the case review with the medical director.

77. Which of the following is generally not included in a case review of a cardiac arrest for which an AED was used?
    a. the time it took to deliver the first shock
    b. appropriate assessment and interventions
    c. following the EMS agency's AED protocol
    d. the outcomes for patients with anterior infarcts versus lateral infarcts

78. Your medical director is going to do a case review with you for the last cardiac arrest call you had. Which component of care is he most likely to discuss with you?
    a. the patient's past medical history
    b. the location of AED training in your community
    c. ACLS integration with BLS providers
    d. the type of medications that the patient was prescribed

79. Which of the following is typically considered a goal of quality improvement regarding AED use?
    a. assessing training and skills needs
    b. making all the links in the "Chain of Survival" stronger
    c. tracking and reporting data relating to respiratory arrest calls
    d. disciplining for incorrect actions or inappropriate defibrillation

80. You have been asked to participate in your EMS agency's quality improvement program. Your role in this program will be to:
    a. act as a liaison between your agency and mutual aid agencies.
    b. help determine appropriate disciplinary action for coworkers who have poor patient skills.
    c. participate in case reviews and help strengthen your link in the "Chain of Survival."
    d. ask each of your patients to complete an evaluation form on your performance after the call.

81. When you assess the pulse of your patient, you find that it is quite irregular. How can you best obtain an accurate count?
    a. Attach the AED and monitor the rhythm.
    b. Count the number of beats for 1 minute.
    c. Listen to the heartbeats with a stethoscope and count for 2 minutes.
    d. Have the most senior crew member assess the pulse.

82. When a patient tells you that he has an implanted defibrillator, this means that:
    a. the patient is at high risk for a cardiac event.
    b. the patient has definitely had a heart attack in the past.
    c. the heart's natural pacemaker does not work anymore.
    d. the patient has had more than one heart attack in the past.

83. Within minutes of assisting a patient with chest pressure to take her nitroglycerin, you reevaluate her blood pressure and find that it has dropped below 100 systolic. The patient still has chest pressure, so what should you do now?
    a. Lay her down and assist her with another nitroglycerin pill.
    b. Do nothing, because a drop in blood pressure is normal after taking nitroglycerin.
    c. Elevate her legs; the blood pressure will come up after a few minutes.
    d. Lay her down, begin transport, and call medical control to advise of the change in blood pressure.

84. After completing a focused history and physical exam of a 58-year-old male with a complaint of chest pain that radiates into the neck and jaw, you discover that before calling EMS, the patient took one dose of nitroglycerin with no relief. Now you are going to:
    a. utilize your local protocol for additional doses of nitroglycerin.
    b. transport the patient with oxygen only, as nitroglycerin did not work.
    c. give the patient a dose of aspirin, provide high-flow oxygen, and transport.
    d. call medical control and request an order for aspirin, as nitroglycerin did not work.

85. Before you assist a patient with nitroglycerin, you must complete each of the following, *except*:
    a. obtain an OPQRST and SAMPLE history.
    b. verify that the patient has a cardiac history.
    c. assure that the blood pressure is accurate.
    d. obtain an order from the patient's physician.

86. Which one of the following group of patient complaints is an indication for the use of nitroglycerin?
    a. chest tightness, weakness, and labored breathing
    b. slurred speech, shortness of breath, and weakness in the left arm
    c. difficulty breathing, wheezing, and tingling in the hand, arms, and face
    d. a brief fainting episode followed by sweating, nausea, and vomiting

87. Your patient is complaining of shortness of breath and a heavy feeling in his chest. He has a history of angina, but tells you that this pain is different. His vital signs are: respirations 36, shallow; pulse 58, irregular; BP 90/50. Which of these findings is a contraindication for the use of nitroglycerin with this patient?
    a. hypotension
    b. the shortness of breath
    c. pain that is not his typical angina pain
    d. pulse is too slow and respirations are too fast

88. You have been ordered by medical control to assist a patient complaining of chest discomfort to take his nitroglycerin for the first time. However, the physician has asked you to explain the possible side effects of the medication. You tell the patient:
    a. that the taste is unpleasant.
    b. that he will experience a burning sensation.
    c. to lean forward, as he might feel nauseated and vomit.
    d. to lie back on the stretcher, as he might feel dizzy or lightheaded.

89. Which of the following statements is most correct regarding the controls on an AED?
    a. All AEDs have the same functions and controls.
    b. All semi-automated AEDs have voice prompts.
    c. Every AED has different functions and control buttons.
    d. Each brand of AED has standardized functions so that they can be used in the same manner.

90. Which of the following tasks is considered maintenance for an AED?
    a. recharging the batteries every day
    b. changing the defibrillation pads after each use
    c. rotating the defibrillation pads on a monthly basis
    d. following the instructions in the user's manual for recommended service

Chapter 18 Answer Form

	A	B	C	D			A	B	C	D
1.	❏	❏	❏	❏		33.	❏	❏	❏	❏
2.	❏	❏	❏	❏		34.	❏	❏	❏	❏
3.	❏	❏	❏	❏		35.	❏	❏	❏	❏
4.	❏	❏	❏	❏		36.	❏	❏	❏	❏
5.	❏	❏	❏	❏		37.	❏	❏	❏	❏
6.	❏	❏	❏	❏		38.	❏	❏	❏	❏
7.	❏	❏	❏	❏		39.	❏	❏	❏	❏
8.	❏	❏	❏	❏		40.	❏	❏	❏	❏
9.	❏	❏	❏	❏		41.	❏	❏	❏	❏
10.	❏	❏	❏	❏		42.	❏	❏	❏	❏
11.	❏	❏	❏	❏		43.	❏	❏	❏	❏
12.	❏	❏	❏	❏		44.	❏	❏	❏	❏
13.	❏	❏	❏	❏		45.	❏	❏	❏	❏
14.	❏	❏	❏	❏		46.	❏	❏	❏	❏
15.	❏	❏	❏	❏		47.	❏	❏	❏	❏
16.	❏	❏	❏	❏		48.	❏	❏	❏	❏
17.	❏	❏	❏	❏		49.	❏	❏	❏	❏
18.	❏	❏	❏	❏		50.	❏	❏	❏	❏
19.	❏	❏	❏	❏		51.	❏	❏	❏	❏
20.	❏	❏	❏	❏		52.	❏	❏	❏	❏
21.	❏	❏	❏	❏		53.	❏	❏	❏	❏
22.	❏	❏	❏	❏		54.	❏	❏	❏	❏
23.	❏	❏	❏	❏		55.	❏	❏	❏	❏
24.	❏	❏	❏	❏		56.	❏	❏	❏	❏
25.	❏	❏	❏	❏		57.	❏	❏	❏	❏
26.	❏	❏	❏	❏		58.	❏	❏	❏	❏
27.	❏	❏	❏	❏		59.	❏	❏	❏	❏
28.	❏	❏	❏	❏		60.	❏	❏	❏	❏
29.	❏	❏	❏	❏		61.	❏	❏	❏	❏
30.	❏	❏	❏	❏		62.	❏	❏	❏	❏
31.	❏	❏	❏	❏		63.	❏	❏	❏	❏
32.	❏	❏	❏	❏		64.	❏	❏	❏	❏

	A	B	C	D		A	B	C	D
65.	❏	❏	❏	❏	78.	❏	❏	❏	❏
66.	❏	❏	❏	❏	79.	❏	❏	❏	❏
67.	❏	❏	❏	❏	80.	❏	❏	❏	❏
68.	❏	❏	❏	❏	81.	❏	❏	❏	❏
69.	❏	❏	❏	❏	82.	❏	❏	❏	❏
70.	❏	❏	❏	❏	83.	❏	❏	❏	❏
71.	❏	❏	❏	❏	84.	❏	❏	❏	❏
72.	❏	❏	❏	❏	85.	❏	❏	❏	❏
73.	❏	❏	❏	❏	86.	❏	❏	❏	❏
74.	❏	❏	❏	❏	87.	❏	❏	❏	❏
75.	❏	❏	❏	❏	88.	❏	❏	❏	❏
76.	❏	❏	❏	❏	89.	❏	❏	❏	❏
77.	❏	❏	❏	❏	90.	❏	❏	❏	❏

CHAPTER

19

Diabetic Emergencies and Altered Mental Status

1. A 30-year-old female with a history of diabetes was found unresponsive. The patient's husband tells you that she does not take insulin because she controls her blood sugar with her diet. What type of diabetes does the patient most likely have?
   a. type 1
   b. type 2
   c. type 3
   d. type 4

2. The adult female patient you are assessing appears dazed. She responds to her name but is confused about the day of the week and other questions you ask her. A neighbor who is on the scene tells you he thinks she is an insulin-dependent diabetic. In an effort to confirm this, you ask your partner to:
   a. perform a prehospital stroke exam.
   b. look in the refrigerator for her insulin.
   c. search the apartment for needles and syringes.
   d. check her blood pressure to see if she is hypotensive.

3. You are dispatched on a call for a sick person who is vomiting. Upon arrival, you form a general impression of a conscious elderly male who is sitting up at his desk complaining of a tingling sensation in his face. In slow speech, he keeps repeating the phrase "I am low." Your next action would be to:
   a. administer oral glucose.
   b. complete a primary assessment.
   c. consider that the patient is having a stroke.
   d. consider that the patient is hyperventilating.

4. You have responded to a call for a fall and find that the patient is in bed. He appears awake, yet stunned. Family members tell you that the patient is an insulin-dependent diabetic who was fine before tripping and falling. What step(s) should you take first?
   a. Perform a rapid trauma exam.
   b. Take C-spine precautions, then assess and manage the ABCs.
   c. Ask a family member to use the patient's glucometer to check his blood sugar.
   d. Apply high-flow oxygen and assist the patient with high-concentration oral glucose.

5. A patient with an altered mental status is taking diabetic medicine and has a history of diabetes. If you are unable to measure the blood sugar or are uncertain, you should:
   a. call for ALS.
   b. assume that the blood sugar is low.
   c. assume that the blood sugar is high.
   d. look for another cause of altered mental status.

6. The mother of an 11-year-old patient who is unresponsive and has a history of diabetes tells you that they checked the blood sugar reading an hour ago and it was 130 mg/dl. No trauma was involved, so you suspect that:
   a. there may have been a medication dosing error.
   b. the patient's glucometer is not properly calibrated.
   c. the cause of the altered mental status is low blood sugar until proven otherwise.
   d. all of the above.

7. You have been called to transport a male teenager who was witnessed drinking alcohol. He appears to be very intoxicated but is cooperative getting into the ambulance. This patient is at high risk for _____, making airway management a high priority.

   a. vomiting
   b. seizures
   c. hypoglycemia
   d. hyperglycemia

8. Select the airway adjunct most appropriate for an adult male who is unresponsive and seizing.

   a. oropharyngeal airway
   b. nasopharyngeal airway
   c. soft-tip suction catheter
   d. rigid-tip suction catheter

9. The family of a 92-year-old woman called EMS because they have seen a change in the woman's mental status since yesterday. Today she seems confused and weak. She has not eaten or drank much today. When you interview the patient, she is slow to answer and her skin is hot and dry when you assess a pulse. With the information you have, which condition do you suspect at this point?

   a. stroke
   b. overdose
   c. infection
   d. hypoglycemia

10. (Continuing with the previous question) You assess breathing and listen to lung sounds, which are clear. The pulse is tachy and regular. The SpO_2 is 98% and the blood sugar reading is 104 mg/dl. Which of the following assessments must be completed to rule out a life-threatening event?

    a. trauma
    b. behavioral
    c. stroke exam
    d. abdominal

11. Orange juice, non-diet sodas, and oral glucose gel in toothpaste-like tubes are all:

    a. dangerous for the patient who has type 1 diabetes.
    b. contraindicated for use in the patient with no history of diabetes.
    c. commercial, oral high-concentration glucose products for diabetic emergencies.
    d. high-concentration glucose products that may be ingested to raise the blood sugar.

12. One method of assisting a conscious diabetic patient with an altered mental status is to place oral high-concentration glucose gel between the cheek and gum. This method works to improve mental status by:

    a. reducing the risk of hypoxia.
    b. stimulating the release of insulin.
    c. increasing a person's sensitivity to insulin.
    d. the rapid absorption of glucose through a highly vascular area.

13. A diabetic patient who had an altered mental status was assisted to eat a tube of high-concentration glucose gel. Approximately 15 minutes later, the patient has become more alert. Management of this patient will now include:

    a. continuing to reassess and beginning transportation.
    b. doing nothing until a blood sugar reading is obtained.
    c. calling for ALS, as the patient is going to need IV glucose.
    d. calling medical control and asking to assist with two additional tubes of glucose.

14. When caring for a patient with a possible diabetic problem, the EMT should call medical direction:

    a. only if ALS is not available.
    b. according to local protocols.
    c. only if the patient appears to be going into respiratory arrest.
    d. after completing a focused history and physical exam and before beginning treatment.

15. The wife of an unresponsive patient who has a history of diabetes tells you that she tried to give her husband orange juice prior to your arrival, but was unsuccessful. The patient has an open airway, is breathing adequately, and has a strong pulse. The management steps for this patient include:

    a. rapid transport, monitoring serial vital signs, and performing a secondary assessment while en route.
    b. applying high-flow oxygen, monitoring vital signs, contacting medical control, and transport.
    c. assisting with oral glucose gel under the tongue, obtaining vital signs, and transport.
    d. assisting with oral glucose gel between the cheek and gum, obtaining vital signs, and performing a focused history and physical exam.

16. When a diabetic gets too much insulin, the effects on the body include:

    a. an increase in mental alertness.
    b. cells becoming filled with glucose.
    c. a significant drop in blood sugar levels.
    d. extreme thirst.

17. For a diabetic patient who meets the criteria, the quick administration of oral glucose by the EMT means that:

    a. a diabetic emergency is being managed appropriately.
    b. blood sugar levels will return to normal within 30 minutes.
    c. the patient may complain of abdominal pain after awakening.
    d. transport to the hospital will not be necessary once the patient awakens.

18. When the blood sugar falls to a hypoglycemic state, the longer a patient remains hypoglycemic the more likely there will be:
    a. urinary incontinence.
    b. a drop in blood pressure.
    c. a fruity smell on the breath.
    d. permanent damage to brain cells.

19. The function of insulin is to:
    a. carry sugar from the blood into the cells.
    b. carry sugar from the cells into the blood.
    c. break down glucagon and create energy.
    d. prevent too much sugar from being released into the bloodstream.

20. The most common cause of seizures in toddlers is:
    a. trauma.
    b. poison ingestion.
    c. drug or alcohol related.
    d. a rapid increase in body temperature.

21. You are assessing a patient with an altered mental status. She is very confused, but is becoming more awake as you obtain vital signs and complete a rapid trauma exam. The patient is wearing a medic alert device that tells you she has seizures. Your primary concern for this patient now is:
    a. to be prepared for another seizure.
    b. to be alert for incontinence and take precautions.
    c. to call medical control and request to assist the patient with oral glucose.
    d. to wait for the patient to become more alert, then assist with oral glucose.

22. When a patient has two or more seizures without a period of consciousness in between, the condition is known as status epilepticus. What makes this a true emergency is that:
    a. the patient can swallow his tongue.
    b. the patient is at risk for traumatic injury.
    c. prolonged seizures can cause brain damage.
    d. prolonged seizures cause extreme states of hypoglycemia.

23. A family has called EMS because Grandpa had fallen several times in the last 2 days. They described him having had a couple of periods of "fogginess and forgetfulness." This patient has an extensive history of heart disease and high blood pressure, and recently he had surgery on his leg for vascular problems. Which of the following do you suspect is the cause of the change over the last 2 days?
    a. infection
    b. mini-strokes
    c. dehydration
    d. new onset of diabetes

24. This morning the wife of an elderly patient had trouble waking her husband, so she called EMS. She tells you he is not a diabetic, but takes medication for high blood pressure, and that this has never happened before. The patient does not respond to you verbally, and you find a complete weakness on the left side of the body during your physical exam. Management of this patient will include:
    a. being prepared for a seizure, administering high-flow oxygen, and observing for vomiting.
    b. obtaining a temperature if possible, administering high-flow oxygen, and treating for shock.
    c. administering high-flow oxygen, providing supportive care, and giving early notice to the hospital for a possible stroke.
    d. administering high-flow oxygen, contacting medical control to assist with oral glucose, and rapid transport.

25. The family of an elderly woman has called EMS because they noticed that during lunch she had a brief period of looking stunned, followed by a change in speech. She now seems better. The patient has no past medical history and takes only vitamins. You suspect that the:
    a. patient had a mini-stroke.
    b. patient is developing dementia.
    c. patient had low blood sugar, which improved after she finished her lunch.
    d. family may not be fully forthcoming because they are trying to get the woman admitted to the hospital for a while.

26. Which of the following conditions in a diabetic patient, left untreated, can cause altered mental status due to hypoglycemia?
    a. infection
    b. wheezing
    c. asthma attack
    d. traumatic injury

27. The roommate of a 23-year-old female returned home from the drug store to find that her friend was difficult to awaken. She was sweaty and hot to the touch as well. Except for the patient becoming suddenly sick during the night, there is no significant past medical history, no medications, and no allergies. Which of the following is most likely the cause of the altered mental status in this patient?
    a. seizure
    b. infection
    c. hypoglycemia
    d. hyperglycemia

28. The EMT should consider altered mental status in an elderly patient to be associated with _____ until proven otherwise.
    a. stroke or TIA
    b. tachycardia
    c. abuse or neglect
    d. hypoxia or hypoglycemia

29. Your crew has been dispatched for a 17-year-old female having a seizure. When you arrive, the patient is not seizing, but is not alert. There is blood and saliva around the mouth and cheeks. The respirations are snoring and gurgling. Which action should be taken first?
    a. Suction the airway.
    b. Determine if the seizure was witnessed.
    c. Open the airway with spinal precautions.
    d. Turn the patient on her side to allow for drainage of her airway.

30. (Continuing with the previous question) The patient's breathing effort has improved and she is opening her eyes. Caregivers tell you that she has a history of seizures and the seizure today is similar to other seizures she has had. Her vital signs are respiratory rate 20, pulse rate 120, and blood pressure 130/80. What treatment is appropriate at this point?
    a. Insert a nasopharyngeal airway.
    b. Continue to suction the airway.
    c. Administer high-flow oxygen by non-rebreather mask.
    d. Place a cervical collar on the patient and immobilize her on a long backboard.

31. A woman called EMS because her mother had fainted and fallen at home. Your general impression is that of a 64-year-old female who is sitting up with no apparent signs of distress or injury. The daughter reports that the patient has a history of hypertension and arthritis, and that she had been well prior to the brief loss of consciousness. Your primary assessment findings are that the patient is unable to talk; she has an open airway with adequate respiratory effort, clear lung sounds, and strong and regular distal pulse; and her skin is pink, warm, and dry. What action would be appropriate next?
    a. Administer oral glucose.
    b. Assess the patient further for signs of stroke.
    c. Search the residence for alcohol or drugs that are commonly abused.
    d. Perform a rapid trauma assessment, while remaining alert for signs of physical abuse.

32. (Continuing with the preceding question) You now administer oxygen and finish obtaining a SAMPLE history and OPQRST information from the daughter as your partner obtains vital signs. The patient is compliant with her medications, has no allergies, and has never had a similar episode. The patient is able to answer questions by moving her head, and she denies any difficulty breathing, pain, or injury. Vital signs are: respiratory rate 16; pulse 66, strong and regular; BP 9/90; SpO$_2$ 100%. The patient has weakness, which requires that you lift her onto the stretcher. As you settle the patient into the ambulance, she begins to speak, but has slurring. What do you suspect is happening to the patient, and what can you do to confirm your suspicions?
    a. The patient has signs and symptoms of a transient ischemic attack. Perform serial reassessments using a stroke scale.
    b. The patient may have an alcohol or substance abuse problem and now the effects of the alcohol or substance are probably wearing off. Take any medications found at the residence to the hospital.
    c. The patient has signs and symptoms of a head injury. Perform an ongoing assessment focusing on mental status and vital signs.
    d. The patient may have a new onset of diabetes and be hypoglycemic. Continue to administer additional oral glucose and watch for signs of improvement.

33. EMS was dispatched for an unresponsive male in his fifties. When you enter the residence, you find the patient on the floor with his eyes closed. He appears disoriented, as he repeatedly waves his right arm in small circles. His airway is clear and he is breathing adequately; his skin is pale, moist, and very cold. He will not respond to you. Family members state that they found him on the floor when they got up this morning and that he is a diabetic. They have a glucagon kit for emergencies, but are not sure how to use it. You confirm that ALS is en route and will arrive within 5 minutes. During that time, what actions should you take?
    a. Administer one tube of oral glucose.
    b. Administer glucagon from the patient's emergency kit.
    c. Administer oxygen, move the patient off the cold floor, and provide warmth.
    d. Administer oxygen and immobilize the patient to keep him from harming himself.

34. You have been dispatched to a call for severe headache. At the residence, you find the patient to be a 24-year-old female who is alert and sitting up, complaining of pain from the worst headache she has ever experienced. The pain started suddenly after she came home from jogging. The patient also has extreme weakness and numbness in the right arm and leg and is unable to stand up. The vital signs are: respiratory rate 22; pulse rate 90, strong and regular; BP 160/110; skin CTC is pink, warm, and moist. Management of this patient will include:

    a. administration of oxygen, protection of the weak and numb extremities, and rapid transport to a stroke center.
    b. observation only of the patient, as she has most likely hyperventilated to cause the presenting symptoms.
    c. fully immobilizing the patient on a long backboard, as her symptoms are consistent with a traumatic head injury.
    d. administering oxygen, determining if the patient is pregnant, providing supportive care, and transporting to the hospital of her choice.

35. The wife of a 71-year-old male calls EMS because she thinks her husband is having a stroke. When you arrive, she tells you that the patient was watching television when the symptoms began. She says that her mother suffered a stroke and that she recognized her husband as having very similar symptoms. As part of the stroke assessment, which of the following will you examine the patient for?

    a. facial droop, arm drift, and abnormal speech
    b. evidence of hypertension and inability to move all extremities
    c. abnormal speech, equal grip strength, and ability to walk a straight line
    d. arm drift or weakness, evidence of headache, or new onset of hearing loss

Chapter 19 Answer Form

	A	B	C	D
1.	❏	❏	❏	❏
2.	❏	❏	❏	❏
3.	❏	❏	❏	❏
4.	❏	❏	❏	❏
5.	❏	❏	❏	❏
6.	❏	❏	❏	❏
7.	❏	❏	❏	❏
8.	❏	❏	❏	❏
9.	❏	❏	❏	❏
10.	❏	❏	❏	❏
11.	❏	❏	❏	❏
12.	❏	❏	❏	❏
13.	❏	❏	❏	❏
14.	❏	❏	❏	❏
15.	❏	❏	❏	❏
16.	❏	❏	❏	❏
17.	❏	❏	❏	❏
18.	❏	❏	❏	❏

	A	B	C	D
19.	❏	❏	❏	❏
20.	❏	❏	❏	❏
21.	❏	❏	❏	❏
22.	❏	❏	❏	❏
23.	❏	❏	❏	❏
24.	❏	❏	❏	❏
25.	❏	❏	❏	❏
26.	❏	❏	❏	❏
27.	❏	❏	❏	❏
28.	❏	❏	❏	❏
29.	❏	❏	❏	❏
30.	❏	❏	❏	❏
31.	❏	❏	❏	❏
32.	❏	❏	❏	❏
33.	❏	❏	❏	❏
34.	❏	❏	❏	❏
35.	❏	❏	❏	❏

CHAPTER

20

Allergic Reaction, Poisoning, and Overdose

1. A patient who is experiencing an allergic reaction might have which of the following findings associated with the upper airway?
   a. stridor
   b. wheezing
   c. bronchospasm
   d. pulmonary edema

2. Which group of symptoms suggests an allergic reaction that has not progressed to anaphylaxis?
   a. wheezing, abdominal cramps, and nausea
   b. hives on the upper arms, sweating, and no distal pulse
   c. blotches and itching on the arms, back, chest, and thighs
   d. pale skin color, dizziness, and rash on the chest and arms

3. You have responded to a call for a 10-year-old having an allergic reaction. The parent tells you that the child developed a rash on the chest, back, and abdomen shortly after taking a new medication. The child was given a Benedryl® (diphenhydramine) tablet when the parent recognized the allergic reaction. This medication is helpful for these symptoms because it is an:
   a. antibiotic.
   b. antihistamine.
   c. anti-inflammatory drug.
   d. over-the-counter medication.

4. You are working with a new partner today. You are returning to service from the last call when you notice that your partner's hands are red and slightly swollen. He tells you that his hands are itchy, but otherwise he feels fine. What should you do next?
   a. Call your supervisor and ask to be placed with another partner.
   b. Suspect a possible latex allergy and go back to the emergency department.
   c. Have your partner wash his hands thoroughly and report the incident to the supervisor.
   d. Go back to the emergency department and try to determine if your last patient has an infectious disease.

5. At a standby for a soccer game, a parent approaches you with her 8-year-old son who has two bee stings on his lower leg. The mother tells you that she removed the stingers but she would like you to look at the child. Which of the following findings would you consider significant, requiring treatment by EMS?
   a. swelling of the lips
   b. the child is crying
   c. local swelling at the site of the sting
   d. redness at the site of the sting

6. Responding to a call for a possible allergic reaction, you find a 36-year-old female who took a new antibiotic prescription two hours ago and now feels very sleepy. Her vital signs are: respirations 20, adequate; pulse 78, regular; BP 114/68; skin CTC is pink, warm, and dry. She denies difficulty breathing, but feels there is something wrong. Management of this patient includes:
   a. treatment for shock and rapid transport.
   b. administration of oxygen, position of comfort, reassessment, and transport.
   c. administration of high-flow oxygen, assistance with an Epi auto-injector, and rapid transport.
   d. calling medical control for permission to let the patient sign off and follow up with her own physician.

7. While playing football, a 16-year-old male disturbed a wasp nest and was stung approximately 10 times. He has redness at the sites and is developing a rash on his chest. He is also complaining of feeling dizzy. You begin airway management with:
   a. high-flow oxygen by non-rebreather mask.
   b. inspecting the mouth for stings and swelling.
   c. assisting the patient to use his epinephrine auto-injector.
   d. removal of any remaining stingers, to prevent further exposure to antigens.

8. While at school, a 14-year-old girl ate a cookie not knowing that it contained a nut to which she has a known allergy. She is complaining of chest tightness and swelling of the tongue, and her respiratory rate is 30. How should you manage the airway?

   a. Lay the patient down with legs elevated and assist ventilations with a bag mask device.
   b. Keep the patient calm and administer oxygen with a nasal cannula at 6 lpm.
   c. Keep the patient calm, place an NPA in the right nostril, and administer high-flow oxygen with a non-rebreather mask.
   d. Allow the patient to stay in a position of comfort, administer high-flow oxygen with a non-rebreather mask, and be prepared to assist her with epinephrine administration.

9. Your unit is dispatched for an unresponsive 28-year-old male. His wife tells you that the patient complained of being bitten or stung by an insect in the lower left leg before collapsing. You quickly determine that he has inadequate breathing and is cyanotic. You begin to manage the airway by:

   a. inserting an OPA and assisting ventilations with a bag mask device.
   b. suctioning as needed and assisting ventilations with a bag mask device.
   c. suctioning the airway, inserting an OPA, and administering high-flow oxygen with a non-rebreather mask.
   d. inserting an NPA, suctioning, and then assisting ventilations with a pocket mask connected to oxygen.

10. _____ is the trade name for the medication in an auto-injector prescribed for severe allergic reactions.

    a. Adrenalin
    b. Benadryl
    c. Epinephrine
    d. EpiPen Jr.

11. _____ is the generic name for the medication in an auto-injector prescribed for severe allergic reactions.

    a. EpiPen.
    b. Adrenalin
    c. Epinephrine
    d. Bronchodilator

12. For a severe allergic reaction with respiratory distress, the administration of epinephrine is a high priority because:

    a. the effects reduce toxicity from antigens.
    b. it is an antidote for many types of allergens.
    c. it relaxes the smooth muscles of the airways.
    d. the effects are similar to that of an anesthetic.

13. Select the proper order of steps in the procedure for the use of an epinephrine auto-injector.

    a. Remove the cap, place the injector tip against the patient's thigh, push the injector, and hold in place for 10 seconds.
    b. Remove the cap and discard it in a sharps container, shake the injector gently, aim the tip into the patient's upper arm, and inject for 15 seconds.
    c. Shake the injector gently, hold the injector with the tip down, place against the patient's thigh, avoiding any area of hives, and inject.
    d. Shake the injector vigorously, record the time, place the injector tip against the patient's upper arm, and dispose of the injector in a sharps container.

14. The form of epinephrine that comes in an auto-injector is a:

    a. gel.
    b. liquid.
    c. spray.
    d. crystal.

15. When assessing a patient who is experiencing an allergic reaction, which of the following findings would prompt you to call medical control immediately?

    a. skin flushing
    b. swelling of the hands
    c. the presence of shock
    d. hives on the arms and legs

16. Which of the following is not an indication for the use of an epinephrine auto-injector?

    a. The patient has a history of multiple allergies.
    b. The patient has signs and symptoms of severe allergic reaction.
    c. Medical direction has authorized the use of the auto-injector online.
    d. Medical direction has authorized the use of the auto-injector offline.

17. For the patient with signs and symptoms of progressive allergic reaction, the EMT should contact medical control:

    a. as soon as possible.
    b. only when signs and symptoms become severe.
    c. only when signs of respiratory distress are present.
    d. only if administration of the first epinephrine auto-injector does not begin to work within 10 minutes.

18. You are treating and transporting the victim of a low-speed MVC. You have the patient fully immobilized because of a suspected spinal injury. On the way to the hospital, you notice that the patient's skin is red where you have placed adhesive tape. How would you manage this patient now?
    a. Ask the patient if she has ever had to use an epinephrine auto-injector.
    b. Leave the patient secured as is and continue to monitor and reassess her.
    c. Call medical control right away and discuss the use of an epinephrine auto-injector.
    d. Remove the adhesive tape and perform a focused physical exam for a possible allergic reaction.

19. Which of the following factors is a good indicator that a mild allergic reaction may progress to a severe allergic reaction?
    a. multiple prior exposures to the antigen
    b. no known prior exposures to the antigen
    c. the amount of body surface area covered with hives
    d. the speed of onset of symptoms from time of exposure

20. An office manager calls EMS because one of the employees has suddenly developed blotchy redness on her face, neck, and arms over the past 2 hours. The employee says that she has had a runny nose and nasal congestion for three days, but the redness is new. She has no other complaints. What do you suspect is wrong with this patient and how will you manage her?
    a. She has signs of a severe reaction and needs epinephrine and rapid transport.
    b. She has signs of a mild allergic reaction, so provide supportive care and transport for evaluation.
    c. There are no significant findings and the patient has no serious complaints, so help her contact her own physician to follow up.
    d. She is progressing to a severe reaction, so be prepared to assist with an epinephrine auto-injector and begin rapid transport.

21. Which of the following statements is most correct about the use of an epinephrine auto-injector for anaphylaxis?
    a. Epinephrine does not work with allergens that have been inhaled.
    b. The use of epinephrine for anaphylaxis will always save the patient's life.
    c. Any patient with signs and symptoms of anaphylaxis needs to be treated with epinephrine.
    d. For best results, epinephrine should be administered within the first 30 minutes after exposure to the allergen.

22. For a patient experiencing anaphylactic shock with hypotension and no respiratory distress, the use of an epinephrine auto-injector is:
    a. contraindicated.
    b. not a BLS treatment.
    c. for medical direction to decide.
    d. a priority and will increase the blood pressure.

23. Select the proper steps in the management of a patient who is experiencing anaphylaxis.
    a. Treat for shock, assist with an epinephrine auto-injector if available, and transport.
    b. Assist with an epinephrine auto-injector if available, administer high-flow oxygen, and transport.
    c. Begin rapid transport to the nearest hospital, administer high-flow oxygen, and assist with an epinephrine auto-injector if available.
    d. Maintain airway support, assist with an epinephrine auto-injector if available, treat for shock, and transport to the nearest hospital.

24. The main goal in the treatment of anaphylaxis is to:
    a. alleviate hives and rash.
    b. relieve abdominal cramping.
    c. relieve itching and swelling.
    d. restore respiratory and cardiac efficiency.

25. Which of the following side effects is typical with the use of epinephrine in anaphylaxis?
    a. seizure
    b. tachycardia
    c. nausea or vomiting
    d. headache or dizziness

26. After assisting a patient who is experiencing anaphylactic shock to administer his own epinephrine auto-injector, you should expect:
    a. breathing effort to improve.
    b. bradycardia.
    c. the blood pressure to drop.
    d. skin that is flushed, warm, and dry.

27. The use of epinephrine in the elderly comes with a precaution because:
    a. it can cause hypertension.
    b. the side effects are long-lasting.
    c. it increases the workload on the heart.
    d. of its incompatibility with other prescribed medications.

28. The dose of epinephrine in an auto-injector is _____ mg for adults and _____ mg for pediatrics.
    a. 0.3, 0.15
    b. 3.0, 1.5
    c. 1.5, 0.3
    d. 0.03, 0.015

29. Epinephrine has several side effects, of which _____ is(are) the most serious.

    a. nausea
    b. anxiety
    c. cardiac dysrhythmias
    d. respiratory depression

30. The effects of epinephrine are:

    a. slow onset and short-lasting.
    b. slow onset and long-lasting.
    c. rapid onset and short-lasting.
    d. rapid onset and long-lasting.

31. Children are at highest risk for exposure to toxic substances by:

    a. injection.
    b. ingestion.
    c. inhalation.
    d. absorption.

32. Carbon monoxide poisoning is an example of an _____ exposure to a toxic substance.

    a. injection
    b. ingestion
    c. inhalation
    d. absorption

33. _____ is a toxic substance that is typically introduced into the body by absorption.

    a. Lead paint
    b. A pesticide
    c. Carbon monoxide
    d. A poisonous mushroom

34. Of the following statements, which is most correct regarding the signs and symptoms of poisoning?

    a. The effects of toxic substances will not be immediately apparent.
    b. Signs and symptoms vary widely and depend on the substance and amount taken into the body.
    c. Any time a toxic substance is taken into the body, the patient will have signs of an altered mental status.
    d. Any patient with a decreased pulse and respiratory rate should be considered for exposure to a toxic substance.

35. The most dangerous toxic substances affect the _____ system(s).

    a. respiratory
    b. nervous
    c. endocrine and gastrointestinal
    d. respiratory, nervous, and endocrine

36. The most significant findings associated with signs and symptoms of poisoning are:

    a. age-related.
    b. headache and seizures.
    c. changes in the size of the pupils.
    d. those that affect the ABCs.

37. The police have called you to transport an intoxicated patient. You assess a 52-year-old male who is conscious, but has slurred speech, smells of alcohol, has filthy clothing, and does not answer your questions appropriately. Management of this patient will include:

    a. performing a secondary assessment and being alert for vomiting or seizures.
    b. getting him on the stretcher and letting him sleep during the transport to the hospital.
    c. obtaining vital signs, assessing for incontinence, and removing his clothing prior to arrival at the hospital.
    d. obtaining vital signs and performing a physical exam while being alert for any other causes of altered mental status.

38. An elderly patient's home health aide has called EMS because she found three empty medication bottles that should be nearly full according to the dates on the bottles. Primary assessment of the patient reveals that she is conscious but confused; she does not recall taking any medications. Her vital signs are: respirations 18, adequate; pulse 60, regular; BP 148/90. What should you do next?

    a. Administer activated charcoal.
    b. Verify the home health aide's credentials.
    c. Obtain a focused history and perform a physical assessment.
    d. Attempt to get the patient to vomit and take the vomitus to the hospital.

39. The father of a toddler calls EMS because he thinks his child has eaten an entire box of throat lozenges. The father is quite upset and the child is crying. What should you do next?

    a. Notify dispatch to send a crisis counselor to the scene.
    b. Call the child's pediatrician and notify her about the incident.
    c. Talk to the father and obtain a focused history, while your partner assesses the child.
    d. Tell the father there is nothing to worry about, as there is no potential danger from ingesting throat lozenges.

40. Two women custodians who used cleaning products in a confined space for approximately 1 hour are now complaining of dizziness and nausea. They deny difficulty breathing, chest pain, or vomiting. Lung sounds are clear and neither of them has red eyes or tearing. The emergency medical care for these patients begins with:

    a. decontaminating the patients.
    b. calling the poison control center for instructions.
    c. locating the material safety data sheet (MSDS).
    d. removing them from the confined area and providing high-flow oxygen.

41. You are obtaining a focused history from a patient with suspected poisoning. Which of the following questions is of least significance for the EMT?
   a. How much was ingested?
   b. When did the poisoning occur?
   c. Has this substance been ingested before?
   d. What, if anything, has been done for treatment so far?

42. Your next-door neighbor calls you and says that her 20-month-old son has eaten an unknown amount of toothpaste; she wants to know what to do. What steps should you take now?
   a. Tell her to flush out the child's mouth and give him milk to drink.
   b. Call poison control and get instructions before going next door to help.
   c. Call 9-1-1 for the neighbor, then go over and begin assessing the child.
   d. Tell her to call 9-1-1, because you really cannot give any advice while off duty.

43. A 16-year-old female is suspected of taking multiple prescriptions in a suicide attempt. She is unresponsive to pain with the following vital signs: respirations 8, shallow and inadequate; pulse 58, regular; BP 100/40. Your first steps in managing this patient include:
   a. hyperventilating the patient with bag mask ventilations.
   b. suctioning and administering high-flow oxygen by a non-rebreather mask.
   c. attempting oropharyngeal airway insertion and assisting ventilations with a bag mask device.
   d. inserting a nasopharyngeal airway and administering high-flow oxygen by a non-rebreather mask.

44. EMS was called to a residence where a party is going on. Friends of the unresponsive patient describe him as having had way too much to drink, and they are unable to wake him. The patient has snoring respirations at a rate of 12 per minute; distal pulse of 60, strong and regular; skin is normal color, warm, and dry. Initial airway management should include:
   a. placing the patient in the recovery position.
   b. suctioning and assisting ventilations with a bag mask device.
   c. inserting an OPA and administering high-flow oxygen by a non-rebreather mask.
   d. inserting an NPA and administering high-flow oxygen by a non-rebreather mask.

45. A forklift operator accidentally splashed liquid chlorine onto his face. He is alert and breathing adequately, but complains of severe burning pain in both eyes. The initial management for this patient includes:
   a. calling medical control for advice prior to touching him.
   b. not touching the patient until the fire department arrives to decontaminate him.
   c. removing the patient's clothing and continuously irrigating the eyes and face.
   d. irrigating the eyes and face for five minutes, administering high-flow oxygen, and rapid transport.

46. The generic name for the antidote used for ingested poisons is:
   a. Super-Char®.
   b. charcola.
   c. Charco aide.
   d. activated charcoal.

47. You are about to assist your partner with administering activated charcoal to a patient who has ingested a poison. What form of medication will you be using?
   a. liquid
   b. oral spray
   c. slow-acting tablets
   d. fast-dissolving capsules

48. A family of five is complaining of symptoms of carbon monoxide poisoning. Before you arrived, the fire department took the family outside into the fresh air. All five patients have severe headache, three are vomiting violently, and two have nausea. Select the correct steps in the management of these patients.
   a. Triage, contact medical control, then treat and transport.
   b. Manage the ABCs, declare a multiple casualty incident, and triage.
   c. Declare a multiple casualty incident, then triage, treat, and transport.
   d. Call dispatch and ask for four more ambulances, then triage and contact medical control.

49. You are treating a patient who ingested a chemical product thinking it was his coffee. He is alert and complaining of burning in his mouth and throat. His vital signs are stable. Your protocols allow you to administer activated charcoal on standing orders, but you think the chemical may be corrosive. What should you do?
   a. Call medical control for instructions.
   b. Have the patient gargle with an antiseptic.
   c. Have the patient flush out his mouth with milk.
   d. Administer the activated charcoal on standing orders.

50. The fire department carried a victim out of a confined space that had noxious fumes in it. The patient is conscious but confused. While you are listening to his breath sounds, he begins to seize. You protect the patient from injury and ask your partner to:
   a. suction and insert an oropharyngeal airway.
   b. call medical control for decontamination instructions.
   c. administer high-flow oxygen and be prepared to assist with ventilations.
   d. call medical control and request an order to administer activated charcoal.

51. A frantic young mother calls EMS because one of her preschool-aged children ingested an entire bottle of baby aspirin, thinking it was candy. The use of activated charcoal in this patient is:
   a. not indicated, because of the child's age.
   b. contraindicated for aspirin ingestion.
   c. indicated and will work for aspirin overdose.
   d. indicated, but probably will not work for aspirin overdose.

52. One hour after ingesting a full bottle of prescription sleeping pills, the patient vomited the pills. Now that the patient has vomited, the use of activated charcoal is:
   a. indicated, as it will help decrease the effects of depression.
   b. indicated, as it will absorb toxins still present in the GI tract.
   c. not indicated, because the patient has eliminated the toxins.
   d. not indicated, because there was not enough time for the toxins to become dangerous.

53. In the prehospital management of a poisoned or overdosed patient, the EMT should contact medical direction early, because:
   a. it takes a while to prepare the activated charcoal.
   b. if you wait too long to give activated charcoal, it will not be effective.
   c. medical control clarifies treatment options recommended by poison control.
   d. only medical control will know how critical the patient can become.

54. After assessing and providing high-flow oxygen to a patient who accidentally ingested too much of a prescription antibiotic, you call medical control to obtain an order to administer activated charcoal. You explain to the patient that the actions of activated charcoal are:
   a. slow.
   b. delayed.
   c. immediate.
   d. long-lasting and require only one dose.

55. You respond to a call for a sick person and upon arrival find a 65-year-old male and his wife who promptly tell you they think they have food poisoning. They are complaining of abdominal cramping, vomiting, and diarrhea. The symptoms began early this morning and the husband's symptoms have gotten worse. They both ate hamburgers last night at a local restaurant. What should you do you next?
   a. Call the fire department to check out a possible high CO exposure.
   b. Obtain vital signs, get a focused history, and perform a physical exam.
   c. Manage the ABCs and call medical control to request an order to assist with activated charcoal.
   d. Find out which restaurant the patients ate at and report it to dispatch for notification to the health department.

Chapter 20 Answer Form

	A	B	C	D		A	B	C	D
1.	❏	❏	❏	❏	29.	❏	❏	❏	❏
2.	❏	❏	❏	❏	30.	❏	❏	❏	❏
3.	❏	❏	❏	❏	31.	❏	❏	❏	❏
4.	❏	❏	❏	❏	32.	❏	❏	❏	❏
5.	❏	❏	❏	❏	33.	❏	❏	❏	❏
6.	❏	❏	❏	❏	34.	❏	❏	❏	❏
7.	❏	❏	❏	❏	35.	❏	❏	❏	❏
8.	❏	❏	❏	❏	36.	❏	❏	❏	❏
9.	❏	❏	❏	❏	37.	❏	❏	❏	❏
10.	❏	❏	❏	❏	38.	❏	❏	❏	❏
11.	❏	❏	❏	❏	39.	❏	❏	❏	❏
12.	❏	❏	❏	❏	40.	❏	❏	❏	❏
13.	❏	❏	❏	❏	41.	❏	❏	❏	❏
14.	❏	❏	❏	❏	42.	❏	❏	❏	❏
15.	❏	❏	❏	❏	43.	❏	❏	❏	❏
16.	❏	❏	❏	❏	44.	❏	❏	❏	❏
17.	❏	❏	❏	❏	45.	❏	❏	❏	❏
18.	❏	❏	❏	❏	46.	❏	❏	❏	❏
19.	❏	❏	❏	❏	47.	❏	❏	❏	❏
20.	❏	❏	❏	❏	48.	❏	❏	❏	❏
21.	❏	❏	❏	❏	49.	❏	❏	❏	❏
22.	❏	❏	❏	❏	50.	❏	❏	❏	❏
23.	❏	❏	❏	❏	51.	❏	❏	❏	❏
24.	❏	❏	❏	❏	52.	❏	❏	❏	❏
25.	❏	❏	❏	❏	53.	❏	❏	❏	❏
26.	❏	❏	❏	❏	54.	❏	❏	❏	❏
27.	❏	❏	❏	❏	55.	❏	❏	❏	❏
28.	❏	❏	❏	❏					

Abdominal Emergencies

1. The abdominal cavity contains hollow organs including the stomach, large intestine, small intestine, and:
   a. liver.
   b. spleen.
   c. kidneys.
   d. gallbladder.

2. The _____ is(are) the layer(s) of serous membrane that cover(s) most of the abdominal organs.
   a. diaphragm
   b. parietal peritoneum
   c. visceral peritoneum
   d. small and large intestines

3. Sometimes pain originating from an abdominal organ is felt in another part of the body. This type of pain is known as _____ pain.
   a. referred
   b. visceral
   c. somatic
   d. parietal

4. During the interview of a patient with a chief complaint of abdominal pain, you learn that the patient has had loose black stool for two days. Which condition do you suspect?
   a. appendicitis
   b. hemorrhoids
   c. bowel obstruction
   d. intestinal bleeding

5. A 54-year-old male is vomiting blood and complains of nausea and abdominal cramping that began six hours earlier. He has a history of peptic ulcer and takes medication for it. His vital signs are respiratory rate 20 non-labored, pulse rate 110 and regular, and BP 100/50. As you prepare to get him on the stretcher, he continues to vomit. What is the safest way to transport the patient?
   a. Lay him on his side and give him an emesis bag.
   b. Sit him on the stretcher and administer oxygen by cannula.
   c. Lay him down, raise his legs, and administer oxygen by non-rebreather.
   d. Sit him on the stretcher and let him bend his knees to relax the peritoneum.

6. A common presentation of a person experiencing pain is a kidney stone is that the patient:
   a. is unable to find any comfortable position.
   b. must lie on their back with their head elevated.
   c. will lie in the fetal position with thighs flexed.
   d. must lie still because movement aggravates their pain.

7. _____ is a condition that does not originate in the abdomen, but can cause abdominal pain.
   a. Stroke
   b. Pneumonia
   c. Febrile seizure
   d. Hypertension

8. A 30-year-old male is complaining of abdominal pain that has been getting worse over the past two days. He vomited last night and feels nauseated today. He is lying very still and will not allow you to touch his stomach due to the pain. Which of the following conditions do you suspect?
   a. reflux
   b. appendicitis
   c. kidney stone
   d. constipation

9. When caring for patients with abdominal emergencies, it is important to not allow them to eat or drink anything because:
   a. ingesting something may cause vomiting.
   b. pain medication works best with an empty stomach.
   c. an empty stomach is preferred when surgery is needed.
   d. a full stomach makes it difficult to make a specific diagnosis.

10. When assessing patients with abdominal pain, the EMT should be especially alert for:
    a. signs of shock.
    b. blood in the stool.
    c. a history of kidney stones.
    d. a history of ectopic pregnancy.

11. You are assessing a 24-year-old woman who suddenly developed sharp lower abdominal pain 30 minutes before calling 9-1-1. She denied having nausea, vomiting, or constipation and has no history of similar pain or being pregnant. Which of the following conditions must be ruled out first?

   a. ectopic pregnancy
   b. urinary tract infection
   c. irritable bowel syndrome
   d. sexually transmitted disease

12. (Continuing with the previous question) You obtain vitals signs, which are respiratory rate 24 non-labored, pulse rate 90 and regular, and BP 110/50. Her skin is pale, warm, and dry. Her abdomen is soft with no masses and tender in the left lower quadrant. You begin treatment:

   a. by treating for shock.
   b. after you complete a secondary assessment.
   c. on the way to the hospital.
   d. by administering high-flow oxygen.

13. A 36-year-old male was working in a warehouse when he suddenly developed extreme pain in the abdomen and groin area on the right side. He is in obvious distress from the pain and is pale and diaphoretic. When you examine his lower abdomen and groin, there appears to be an unusual mass, which the patient states was not there before. What do you suspect is the problem?

   a. He has cancer.
   b. He pulled a groin muscle.
   c. He has an inguinal hernia.
   d. He has a bowel obstruction.

14. (Continuing with the previous question) The patient is feeling dizzy and has nausea in addition to the profound pain. His vital signs are respirations 22 non-labored, pulse rate 100 and regular, and BP 140/90. What is the emergency care for this condition?

   a. Apply ice to the affected area.
   b. Immobilize the patient on a long backboard.
   c. Administer high-flow oxygen and treat for shock.
   d. Let the patient take any comfortable position on the stretcher.

15. Eating fatty foods causes the _____ to contract and can cause abdominal pain for some people.

   a. colon
   b. stomach
   c. appendix
   d. gallbladder

16. For the patient complaining of nausea and indigestion, the EMT should first suspect and assess for _____ to avoid missing a possible life-threatening condition.

   a. bowel obstruction
   b. acute coronary syndrome
   c. abdominal aortic aneurysm
   d. appendicitis

17. Your ambulance has responded to a call for an unconscious patient. When you enter the residence, there is a bad smell, which you recognize immediately as GI bleeding. A woman brings you to a bed where her husband is lying. She states that he passed out briefly, has had diarrhea since last night, and complained of abdominal pain. The patient is pale and cool to the touch. What do you assess first?

   a. pulse
   b. blood sugar
   c. mental status
   d. blood pressure

18. (Continuing with the previous question) The patient's vital signs are respiratory rate 16 shallow, pulse rate 118 and regular, and BP 88/40. His SpO_2 is 94 percent and blood sugar is 86 mg/dl. Your partner has administered oxygen by a non-rebreather mask and called for ALS. What action should be taken next?

   a. Begin rapid transport.
   b. Lay the patient on the stretcher and raise his legs.
   c. Estimate the amount of blood lost and notify the hospital.
   d. Take another set of vital signs while waiting for ALS to arrive.

19. A 72-year-old female called 9-1-1 from home. When you arrive, she is lying in bed and tells you that her stomach is bloated and she is very uncomfortable. She is being treated for stomach cancer and is taking pain medication, which has not helped her discomfort. Her last bowel movement was three days ago and she feels that is her problem. What action should be taken next?

   a. Assess her abdomen.
   b. Administer high-flow oxygen.
   c. Complete the primary assessment.
   d. Transport her to the hospital of her choice.

20. (Continuing with the previous question) While en route to the hospital, the patient's discomfort worsens. What action should be taken next?

   a. Reassess vital signs.
   b. Instruct the ambulance driver to go faster.
   c. Instruct the ambulance driver to divert to the nearest hospital.
   d. Keep the patient still and provide warmth with extra blankets.

21. A 75-year-old male has a sudden onset of severe non-traumatic back pain. He has a history of high blood pressure and arthritis and is compliant with his medication. His vital signs are respiratory rate 20 non-labored, pulse rate 78 and regular, and BP 94/48. His back has no sign of injury and his abdomen has a pulsing mass in the midline. What condition do you suspect is most likely the problem?

   a. pancreatitis
   b. gallstones
   c. arthritic pain
   d. leaking aortic aneurysm

22. (Continuing with the previous question) After administering oxygen, you and your partner gently load the patient onto the stretcher and into the ambulance. En route to the hospital, the patient begins to vomit. What action do you take next?

    a. Reassess vital signs.
    b. Remove the oxygen mask.
    c. Examine the vomitus for blood.
    d. Ask the driver to stop the ambulance.

23. When you physically assess a patient's abdomen by pressing on it then quickly removing your fingers and the patient displays extreme discomfort during the release, _____ is present.

    a. shock
    b. referred pain
    c. colorectal cancer
    d. rebound tenderness

24. _____ is an example of a metabolic problem that can cause abdominal pain.

    a. Pneumonia
    b. Myocardial infarction
    c. Diabetic ketoacidosis
    d. Spontaneous pneumothorax

25. _____ is a general term for the inflammation of any part or parts of the large or small bowel due to infection.

    a. Hemorrhoid
    b. Appendicitis
    c. Gastroenteritis
    d. Bowel obstruction

Chapter 21 Answer Form

	A	B	C	D
1.	❑	❑	❑	❑
2.	❑	❑	❑	❑
3.	❑	❑	❑	❑
4.	❑	❑	❑	❑
5.	❑	❑	❑	❑
6.	❑	❑	❑	❑
7.	❑	❑	❑	❑
8.	❑	❑	❑	❑
9.	❑	❑	❑	❑
10.	❑	❑	❑	❑
11.	❑	❑	❑	❑
12.	❑	❑	❑	❑
13.	❑	❑	❑	❑

	A	B	C	D
14.	❑	❑	❑	❑
15.	❑	❑	❑	❑
16.	❑	❑	❑	❑
17.	❑	❑	❑	❑
18.	❑	❑	❑	❑
19.	❑	❑	❑	❑
20.	❑	❑	❑	❑
21.	❑	❑	❑	❑
22.	❑	❑	❑	❑
23.	❑	❑	❑	❑
24.	❑	❑	❑	❑
25.	❑	❑	❑	❑

CHAPTER 22

Hematologic and Renal Emergencies

1. _____ is the condition of having a low number of healthy red blood cells.
   a. Anemia
   b. Leukemia
   c. Hemophilia
   d. Hypoxia

2. Sickle cell disease is a disorder, which causes the production of:
   a. too few red blood cells.
   b. too many red blood cells.
   c. too few white blood cells.
   d. abnormally shaped red blood cells.

3. Patients with sickle cell anemia:
   a. are contagious.
   b. have inherited it.
   c. develop the condition as a child.
   d. develop the condition as a young adult.

4. A patient experiencing a sickle cell crisis will most likely:
   a. have internal bleeding.
   b. require a bone marrow transplant.
   c. feel short of breath and have severe abdominal pain.
   d. develop shock from abnormal blood vessel dilation.

5. People with sickle cell disease are at increased risk for developing:
   a. cancer.
   b. diabetes.
   c. hypothermia.
   d. an infection.

6. _____ is the measure of the number of red blood cells per unit of blood volume.
   a. Hematocrit
   b. Hemoglobin
   c. End tidal CO_2
   d. Pulse oximetry

7. _____ is what gives blood cells their red color and ability to carry oxygen.
   a. Albumin
   b. Estrogen
   c. Hematocrit
   d. Hemoglobin

8. If you have _____, you may bleed longer than normal after an injury.
   a. anemia
   b. leukemia
   c. hemophilia
   d. sickle cell disease

9. The majority of blood cells are formed in the:
   a. liver.
   b. spleen.
   c. kidney.
   d. bone marrow.

10. Hemophilia is a rare condition predominantly found in:
    a. men.
    b. women.
    c. Hispanics.
    d. Black Americans.

11. The blood of a person with hemophilia:
    a. will not clot normally.
    b. has too many red blood cells.
    c. has too few red blood cells.
    d. does not have enough platelets.

12. You have been dispatched to an elementary school for a traumatic injury. In the nurse's office, a 7-year-old boy is bleeding from a laceration on his lower leg. The nurse tells you that the boy is a hemophiliac who has a minor cut with bleeding that is not stopping or slowing. This has happened in school before and he had to go to the hospital by ambulance at that time. Care for this type of wound includes:
    a. treating for shock.
    b. waiting for the parent(s) to arrive.
    c. applying direct pressure and ice.
    d. assisting the patient with administering factor replacement therapy.

13. Mature red blood cells circulate _____ days before they are absorbed by the body.
    a. 30
    b. 90
    c. 120
    d. 180

14. An average weight adult male has approximately _____ liters of blood.
    a. 5 to 6
    b. 7 to 8
    c. 9 to 10
    d. 11 to 12

15. When the body is fighting an infection, the count of _____ in the blood will increase.
    a. plasma
    b. red blood cells
    c. white blood cells
    d. platelets

16. The main function of _____ is to prevent bleeding.
    a. plasma
    b. red blood cells
    c. white blood cells
    d. platelets

17. _____ is/are the pale and yellowish part of blood and contains clotting elements.
    a. Plasma
    b. Red blood cells
    c. White blood cells
    d. Platelets

18. The most common emergency from peritoneal dialysis is a/an _____. The patient presents with severe pain and often signs of early shock.
    a. stroke
    b. infection
    c. hemorrhage
    d. myocardial infarction

19. An assisted living facility has requested transport for an 89-year-old male who is unable to pass urine. His medical history includes diabetes, hypertension, enlarged prostate, and recent kidney stone. He is very uncomfortable and his vital signs are respiratory rate 22 regular, pulse rate 66 irregular, and BP 148/76. Which of the following is most likely the cause of his urine retention?
    a. hypertension
    b. enlarged prostate
    c. a new kidney stone
    d. diabetic related

20. A 68-year-old male passed out at home 1 hour after returning home from dialysis treatment. He is awake when you arrive and denies having difficulty breathing or chest pain. What is the most probable cause of the syncope?
    a. hypotension
    b. occluded fistula
    c. air embolism
    d. internal bleeding

21. _____ is the procedure for filtering waste products from the blood of some kidney disease patients.
    a. Hemocysteine
    b. Hemodialysis
    c. Hemapheresis
    d. Hysteroscopic

22. A 32-year-old male with renal failure has acute and severe flank pain that radiates into the lower abdominal quadrant. He tells you that he has nausea and has vomited. What condition is most likely?
    a. appendicitis
    b. kidney stone
    c. urinary tract infection
    d. he is overdue for dialysis

23. (Continuing with the previous question) Which of the following treatments would be most helpful?
    a. oxygen
    b. pain management
    c. position of comfort
    d. rapid transport to the hospital

24. The EMT taking care of a dialysis patient with an acute problem must remember:
    a. to avoid taking a blood pressure in an arm with a fistula.
    b. that patients with renal failure cannot lie flat on their back (supine).
    c. that patients with renal failure have altered pain perception.
    d. that dialysis patients are overweight and require bariatric equipment.

25. Your ambulance has been dispatched to a local nursing home to transport a 78-year-old female with cloudy urine, which is visible in the urinary catheter and bag. When you assess her vital signs, her skin appears hot and dry with good color. The staff reports that she is confused today, but has not complained of having pain. You suspect that the patient:
    a. has renal failure.
    b. is dehydrated.
    c. has a urinary tract infection.
    d. is developing kidney stones.

Chapter 22 Answer Form

	A	B	C	D			A	B	C	D
1.	❏	❏	❏	❏		14.	❏	❏	❏	❏
2.	❏	❏	❏	❏		15.	❏	❏	❏	❏
3.	❏	❏	❏	❏		16.	❏	❏	❏	❏
4.	❏	❏	❏	❏		17.	❏	❏	❏	❏
5.	❏	❏	❏	❏		18.	❏	❏	❏	❏
6.	❏	❏	❏	❏		19.	❏	❏	❏	❏
7.	❏	❏	❏	❏		20.	❏	❏	❏	❏
8.	❏	❏	❏	❏		21.	❏	❏	❏	❏
9.	❏	❏	❏	❏		22.	❏	❏	❏	❏
10.	❏	❏	❏	❏		23.	❏	❏	❏	❏
11.	❏	❏	❏	❏		24.	❏	❏	❏	❏
12.	❏	❏	❏	❏		25.	❏	❏	❏	❏
13.	❏	❏	❏	❏						

CHAPTER 23

Behavioral and Psychiatric Emergencies and Suicide

1. A friend of a 21-year-old female called 9-1-1 because the woman is depressed over a recent breakup and took 10 sleeping pills in an effort to kill herself. When you arrive and interview the patient, she tells you that she vomited the pills and now regrets what she has done. This type of incident is referred to as a:
   a. panic attack.
   b. suicide gesture.
   c. suicide attempt.
   d. bipolar reaction.

2. Abnormal behavior that results from a crisis in a person's life is interpreted as a/an:
   a. emotion.
   b. adaptive behavior.
   c. emotional disorders.
   d. behavioral emergency.

3. A strong feeling that is typically accompanied by physical findings such as increased heart rate is a/an:
   a. emotion.
   b. mental disorder.
   c. behavioral disorder.
   d. psychiatric disorder.

4. Research shows that after a divorce or marital separation, the risk of suicide for men is twice that of women, primarily because:
   a. men tend to be more violent.
   b. women remarry quicker than men.
   c. woman have better support systems.
   d. women are mentally stronger than men.

5. The EMT is responsible for knowing local protocols and _____ regarding treatment of persons with mental illness.
   a. state laws
   b. definitive care
   c. crisis intervention procedures
   d. making a specific field diagnosis of a behavioral condition

6. Which of the following statements reported by a patient would indicate that she is currently experiencing a behavioral emergency?
   a. I am feeling overwhelmed.
   b. I am a recovering alcoholic.
   c. I am taking medication for depression.
   d. There is a history of schizophrenia in my family.

7. The sudden death of a parent, a sudden change in the course of an acute disease, or the inability to accept a new role in life, such as becoming a parent, are all examples of:
   a. phobias.
   b. personality disorders.
   c. the need for crisis intervention.
   d. reasons for psychological crisis.

8. _____ is any acute, severe disruption in the balance of an individual or group.
   a. Crisis
   b. Anxiety
   c. Distress
   d. Emotion

9. Which of the following statements is most correct regarding the potential for a crisis situation?
   a. The reaction to a crisis will be the same for each individual.
   b. Every illness or injury is associated with some type of psychological stress.
   c. The patient in crisis usually has a history of drug or alcohol dependency.
   d. A person with a previous emotional illness is most likely to lapse into a crisis situation.

10. Which of the following characteristics is typically an unassociated risk factor for suicide?
    a. paranoia
    b. serious illness
    c. lack of self-esteem
    d. the loss of a significant loved one

11. A patient who makes a suicide gesture:
    a. is not really serious about suicide.
    b. typically uses a violent method of self-destruction.
    c. is most likely to be noncompliant with medications.
    d. must be treated and transported for evaluation by a psychiatrist.

12. One of the most common behavioral disorders that can lead to suicide and other psychological and medical disorders is:
    a. anxiety.
    b. dementia.
    c. depression.
    d. bipolar disorder.

13. _____ involves increased medical and legal considerations for the EMT.
    a. Treating a victim of assault
    b. Caring for the victim of a rape
    c. Physically restraining a patient
    d. Attempted resuscitation of a victim of suicide

14. When the EMT is assessing and treating a patient who is impaired due to alcohol intoxication, the EMT is responsible for:
    a. arranging transportation to a detoxification facility.
    b. classifying the impairment as behavioral or psychiatric in nature.
    c. transporting the patient to a facility capable of providing a psychiatric evaluation.
    d. following both local protocols and state laws regarding persons with an altered mental status.

15. When entering a crime scene to care for a patient who is experiencing a behavioral emergency, the first priority is to:
    a. protect yourself.
    b. preserve the crime scene.
    c. preserve any evidence found on the patient.
    d. get the patient into the ambulance quickly.

16. A behavioral emergency can be caused by organic or emotional problems and should be treated:
    a. as nonurgent.
    b. as a physical problem.
    c. promptly, but without rushing the patient.
    d. as though the patient will require restraints.

17. Each of the following is a common misconception about behavioral illnesses, *except*:
    a. all mental patients are unstable.
    b. all mental patients are dangerous.
    c. abnormal behavior is always weird.
    d. behavioral illnesses often have an organic cause.

18. When managing a patient who is experiencing a behavioral emergency, it is necessary to:
    a. begin crisis intervention after the primary assessment.
    b. allow the police to be included in all phases of the call.
    c. begin crisis intervention after the secondary assessment.
    d. assess for physical causes that may mimic a behavioral emergency.

19. A factor most likely to cause an individual to become violent on the scene of an EMS call is the:
    a. age of the patient.
    b. gender of the patient.
    c. history of depression.
    d. patient's perception of the EMT.

20. A sign indicating that a patient may become violent is:
    a. memory loss.
    b. the patient raising his tone of voice.
    c. unusual odors on the breath.
    d. the appearance of being withdrawn.

21. A patient who is acting out in a hostile and violent manner is most likely:
    a. at high risk for suicide.
    b. experiencing depression.
    c. to be a disturbed teenager looking for attention.
    d. making an attempt to gain control of the situation.

22. The use of physical restraints on a patient who is displaying violent behavior is:
    a. dangerous for the patient and the rescuers.
    b. no longer a legal or moral treatment option.
    c. an acceptable method of calming the patient.
    d. necessary with all patients who are at risk for violence.

23. The police have called your crew to transport a teenager who punched his mother in the face. The patient is talking continuously in a loud tone and frequently using vulgar language. He is in handcuffs and an officer is accompanying you. Your approach to calming this patient should include:
    a. transporting both patients in the same ambulance.
    b. obtaining vital signs only.
    c. not attempting to touch the patient if that is his desire.
    d. telling the patient what he wants to hear.

24. In managing a patient with an acute attack of anxiety, the EMT can help calm the patient by:
    a. keeping eye contact whenever possible.
    b. keeping a distance of a minimum of 6 feet.
    c. explaining to the patient that she is overreacting.
    d. telling the patient that you are here to help and that she can expect help from you.

25. You are faced with the problem of having to transport a patient against his will, because he poses a possible danger to himself or others. It is necessary to:
    a. display authoritative and threatening actions.
    b. impose a physical assessment on the patient.
    c. follow local protocols together with medical control.
    d. assure the patient that he will not be able to harm anyone while in your care.

26. The patient who is experiencing a behavioral emergency may become violent as a result of an action that would not normally lead to violence. Therefore, the EMT who responds to care for such a patient should:
    a. remain calm and professional at all times.
    b. not let the patient verbally express any anger or frustration.
    c. restrain every patient who is experiencing a behavioral emergency.
    d. request a police escort for every transport that involves behavioral emergency.

27. While performing a physical exam on a patient, which of the following findings would cause you to suspect that the patient has a history of a behavioral or psychiatric disorder?
    a. The patient has urinated on himself.
    b. The patient has a strong odor of alcohol.
    c. The patient has a strong odor of cigarettes.
    d. The patient shows an abnormal lack of regard for personal hygiene.

28. Generally, the time you spend with a patient who is experiencing a behavioral emergency will be:
    a. the same as with any other patient.
    b. longer, because of the time it takes to restrain the patient.
    c. longer, because of the special needs of this type of patient.
    d. shorter, because the patient will usually refuse to be touched.

29. In the management of a patient who intentionally took an overdose of medication, with the intent to harm himself, the EMT should:
    a. listen carefully to what the patient wants to say.
    b. avoid asking the patient if this is his first attempt at suicide.
    c. be indirect and nonspecific with communications and actions.
    d. not allow the patient to discuss his problems until the police are present.

30. Statistics show that _____ make more suicide attempts and that _____ are more successful at suicide.
    a. females, males
    b. males, females
    c. teenagers, females
    d. the elderly, males

Chapter 23 Answer Form

	A	B	C	D			A	B	C	D
1.	❏	❏	❏	❏		16.	❏	❏	❏	❏
2.	❏	❏	❏	❏		17.	❏	❏	❏	❏
3.	❏	❏	❏	❏		18.	❏	❏	❏	❏
4.	❏	❏	❏	❏		19.	❏	❏	❏	❏
5.	❏	❏	❏	❏		20.	❏	❏	❏	❏
6.	❏	❏	❏	❏		21.	❏	❏	❏	❏
7.	❏	❏	❏	❏		22.	❏	❏	❏	❏
8.	❏	❏	❏	❏		23.	❏	❏	❏	❏
9.	❏	❏	❏	❏		24.	❏	❏	❏	❏
10.	❏	❏	❏	❏		25.	❏	❏	❏	❏
11.	❏	❏	❏	❏		26.	❏	❏	❏	❏
12.	❏	❏	❏	❏		27.	❏	❏	❏	❏
13.	❏	❏	❏	❏		28.	❏	❏	❏	❏
14.	❏	❏	❏	❏		29.	❏	❏	❏	❏
15.	❏	❏	❏	❏		30.	❏	❏	❏	❏

SECTION

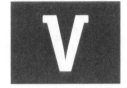

TRAUMA

24

Bleeding and Shock

1. The primary function of the circulatory system is to:
   a. prevent obstruction in circulation to the heart.
   b. provide a continuous source of nutrients to tissues.
   c. prevent the formation of diseased states of the body.
   d. maintain pressure within the inner walls of the blood vessels.

2. The fluid that transports cells and nutrients to all body tissues is:
   a. lymph.
   b. plasma.
   c. platelet.
   d. marrow.

3. Blood is involved in all of the following functions, *except*:
   a. nutrition.
   b. fluid balance.
   c. temperature regulation.
   d. nerve impulse regulation.

4. A woman called 9-1-1 after she accidentally cut her arm with a utility knife. She has wrapped a cloth around the arm and it is soaked through with dark red blood. You suspect that the bleeding is:
   a. venous.
   b. arterial.
   c. capillary.
   d. life-threatening.

5. A 23-year-old male put his hand through a glass door; the injury resulted in bleeding that is pulsating and difficult to control. You recognize this as _____ bleeding.
   a. arterial
   b. venous
   c. internal
   d. capillary

6. A 12-year-old boy injured his wrist while skateboarding. While splinting his arm, you notice bloodstains on the knees of his jeans. Your partner exposes the patient's knees and finds abrasions on both legs. This type of bleeding is typically:
   a. arterial.
   b. venous.
   c. capillary.
   d. difficult to control.

7. The method of using elevation to control external bleeding works best when:
   a. the wound is below the waist.
   b. ice has been applied to the wound.
   c. the wound is raised above the level of the heart.
   d. the wound is more than 2 inches in length or diameter.

8. Bleeding from a deep gash on the forearm is pulsing and flowing rapidly. Direct pressure is not slowing the bleeding. What step should be taken next to control bleeding?
   a. Apply an ice pack.
   b. Elevate the extremity.
   c. Pack the wound with gauze.
   d. Apply a hemostatic dressing.

9. A tourniquet applied on an extremity to control a life-threatening bleed is:
   a. used on lower extremities only.
   b. used on upper extremities only.
   c. no longer used in the prehospital setting.
   d. a method of last resort to control bleeding in the prehospital setting.

10. Standard precautions refer to:
    a. keeping immunizations current.
    b. the belief that all blood and body fluids are potentially infectious.
    c. health care providers washing their hands after every patient contact.
    d. everyone washing their hands before and after every patient contact, to decrease the incidence of disease.

11. _____ is the most common serious infectious disease that is transmitted by exposure to external bleeding.
    a. HIV
    b. Hepatitis
    c. Meningitis
    d. Tuberculosis

12. Which of the following is not considered a significant exposure as a result of managing a hemorrhage?
    a. spray into the mouth
    b. splatter into the eye(s)
    c. contact with broken skin
    d. soaking the uniform pant leg

13. While standing by at a soccer tournament, you witness a player run face-first into the goal. He appears to have broken his nose and is bleeding steadily. After several minutes of pinching the nostrils, you are unsuccessful in controlling the bleeding, and now the patient is complaining of nausea. How would you manage the airway now?
    a. Suction the nose and mouth.
    b. Pack the nostrils and apply an ice pack.
    c. Tilt the head back and apply an ice pack to the nose.
    d. Tilt the head forward and have the patient spit out the blood.

14. You are transporting a large female, who is immobilized, to a long backboard. She complained of neck pain after her vehicle was struck from behind. During the ride in, she develops nausea and states that she is going to vomit. The next action to take should be to:
    a. turn on the suction and begin suctioning.
    b. take off her collar and loosen the straps on the board.
    c. tell the driver to use the lights and siren and hurry to the ED.
    d. loosen the stretcher straps enough to be able to tilt the board.

15. A worker fell from a height of approximately 40 feet. You have determined that he is apneic and pulseless and direct your partner to perform manual spinal immobilization. You insert an OPA and attempt to ventilate him with a bag mask device while another rescuer starts compressions. The ventilations are poor with no chest rise. You attempt to correct the problem by:
    a. suctioning the airway.
    b. improving the mask seal.
    c. tilting the head and lifting the jaw.
    d. stopping compressions to assess the airway.

16. An 81-year-old female is bleeding from the back of her head. She states she lost her balance and fell while in the kitchen. There is blood on the edge of a table and drops of blood on the floor. She used an entire roll of paper towels in an attempt to stop the bleeding but was unsuccessful and called 9-1-1. The blood is flowing steady from a patch of matted hair on the scalp. The first step in the management of this type of wound is to:
    a. apply direct pressure using a dressing.
    b. apply a dressing with an ice pack inside.
    c. determine if the patient is taking a blood thinner.
    d. wash the wound and estimate the size of the laceration.

17. The fire department has extricated the driver of a vehicle that struck a pole. The airbag deployed, but he was not wearing a seat belt. He has a large bruise on his forehead and a deformed ankle. The patient has an altered mental status and his vital signs are: respirations 18, adequate; pulse 120, weak and regular; blood pressure 80/40. Which injury do you suspect is the cause of shock?
    a. head injury
    b. ankle injury
    c. spinal injury
    d. internal bleeding

18. A 19-year-old male was stabbed in the upper-right quadrant of his abdomen by another teenage male, who used a 3-inch knife. Which organs are most likely to be injured?
    a. liver, large intestine, and lung
    b. heart, aorta, diaphragm, and spleen
    c. stomach, appendix, and small intestine
    d. diaphragm, liver, large intestine, and lung

19. Early signs indicating that a patient has intraabdominal bleeding include:
    a. hypertension, headache, and nausea.
    b. hyperventilation, hypoxia, and constipation.
    c. bradycardia, hypotension, and irregular pulse.
    d. sustained tachycardia and normal or low blood pressure.

20. Which of the following signs is not a reliable finding associated with internal bleeding?
    a. tarry stool
    b. bowel sounds
    c. rigid abdomen
    d. blood in the urine

21. The mother of a 12-year-old male has called you because her son fainted. Your primary assessment finds a patient who is conscious, pale, and moist with a weak, rapid pulse. The patient denies any recent injury or illness and his mother agrees; also, he has no significant past medical history and takes no medications. Your initial treatment plan is to:

    a. prepare for vomiting.

    b. consider the use of MAST/PASG.

    c. administer high-flow oxygen and treat for shock.

    d. perform a focused physical exam of the abdomen.

22. A 52-year-old male patient with symptoms of nausea, dizziness, and vomiting blood has a history of gastric reflux. His vital signs are: respirations 24, adequate; pulse 120, regular; BP 96/50; skin CTC cool, moist, and pasty-looking. Management of this patient should include:

    a. oxygen by cannula, observation for vomiting, and routine transport.

    b. high-flow oxygen, position of comfort, warmth, and routine transport.

    c. supine position with legs flexed for comfort, high-flow oxygen, and rapid transport.

    d. supine position, high-flow oxygen, warmth, rapid transport, and call for ALS.

23. After falling approximately 25 feet from a roof, a construction worker was unconscious for approximately 30 seconds. He is now alert and complaining of severe low back pain. There is blood trickling out of his left ear. The bleeding from this injury should be managed by:

    a. packing the ear with sterile gauze.

    b. direct pressure and elevation of the head.

    c. a sterile dressing taped over the outside of the ear.

    d. turning the patient on his left side to allow drainage.

24. A driver who was involved in a moderate-speed MVC appears to have struck his face on the steering wheel during the incident. There is blood draining from his nose. Bleeding should be controlled by which method?

    a. direct pressure

    b. pressure dressing

    c. use of a pressure point

    d. packing the nose with a sterile dressing

25. The skin signs of a patient experiencing hypoperfusion include:

    a. cold, white, and dry.

    b. cool, pale, and moist.

    c. hot, cyanotic, and dry.

    d. hot, flushed, and moist.

26. Severe hemorrhage results in the loss of _____, causing a decrease in oxygenation of the body tissues.

    a. plasma

    b. platelets

    c. red blood cells

    d. white blood cells

27. When the adult body senses a loss of blood volume, one of the body's first responses is:

    a. fainting.

    b. respiratory distress.

    c. an increased pumping rate of the heart.

    d. to initiate a process that leads to kidney failure.

28. A woman has called EMS because her husband fainted this morning. He is lying in bed and appears very weak and pale. There is a strong odor of stool, and the wife confirms that the patient has had diarrhea and vomiting during the night and all morning. The vital signs are: respirations 24, labored; pulse 110, regular but weak; BP 70/40. After you administer high-flow oxygen, the next steps in the emergency medical care of this patient include:

    a. providing rapid transport only.

    b. attaching the AED, requesting an ALS intercept, and beginning rapid transport.

    c. requesting ALS and preparing the patient for transport while waiting for ALS to arrive.

    d. elevating the legs, providing warmth, beginning rapid transport, and requesting ALS intercept.

29. Dispatched for a traumatic injury, you arrive on the scene to find a 50-year-old male who has nearly cut off one of his fingers with a chainsaw. He is pale and has beads of sweat on his forehead. A family member has a cold wet bandage on the finger and has controlled the bleeding. Your primary assessment of this patient prompts you to treat this patient for _____ shock.

    a. cardiogenic

    b. psychogenic

    c. compensating

    d. decompensating

30. The rider of a motorcycle was traveling at a moderate speed when she was cut off by a car and knocked to the ground. The patient is conscious now, but bystanders report that she was unconscious for about a minute. Her helmet is cracked and both of her thighs appear to have closed fractures. Her airway is clear; skin is pale, moist, and cool; and her vital signs are: respirations 18, adequate; pulse 126, regular; BP 80/40. Your management of this patient will be to treat for:

    a. compensating shock due to the head injury.

    b. decompensating shock due to the head injury.

    c. compensating shock due to the internal bleeding.

    d. decompensating shock due to the internal bleeding.

31. Each additional minute spent on the scene for a patient with life-threatening traumatic injuries:
   a. increases the trauma score.
   b. increases the criteria for rapid transport.
   c. reduces the patient's chance for survival.
   d. reduces the time it takes for ALS to reach the patient.

32. The decision to provide rapid transport for a trauma patient is typically based on:
   a. the MOI.
   b. signs of shock.
   c. external bleeding.
   d. signs of shock and/or the MOI.

33. When you suspect that a patient is bleeding internally, the interventions you provide will be rapid because definitive care is:
   a. often surgical.
   b. accomplished on scene.
   c. available at any hospital.
   d. performed en route to the hospital.

34. Abdominal trauma is the second leading cause of trauma death because:
   a. most abdominal trauma occurs in children.
   b. blunt trauma to the abdomen is always overlooked.
   c. significant blood loss occurs before signs of distention are apparent.
   d. injury to solid organs can produce severe bleeding that progresses rapidly.

35. The severity of a hemorrhage can best be determined by which of the following factors?
   a. arterial versus venous bleeding
   b. internal versus external bleeding
   c. how much blood has been lost
   d. the age and height of the patient

Chapter 24 Answer Form

	A	B	C	D			A	B	C	D
1.	❏	❏	❏	❏		19.	❏	❏	❏	❏
2.	❏	❏	❏	❏		20.	❏	❏	❏	❏
3.	❏	❏	❏	❏		21.	❏	❏	❏	❏
4.	❏	❏	❏	❏		22.	❏	❏	❏	❏
5.	❏	❏	❏	❏		23.	❏	❏	❏	❏
6.	❏	❏	❏	❏		24.	❏	❏	❏	❏
7.	❏	❏	❏	❏		25.	❏	❏	❏	❏
8.	❏	❏	❏	❏		26.	❏	❏	❏	❏
9.	❏	❏	❏	❏		27.	❏	❏	❏	❏
10.	❏	❏	❏	❏		28.	❏	❏	❏	❏
11.	❏	❏	❏	❏		29.	❏	❏	❏	❏
12.	❏	❏	❏	❏		30.	❏	❏	❏	❏
13.	❏	❏	❏	❏		31.	❏	❏	❏	❏
14.	❏	❏	❏	❏		32.	❏	❏	❏	❏
15.	❏	❏	❏	❏		33.	❏	❏	❏	❏
16.	❏	❏	❏	❏		34.	❏	❏	❏	❏
17.	❏	❏	❏	❏		35.	❏	❏	❏	❏
18.	❏	❏	❏	❏						

CHAPTER
25

Soft-Tissue Injuries and Musculoskeletal Care

1. When a significant portion of a person's skin is involved in a burn injury, that person is at high risk for _____ shock.
   a. spinal
   b. cardiogenic
   c. anaphylactic
   d. hypovolemic

2. In order from the surface to the underlying muscle or tissue, the layers of the skin are:
   a. hypodermis, epidermis, and dermis.
   b. epidermis, hypodermis, and dermis.
   c. epidermis, dermis, and subcutaneous tissues.
   d. dermis, epidermis, and subcutaneous tissues.

3. The subcutaneous tissue:
   a. supports the production of calcium.
   b. aids in the production of male hormones.
   c. helps to maintain the growth of hair and nails.
   d. attaches the skin to the underlying bone or muscle.

4. You are evaluating a 16-year-old male who ripped open an area of skin on the inside of his upper arm. The injury is approximately 4 inches long. You see fat or adipose tissue and recognize this as part of the:
   a. dermis.
   b. epidermis.
   c. sebaceous glands.
   d. subcutaneous tissue.

5. First responders have immobilized a 23-year-old male who was knocked off an ATV after striking a tree. They report that he is complaining of neck and back pain, and he has a large contusion on his forehead and a very large hematoma on his left flank. Before you begin your examination, you put on your minimum level of PPE, which includes:
   a. gloves.
   b. gloves and a mask.
   c. gloves and eye protection.
   d. gloves, eye protection, and a mask.

6. An 8-year-old child who fell while skateboarding has sustained abrasions on both knees and his left elbow, but has no other injuries. Before treating his injuries, at a minimum you put on:
   a. gloves.
   b. gloves and a mask.
   c. gloves and eye protection.
   d. gloves, eye protection, and a mask.

7. The victim of an assault has contusions and lacerations on her face and scalp. Her nose is bleeding and she is spitting blood. You take standard precautions that include:
   a. gloves and a gown.
   b. placing an oxygen mask on the patient.
   c. gloves, eye protection, and a mask.
   d. gloves and a face mask for the patient.

8. You are dispatched to the parking lot of the local supermarket for a traumatic injury. Upon arriving, you find a toddler crying. His mother says his fingers were accidentally slammed in the car door. Two fingers are purple under the nails, but the skin is not broken and the fingers do not appear to be broken. This injury can be described as:
   a. closed.
   b. splintering.
   c. compound.
   d. complicated.

9. When a soft-tissue injury results in leakage of fluid from capillaries or larger vessels, the condition is called:
   a. painful.
   b. edema.
   c. life-threatening.
   d. simple compression.

10. Shortly after the accident occurred, EMS was called for a 30-year-old male who walked into a door and struck his forehead. The patient has no altered mental status, but developed swelling, pain, and tenderness at the site. The skin is intact and there is no bleeding, so you determine that this type of injury is a/an:

    a. contusion.
    b. hematoma.
    c. ecchymosis.
    d. possible fracture.

11. An elderly patient tripped on a curb and fell on her face. She has a hematoma and swelling under the left eye. There is no external bleeding, and she denies neck or back pain or losing consciousness. In addition to the closed soft-tissue injury, you must suspect:

    a. facial fractures.
    b. that she is confused about why she fell.
    c. that she is lying about the loss of consciousness.
    d. that this type of blood loss can progress to shock.

12. A babysitter calls EMS for an eye injury. While having a pillow fight, one of the children in her care was struck in the eye. The 8-year-old boy has blood present in the sclera (white part) of the left eye. He denies any pain or vision disturbance. The parents are on their way home. Which actions do you take next?

    a. Apply cold over the closed eye and lay the patient down.
    b. Cover both eyes with a dressing and transport the patient.
    c. Apply heat over the closed eye and keep the patient sitting up.
    d. Do not touch the eye, but offer to transport the patient for evaluation.

13. A neighbor knocks on your station door and shows you her thumb. She was cleaning a window when it came down hard on her hand, and now her thumb is swollen and throbbing with pain. She can move and bend it and wants some advice on how to care for it right now; she does not want to go to the hospital. In addition to recommending that she see her physician, you advise her to:

    a. apply cold and elevation.
    b. keep it dry until it has been x-rayed.
    c. let you splint it and transport her to the ED.
    d. apply heat first, then alternate cold and heat.

14. Your crew is dispatched to assist a nonambulatory patient with getting back to bed. While assisting the patient, you note one of the following conditions that warrants a trip to the hospital for evaluation. Which is it?

    a. an abdominal hernia
    b. abnormal spinal curvature
    c. peripheral edema in both legs
    d. a lower extremity that is red and hot

15. While cooking on a stove, a woman accidentally dumped a pot of boiling water on her right leg. She has redness and blisters on the front of the entire upper leg. The severity of this burn is:

    a. mild.
    b. severe.
    c. moderate.
    d. complicated.

16. Superficial, partial thickness, and full thickness are all classifications of burns by the:

    a. depth.
    b. source.
    c. location.
    d. severity.

17. While attempting to light a gas grill, a woman lit a match and experienced a sudden burst of flame. She singed her eyebrows, bangs, and arm hairs. She was left with painful reddened skin on the front of both arms and her face. This burn can be classified as a:

    a. superficial burn involving 18 percent BSA.
    b. superficial burn involving 13½ percent BSA.
    c. partial-thickness burn involving 18 percent BSA.
    d. partial-thickness burn involving 27 percent BSA.

18. You have been called to care for the victim of a flash burn. The scene is safe and the patient is sitting down with coworkers who are helping him cool his face with a wet cloth. His entire face and neck are red and he states that he cannot see and that his eyes and face hurt. This burn can be classified as:

    a. superficial.
    b. fourth degree.
    c. full thickness.
    d. partial thickness.

19. A superficial or first-degree burn:

    a. is the most painful type of burn.
    b. involves the outer surface of the skin only.
    c. is characterized as having unbroken blisters.
    d. typically causes painful muscle contractions.

20. When a toddler was lowered into the bathtub, he began screaming. The parents did not test the bath water. The parents call EMS, and when you arrive the child has stocking burns on the legs just below the knees and red spots (splashing) on the thighs. There is severe redness and blisters are beginning to form. This type of burn can be classified as:

    a. child abuse.
    b. partial thickness only.
    c. second and third degree.
    d. superficial and partial thickness.

21. A thermal burn that damages the epidermis and a portion of the dermis, excluding the muscle tissue, is classified as _____ degree.
    a. first
    b. second
    c. third
    d. fourth

22. Persons who suffer a burn injury are at risk for infection:
    a. with any burn.
    b. only with third-degree burns.
    c. when the severity is full thickness or greater.
    d. when the severity is partial thickness or greater.

23. While lighting firecrackers, a 10-year-old male burned his hands, face, and neck. His airway and breathing are clear and adequate, but his face and neck are red and peppered with black powder. Fortunately, his eyes and vision were not affected. His hands are red and blistered and two fingers appear fused together with blisters. Which of his burns is considered the most serious?
    a. first-degree burns on the face
    b. first-degree burns on the neck
    c. partial-thickness burns on the hands
    d. each of these burns is equally serious because of the location

24. A second-degree burn is typically very painful and requires pain management. This is because of the affected:
    a. nerves.
    b. sweat glands.
    c. blood vessels.
    d. sebaceous glands.

25. Which of the following structures is not typically affected by a partial-thickness burn?
    a. nerves
    b. hair follicles
    c. blood vessels
    d. subcutaneous fat

26. A full-thickness burn affects:
    a. every layer of the skin.
    b. only the dermis and epidermis.
    c. more than 30 percent BSA in adults.
    d. more than 15 percent BSA in children.

27. A furnace exploded, creating a blast that has injured a 32-year-old male. His hands and one arm are critically burned into the soft tissue and muscle. He is conscious but confused and has hearing loss and audible wheezing. Which of his injuries is an immediate life-threatening condition?
    a. inhalation injuries
    b. acute hearing loss
    c. full-thickness burns
    d. altered mental status

28. A firefighter came to the emergency department a couple of hours after working at a fire. On the back of his right calf, he has a burn that apparently resulted from an ember that settled into his boot while he was working. He did not realize he had an injury until he showered, when he noticed that the area involved was dark and felt rough and dry. What type of burn does he have?
    a. first degree
    b. second degree
    c. third degree
    d. first, second, and third degree

29. A worker at a construction site was working with cement and did not realize that the gloves he was wearing were too porous for the job. EMS was called when he removed his gloves and saw that his fingers were graying white with the skin peeling. His palms were red and had no skin. What type of burn is this?
    a. third degree
    b. a thermal burn
    c. second degree
    d. second and third degree

30. Which of the following characteristics describes a full-thickness burn?
    a. burned or singed hair
    b. an associated fracture
    c. a complication with the airway
    d. damaged blood vessels, fat, or muscle

31. You arrive at one of the local nursing homes for a burn injury call. The victim is an elderly resident who has a burn on the left arm. An electric heating pad was being used for a preexisting injury to the elbow and was accidentally left on overnight. Approximately two-thirds of the arm is blistered and oozing. The center area of the burn is dry and leathery. This burn can be classified as critical because of the:
    a. age of the patient.
    b. location of the burn.
    c. amount of BSA involved.
    d. type or source of the burn.

32. The mother of a toddler called EMS because her daughter was splashed on the arms with very hot water. The mother tried to calm the child's crying by rubbing butter on the superficial splatter areas on the arms, with no success. With the help of the mother, you:
    a. wrap and immobilize both arms in splints.
    b. use ice cubes to cool and wipe off the butter.
    c. rinse the burned areas with cool water for several minutes.
    d. apply a second coat of butter and wrap the arms in sterile dressings.

33. Before providing the correct emergency care for a burn, the EMT needs to determine the:
    a. age of the patient.
    b. source of the burn.
    c. weight of the patient.
    d. medications the patient is taking.

34. Emergency care for sunburn that involves the entire posterior surface of the body includes:
    a. applying ice.
    b. cooling the burn.
    c. applying a commercial soothing ointment.
    d. not touching the burn and transporting rapidly.

35. A customer at the town garden center had lime powder spill onto his skin and clothing while lifting a bag into his cart. He is now complaining of a burning sensation. To stop the burning process prior to flushing him with water, you carefully brush off as much of the powder as you can and then instruct the patient to:
    a. remove his clothing, socks, and shoes.
    b. lie face down while you hose him off.
    c. lie on his back while you hose him off.
    d. close his eyes and hold his breath while you hose him off.

36. An adult who was exposed to a flash burn received partial-thickness burns over her entire chest, abdomen, anterior legs, and arms. You do not have enough sterile burn dressing to cover the entire area. What do you do next?
    a. Leave the area uncovered.
    b. Wrap the injured area with plastic cling wrap.
    c. Cover the area with a clean dry sheet.
    d. Cover the area with a clean wet sheet.

37. A woman sustained partial-thickness burns on both hands and arms while putting out a stovetop grease fire. The firefighters are bringing her out of the apartment as you arrive. As you begin your assessment, your partner helps you cut away the patient's sleeves and remove her rings and watch. You do this because:
    a. it helps to prevent blisters.
    b. it helps to prevent swelling.
    c. this will help the healing process.
    d. those items can retain heat and continue to burn the patient.

38. A full-thickness extremity burn that is circumferential should be treated as:
    a. a life-threatening emergency.
    b. a limb-threatening emergency.
    c. the same as any other burn.
    d. a fracture and be fully immobilized.

39. While working in a lab, a janitor spilled a chemical container and a coworker received severe burns to both lower legs. After cutting away his clothing, you see that the affected skin is white, dry, and leathery, with skin peeling away. The first step in the care of this burn is to:
    a. prevent shock.
    b. administer oxygen.
    c. decontaminate with flushing.
    d. determine the severity of the burn.

40. The function of a bandage is to:
    a. hold a dressing in place.
    b. reduce arterial blood flow.
    c. occlude venous blood flow.
    d. reduce the risk of a hematoma.

41. Large blisters resulting from steam burns are best managed by:
    a. covering with dressings to keep them from rupturing.
    b. rupturing the blisters first, then wrapping them with bandages.
    c. splinting whenever possible, with dressings over the splint.
    d. wrapping first with dressings, then rupturing the blisters with pressure.

42. The use of a bandage will substantially aid in:
    a. stopping arterial blood flow.
    b. preventing movement at the injury site.
    c. reducing the risk of contamination and infection.
    d. all of the above.

43. A traumatic injury at a work site has left a 45-year-old male with a large laceration across the lower abdomen. When you cut away the clothing, you see abdominal contents protruding and you quickly apply a bandage over the evisceration. The goal of application of this type of dressing is to:
    a. retain moisture and warmth.
    b. prevent nausea and vomiting.
    c. absorb any blood lost from abdominal organs.
    d. absorb any contents spilled from abdominal organs.

44. You are making a pressure bandage for bleeding from an open wound on an extremity. Which of the following pieces of equipment may be used when manual pressure is not enough?
    a. BP cuff
    b. pillow splint
    c. traction splint
    d. padded-board splint

45. Before a pressure bandage is applied to control bleeding, the EMT should:
   a. apply oxygen.
   b. apply an ice pack.
   c. locate the pressure point.
   d. use direct pressure and elevation.

46. In which of the following situations would you suspect a potentially serious airway injury associated with a burn?
   a. a mechanic who is in severe pain after splashing fuel into his eyes
   b. a carpenter who received a high-voltage shock and is conscious
   c. a customer who burnt her lips and tongue on an extremely hot coffee
   d. a firefighter who is wheezing after working in an overhaul after a fire

47. A major complication commonly associated with an improperly applied dressing includes:
   a. death.
   b. loss of limb.
   c. patient discomfort.
   d. increased tissue damage.

48. After unsuccessfully attempting to control an arterial bleed from the lower leg with every method you have been trained to use, you now decide to apply a tourniquet. Which of the following items should be used to control the bleeding?
   a. a strand of string
   b. a wide band of cloth
   c. a piece of rope or wire
   d. a 2-inch or 3-inch tape wrapped around the upper leg

49. You and your partner are attempting to control suspected arterial bleeding from the upper arm. Continuous direct pressure, elevation, and a pressure dressing appear to have stopped the bleeding. In an effort to prevent the bleeding from starting again, you:
   a. apply a tourniquet.
   b. maintain pressure and apply an ice pack.
   c. remove the soaked dressing and apply a clamp on the artery.
   d. remove the soaked dressing and apply a hemostatic dressing.

50. The victim of an assault has been sliced on the face from the ear to the tip of her nose and stabbed in the leg with a 3-inch pocketknife, which is still in the wound. She is alert and spitting blood. Which action do you take first?
   a. Manage the ABCs.
   b. Stabilize the knife wound.
   c. Put on your eye protection and gloves.
   d. Apply direct pressure to the facial wound.

51. Moving or removing an object that has impaled the foot can result in:
   a. nausea and vomiting.
   b. acute hypovolemic shock.
   c. an increased risk of infection and bleeding.
   d. damage to blood vessels, nerves, and muscles.

52. The objective of managing an amputated body part is to:
   a. prevent damage to the exposed nerves.
   b. control bleeding of the stump and the amputated part.
   c. prevent blood vessels from closing and becoming damaged.
   d. control bleeding of the stump and save the part for possible reattachment or reimplantation.

53. The use of dry ice in the emergency care of an amputated body part is not recommended because:
   a. it can actually burn the tissue.
   b. there is no way to control the bleeding of the part.
   c. it is difficult to wrap or seal the part with dry ice.
   d. dry ice is not an effective method of cooling or freezing.

54. While working in a machine shop, an employee took off his hard hat to wipe his brow and face. Just then, a forklift came by and knocked over a metal sheet that struck the worker in the back of the leg, completely tearing off a large piece of skin. When you arrive, coworkers have controlled the bleeding with bandages and have the skin in a plastic bag with ice cubes. You begin to assess the patient and ask your partner to:
   a. try to thaw any parts of the amputated part that may have frozen.
   b. take the amputated part out of the ice and place it in a dry sterile dressing.
   c. place the bag with the amputated part in the ambulance so it is not left behind.
   d. wrap the amputated part in a sterile, moist gauze pad and place it in another plastic bag, and then place the bag on ice.

55. A worker in an industrial setting has splashed a chemical into his eyes. Before you arrived, coworkers got him to an eyewash station and began flushing. The patient tells you that he cannot see and that he has a great deal of pain. When you examine his eyes, you see that he is wearing contact lenses. Management for this injury includes:
   a. calling for ALS, as the patient is going to need analgesia.
   b. removing the lenses or assisting the patient to do so.
   c. not touching the eyes or lenses and continuing to flush the eyes.
   d. not touching the eyes or lenses and beginning transport to the hospital.

56. The police have called you to care for one of their officers. During the arrest of a person who was combative, they used pepper spray and one officer was sprayed in the face. Treatment for this exposure begins with:
    a. wiping off any wet spray that is left on the skin and flushing with milk.
    b. instructing the officer to spit, blow his nose, and not rub the eyes or face.
    c. sponging off the exposed area without rubbing and flushing the eyes with water.
    d. moving the officer to a sink and flushing the entire head, face, and neck with cold water.

57. A golfer who was struck by lightning is lying in the wet grass on the fairway. As you approach, he appears to be unresponsive and a witness tells you he was struck and thrown backward. The first step in emergency care for this patient is to:
    a. start CPR if he has no pulse.
    b. immobilize him to a long backboard.
    c. assess for entrance and exit wounds.
    d. get the patient out of the rain and into the ambulance.

58. A homeowner who was last seen digging in the front yard, by his wife, was found collapsed on the ground. Dispatch is unable to determine if the patient is breathing because the caller is hysterical. As you approach the patient, it becomes clear that he struck an underground wire with his shovel. The next step in the care of this patient is to:
    a. start CPR if he has no pulse.
    b. back off and call the power company.
    c. move the patient onto a long backboard.
    d. let the fire department extricate the patient from his present location.

59. The weekend handyman was attempting to do his own wiring in the basement fuse box when the power went out. His wife called EMS because he was knocked out. When you get to him, he is responsive to pain, is breathing adequately, and has a strong distal pulse. There are obvious black burns on his hands and you look for an exit wound first on his:
    a. feet.
    b. head.
    c. back.
    d. face.

60. Which type of burn can cause the most injury to the lower airways?
    a. arc
    b. flash
    c. steam
    d. chemical

61. An ATV rollover crash involving a 20-year-old male has left him conscious, but not alert. He has an open wound across the nose and the left eyeball has been knocked out of the socket. Care for this injury includes:
    a. continuous flushing of the eye to keep it moist.
    b. replacing the eyeball in the socket and covering it with a dressing.
    c. covering the eye with a moist dressing without replacing it in the socket.
    d. replacing the eyeball in the socket and covering both eyes with a dressing.

62. A circumferential partial- or full-thickness burn to the upper torso is considered a serious injury to the respiratory system because:
    a. of the BSA involved.
    b. of the increased risk of heart attack.
    c. it impedes the ability of the chest wall to expand.
    d. of the rapid onset of shock associated with this area of the body.

63. The three sources of electrical burns are:
    a. first, second, and third degree.
    b. arc, contact, and flash burns.
    c. open, closed, and partial penetration.
    d. superficial, partial thickness, and full thickness.

64. A couple was painting their apartment when the husband stood up under a ladder and cut open his head. You see evidence of a lot of bleeding, and when you assess the wound you see a 6-inch flap of skin folded down over the right ear. You manage this wound by:
    a. replacing the flap and applying a dry sterile bandage.
    b. palpating the skull for a fracture and evidence of brain tissue.
    c. leaving the flap down and applying compression with a dry sterile bandage.
    d. taping the flap down with an occlusive dressing and covering it with a trauma bandage.

65. (Continuing with the preceding question) After you have finished applying a dressing and bandage, you see that the bleeding has not stopped and has soaked the dressing. What steps can you take next?
    a. Apply pressure to the nearest pressure point.
    b. Sit the patient down and apply direct pressure over the wound.
    c. Remove the first dressing and rewrap with a pressure dressing.
    d. Lay the patient down and elevate his legs while holding pressure on the wound.

66. Cartilage, tendons, and ligaments are connective tissues associated with the:
    a. production of blood cells.
    b. beating of the heart muscle.
    c. movement of the skeletal system.
    d. movement of food through the digestive system.

67. The bones of the hands that make up the fingertips are the:
   a. tarsals.
   b. carpals.
   c. phalanges.
   d. metacarpals.

68. The shoulder girdle is comprised of the:
   a. clavicle, humerus, and scapula.
   b. manubrium, clavicle, and scapula.
   c. acromion process, scapula, and manubrium.
   d. acromioclavicular (A/C) joint, clavicle, and cervical spine.

69. When the EMT describes a musculoskeletal injury in a verbal or written report, the information that should be included are the anatomical area involved, the level of discomfort, a description of the painful or swollen deformity, and:
   a. whether it was an open or closed injury.
   b. the name of each bone involved.
   c. a diagnosis of a fracture or sprain.
   d. the name of each muscle involved.

70. On a Saturday morning, you are dispatched to the local elementary school for a traumatic injury. While playing basketball, a 32-year-old male injured his ankle. He states that he landed hard and felt his ankle crack and is now having severe pain. The ankle is grossly deformed and there is blood under the skin in the area of the injury. This injury can be described as:
   a. closed.
   b. open.
   c. sprained.
   d. strained.

71. As the standby ambulance crew at a high school football game, you are signaled to come over to an injured player. The player is writhing in pain as the trainer shows you his kneecap, which appears to be displaced. The area is swollen and deformed and a hematoma is developing. This injury is:
   a. closed.
   b. open.
   c. the type that requires ALS.
   d. the type that cannot be splinted.

72. Splinting a long-bone fracture in _____ will prevent further damage to blood vessels, bones, and muscles.
   a. a straight position
   b. an elevated position
   c. a position of comfort
   d. the position it is found

73. When splinting a dislocation, the EMT should immobilize the injury in the _____ while maintaining a good blood supply distal to the injury.
   a. straight position
   b. elevated position
   c. lowered position
   d. position of comfort for the patient

74. When splinting a long-bone fracture, the key objective is to carefully splint the extremity:
   a. within 30 minutes of the time of the injury.
   b. within 15 minutes of the time of the injury.
   c. to minimize the opportunity for the patient to self-splint.
   d. without allowing the bone to protrude through the skin.

75. You have just finished applying a sling and swathe on a teenager who flipped over the handlebars of his bike and appears to have dislocated or fractured his right shoulder. The goal in splinting this type of injury is to:
   a. immobilize the elbow and wrist joint.
   b. eliminate the patient's pain completely.
   c. immobilize the shoulder and elbow joint.
   d. return the shoulder to a position of function.

76. The ongoing assessment of an extremity that was splinted because of a possible fracture includes:
   a. reassessing vital signs every 5 minutes.
   b. applying ice to reduce the pain and swelling.
   c. noting and managing any diminishment in distal pulses, motor function, and sensation.
   d. reassessing the blood pressure every 15 minutes.

77. An elderly patient who uses a walker fell in her apartment and now has pain in her thigh and is unable to get up. Your partner is holding stabilization on her femur, which appears deformed and swollen. Before applying a traction splint, you:
   a. assess proximal pulse, motor function, and sensation.
   b. assess distal pulse, motor function, and sensation.
   c. move the patient onto a long backboard.
   d. determine if the injury is a sprain or strain rather than a fracture.

78. You are en route to the hospital with a patient who has a painful, swollen deformity of the wrist that you splinted on the scene. You reassess and discover that the patient's fingers are tingling and becoming numb. The cause of this complication is most likely:
   a. that the splint has been applied too loosely.
   b. that the splint has been applied too tightly.
   c. an early sign of permanent nerve damage.
   d. an early indicator of permanent motor function injury.

79. When a splint is incorrectly applied, which of the following conditions is most likely to occur?
    a. increased bleeding
    b. increased swelling and pain
    c. increased circulation distal to the injury
    d. increased circulation proximal to the injury

80. The EMT is trained to fully immobilize a patient with a serious MOI who complains of neck or back pain to a long backboard. Upon arrival at the ED and after examination by the physician, the most common complication associated with this type of splinting is:
    a. that the chest straps were too loose.
    b. that the cervical collar was incorrectly applied.
    c. a decrease in motor function of the lower extremities.
    d. increased back pain due to lying on a long backboard for a long time.

81. After a prolonged extrication, a driver who was trapped in his vehicle is freed. He is alert and his vital signs are good; his only injury is to the left upper arm, which is painfully swollen and deformed. The distal pulse is absent and his fingers feel numb. The transport to the hospital will take 40 minutes. What steps do you take next?
    a. Splint the injury on the scene.
    b. Splint the injury during the transport.
    c. Apply an ice pack and do not splint.
    d. Let the patient put the arm in a position of comfort.

82. Friends have asked you out for a day hike. Shortly after you begin the hike, one of them severely twists an ankle. You begin to look for something to make a splint, but the injured friend insists on walking out, so you explain that the longer you wait to splint the injury, the more likely it is that she will suffer a/an:
    a. decreased blood loss.
    b. increased swelling and pain.
    c. lower risk of loss of function.
    d. less stiffness and more flexibility.

83. You have responded to a call for a traumatic injury. When you arrive, a man waves you in and tells you that his neighbor injured her hand while cleaning the lawn mower. The patient is holding a cloth around her hand, which is deformed and bleeding, as she runs toward the ambulance. She is pleading for you to quickly take her to the hospital, which is only 5 minutes away. You explain to the patient that you need to assess and manage the injury before transporting because:
    a. you can stop the bleeding.
    b. she will bleed to death if you don't.
    c. this will prevent the patient from going into shock.
    d. doing so will minimize the opportunity for further injury.

84. Which of the following types of splint is commonly used for musculoskeletal injuries involving the shoulder, humerus, elbow, and forearm?
    a. air splint
    b. rigid splint
    c. traction splint
    d. sling and swathe

85. After falling on an outstretched hand, a 14-year-old male appears to have a dislocation of the right elbow. This type of injury is serious and requires cautious management during immobilization due to the:
    a. age of the patient.
    b. potential for excessive blood loss.
    c. proximity of the radial artery to the injury site.
    d. proximity of the brachial artery to the injury site.

86. Each of the following is an advantage of splinting a painful, swollen, or deformed extremity, except:
    a. splints help to reduce muscle damage.
    b. splints can easily be made from many different materials.
    c. splinting helps to prevent excessive bleeding at the injury site.
    d. splinting can keep a closed fracture from becoming an open fracture.

87. A skier has fallen and has an open fracture of the lower leg. There is bleeding and a bone end is visible. After assessing distal pulse, motor function, and sensation, the next steps in the management of this injury are to:
    a. splint the leg and then control the bleeding.
    b. control bleeding with a compression bandage, then splint.
    c. rinse off the bone end, splint the leg, and then apply a pressure bandage.
    d. place a temporary tourniquet on the upper leg, then splint and release the tourniquet.

88. In the management of a painful, swollen, and deformed extremity, the EMT can minimize swelling of the injury site by:
    a. applying an ice pack.
    b. applying a heat pack.
    c. elevating the patient's head when the patient is lying on the stretcher.
    d. frequently raising and lowering the extremity to promote improved circulation.

89. After tripping and falling, an elderly patient tells you that her chest hurts in the area under her left arm. She is sitting still and leaning toward the left side. She has pain with each respiration and is taking shallow breaths. You suspect:

a. a pneumothorax and call for ALS.

b. rib fractures and splint her with a sling and swathe.

c. rib fractures and immobilize her to a long backboard.

d. cardiac chest pain and respiratory distress and assist her with nitroglycerin.

90. While cleaning a handgun, the owner accidentally discharged the weapon, causing the bullet to go through his right palm. Which bones do you suspect are involved?

a. carpals and tarsals

b. tarsals and metatarsals

c. carpals and metacarpals

d. metacarpals and metatarsals

Chapter 25 Answer Form

	A	B	C	D		A	B	C	D
1.	❏	❏	❏	❏	33.	❏	❏	❏	❏
2.	❏	❏	❏	❏	34.	❏	❏	❏	❏
3.	❏	❏	❏	❏	35.	❏	❏	❏	❏
4.	❏	❏	❏	❏	36.	❏	❏	❏	❏
5.	❏	❏	❏	❏	37.	❏	❏	❏	❏
6.	❏	❏	❏	❏	38.	❏	❏	❏	❏
7.	❏	❏	❏	❏	39.	❏	❏	❏	❏
8.	❏	❏	❏	❏	40.	❏	❏	❏	❏
9.	❏	❏	❏	❏	41.	❏	❏	❏	❏
10.	❏	❏	❏	❏	42.	❏	❏	❏	❏
11.	❏	❏	❏	❏	43.	❏	❏	❏	❏
12.	❏	❏	❏	❏	44.	❏	❏	❏	❏
13.	❏	❏	❏	❏	45.	❏	❏	❏	❏
14.	❏	❏	❏	❏	46.	❏	❏	❏	❏
15.	❏	❏	❏	❏	47.	❏	❏	❏	❏
16.	❏	❏	❏	❏	48.	❏	❏	❏	❏
17.	❏	❏	❏	❏	49.	❏	❏	❏	❏
18.	❏	❏	❏	❏	50.	❏	❏	❏	❏
19.	❏	❏	❏	❏	51.	❏	❏	❏	❏
20.	❏	❏	❏	❏	52.	❏	❏	❏	❏
21.	❏	❏	❏	❏	53.	❏	❏	❏	❏
22.	❏	❏	❏	❏	54.	❏	❏	❏	❏
23.	❏	❏	❏	❏	55.	❏	❏	❏	❏
24.	❏	❏	❏	❏	56.	❏	❏	❏	❏
25.	❏	❏	❏	❏	57.	❏	❏	❏	❏
26.	❏	❏	❏	❏	58.	❏	❏	❏	❏
27.	❏	❏	❏	❏	59.	❏	❏	❏	❏
28.	❏	❏	❏	❏	60.	❏	❏	❏	❏
29.	❏	❏	❏	❏	61.	❏	❏	❏	❏
30.	❏	❏	❏	❏	62.	❏	❏	❏	❏
31.	❏	❏	❏	❏	63.	❏	❏	❏	❏
32.	❏	❏	❏	❏	64.	❏	❏	❏	❏

	A	B	C	D			A	B	C	D
65.	❏	❏	❏	❏		78.	❏	❏	❏	❏
66.	❏	❏	❏	❏		79.	❏	❏	❏	❏
67.	❏	❏	❏	❏		80.	❏	❏	❏	❏
68.	❏	❏	❏	❏		81.	❏	❏	❏	❏
69.	❏	❏	❏	❏		82.	❏	❏	❏	❏
70.	❏	❏	❏	❏		83.	❏	❏	❏	❏
71.	❏	❏	❏	❏		84.	❏	❏	❏	❏
72.	❏	❏	❏	❏		85.	❏	❏	❏	❏
73.	❏	❏	❏	❏		86.	❏	❏	❏	❏
74.	❏	❏	❏	❏		87.	❏	❏	❏	❏
75.	❏	❏	❏	❏		88.	❏	❏	❏	❏
76.	❏	❏	❏	❏		89.	❏	❏	❏	❏
77.	❏	❏	❏	❏		90.	❏	❏	❏	❏

CHAPTER
26

Chest and Abdominal Trauma

1. A 24-year-old male working in a warehouse was crushed between a corner of the building and a load from a forklift. The injury is on the lower-left side of the chest. There is bruising and the patient is having difficulty breathing. Which underlying organ is most likely affected?

   a. liver
   b. spleen
   c. gallbladder
   d. diaphragm

2. (Continuing with the previous question) When you palpate the injured area, you feel and hear a crackling. This is referred to as:

   a. crepitus
   b. flail segment
   c. tamponade
   d. pneumothorax

3. An unrestrained driver of an older motor vehicle hit and bent the steering wheel when he crashed into a power pole at high speed. His chest appears bruised and deformed on the left side. Upon closer exam, there appears to be a free-floating segment of the chest wall with no external bleeding at the site. This injury should be managed by:

   a. applying an occlusive dressing.
   b. encircling the chest wall using wide tape.
   c. splinting the upper-left arm to the chest wall.
   d. taping a large dressing over the free-floating segment.

4. When managing a penetrating injury to the chest, the EMT will use an occlusive dressing, which:

   a. provides an airtight seal.
   b. decreases cardiac preload.
   c. controls severe hemorrhage.
   d. prevents subcutaneous emphysema.

5. On a transport to the emergency department, you learn that a patient you treated last week for a gun shot wound (GSW) to the chest died from a pericardial tamponade. You recall that this injury can quickly result in death because:

   a. of the loss of pulse pressure.
   b. it impairs the filling of the heart.
   c. it causes the vena cava to kink.
   d. of the increase in tracheal deviation.

6. The victim of a stabbing has a wound to the chest and is having difficulty breathing. While you remove his shirt, you hear a sucking sound each time he:

   a. inhales.
   b. coughs.
   c. exhales.
   d. tries to speak.

7. While at a construction site, a worker dropped his nail gun, which accidentally discharged. A coworker was struck with a nail that entered his chest near the right border of the sternum. There is no exit wound, and the patient is complaining of difficulty breathing. The first treatment step for this patient is to:

   a. apply an occlusive dressing.
   b. assist ventilations with a bag mask device.
   c. determine if the nail was galvanized.
   d. apply a bulky bandage and direct pressure.

8. The victim of an assault is a 20-year-old female who was stabbed with a 12-inch knitting needle. The penetration is 4 inches into the upper-left quadrant of her abdomen. Care for this wound includes:

   a. stabilizing the object in place with bulky dressings.
   b. applying an occlusive dressing and direct pressure.
   c. immobilizing the object, but allowing the wound to drain.
   d. removing the object in the opposite direction of entry and applying direct pressure.

9. The police secured the scene at a residence where there was a domestic violence incident. The patient is a 30-year-old male who was reported as being stabbed in the upper back, over the scapula, with a fork. The bleeding is minor, but it continues to trickle. The patient denies difficulty breathing or any other injuries. Care for this wound includes:

   a. occlusive dressing.
   b. direct pressure and bandage.
   c. direct pressure and sitting the patient upright.
   d. pressure bandage with patient lying on his back.

10. A motorcycle rider lost control of his bike on a curve, hit a guardrail, and tore open his lower abdomen. The lower-right quadrant has an evisceration with a portion of the small bowel exposed. This wound should be managed by:

    a. applying a pressure dressing.
    b. covering with a dry dressing and applying direct pressure.
    c. covering the bowel with a moist sterile dressing and keeping the area warm.
    d. rinsing the bowel, then scooping it back into the abdomen and covering it with a bulky dressing.

11. The police have called EMS for a gun shot wound (GSW) from a drive-by shooting. The patient is a 25-year-old woman who was shot in the stomach. There is an entrance wound in the upper-left quadrant, but no exit wound. In addition to wounds involving abdominal organs, what is another primary associated injury that must be considered immediately?

    a. hypothermia
    b. spinal cord injury
    c. open head injury
    d. closed head injury

12. Police called EMS for the victim of a stabbing. When you arrive, the police officers take you to a young woman who is unresponsive with labored breathing. She is lying on a couch with a 6-inch knife protruding from her abdomen. The knife appears to be pointed up toward the chest and you suspect serious internal injuries. Which of the following is a potential injury associated with this type of MOI?

    a. cervical injury
    b. perforated rectum
    c. perforated heart
    d. lacerated trachea

13. You are called to a local baseball field for a traumatic injury with difficulty breathing. A player was struck in the chest by a full swing of a bat. He is alert, anxious, spitting up blood, and working to breathe. Lung sounds are present in the apices, but decreased in both bases. He has an unstable rib segment and you suspect a hemothorax. Emergency care for this injury begins with:

    a. calling ALS for help with chest decompression.
    b. immobilizing the C-spine and beginning rapid transport.
    c. splinting the ribs, assisting ventilations, and watching for vomiting.
    d. stabilizing the flail section, administering high-flow oxygen, and assisting ventilations if necessary.

14. Teenagers at a backyard pool party were playing with a Frisbee when an 18-year-old girl slipped and fell backward into a glass door. She did not lose consciousness, but she has multiple lacerations on her back, arms, and legs. Upon closer examination, you find a large piece of glass remaining in a wound in her right flank area. Management of her wounds includes:

    a. controlling bleeding, bandaging, and stabilizing the glass in place.
    b. removing all the glass, controlling the bleeding, and immobilizing her on a long backboard.
    c. removing only the largest pieces of glass and immobilizing her on a long backboard.
    d. administering high-flow oxygen and keeping the patient still until advanced life support arrives.

15. A motorcyclist struck and crashed into the guardrail on a curved exit ramp of a highway. He is wearing leather gear that was slashed open in the torso. When you open the jacket, there is bleeding coming from an opening in his abdomen. When you open his clothing to examine the injury, you see a section of his large intestine bulging out of the opening. How should this injury be managed?

    a. Cover the opening with an occlusive dressing.
    b. Cover with a dry dressing and apply direct pressure.
    c. Cover with a moist sterile dressing and keep the area warm.
    d. Rinse the intestine with saline and irrigate frequently during transport.

16. An unresponsive passenger was extricated from a vehicle with significant damage as a result of a crash. In your primary assessment, you determine that she is apneic, pulseless, and has part of an umbrella handle impaled in her chest on the right side of her sternum. What action should be taken next?
    a. Stabilize the impaled object.
    b. Remove the impaled object and begin CPR.
    c. Attach AED electrodes and analyze the patient's heart rhythm.
    d. Begin ventilations while your partner stabilizes the impaled object.

17. An elderly male fell out of bed the day before and did not tell his family right away. Today the family called 9-1-1 because the patient has blood in his urine and his doctor wants him transported to the emergency department for evaluation. His vital signs are respiratory rate 20 and regular; pulse rate 124 and regular; BP 106/78; and skin is pale, warm, and dry. What type of injury might cause this patient's hematuria?
    a. ruptured spleen
    b. injured kidney
    c. lacerated liver
    d. ruptured abdominal aorta

18. Non-penetrating abdominal trauma often goes unrecognized because:
    a. the mechanism of injury is not fully appreciated.
    b. signs and symptoms of shock will not appear right away.
    c. non-penetrating trauma is not as painful as penetrating trauma.
    d. non-penetrating trauma produces different signs and symptoms.

19. A 16-year-old female was assaulted during a domestic dispute and is complaining of abdominal pain after being punched. When you exam her abdomen, there is some discoloration around the umbilicus, there is no distension, but the muscles are rigid and when you palpate and release she cries out in pain. This response to your exam:
    a. is called rebound tenderness.
    b. indicates the patient is pregnant.
    c. is going to need emergency surgery.
    d. is an overreaction associated with assaults from domestic violence.

20. (Continuing with the previous question) The patient's vital signs are respiratory rate 22 and shallow, pulse rate 110 and regular, and BP 108/64. You administer high-flow oxygen and place her _____ for transport.
    a. sitting with legs flexed
    b. head down and legs elevated
    c. in any position she is comfortable
    d. on her left side with legs flexed

21. Which of the following is most accurate about listening to bowel sounds?
    a. To listen accurately takes at least 1 minute.
    b. The absence of bowel sounds is normal in elderly patients.
    c. The presence of bowel sounds may indicate an obstruction.
    d. Listening to bowel sounds in the prehospital setting is typically not helpful.

22. An 18-year-old male sustained blunt trauma to the testicles as a result of a fall. The injury is closed and the patient wants to be transported by ambulance. Care for this type of injury includes:
    a. transport only.
    b. applying a heat pack.
    c. applying a padded ice pack.
    d. padding with trauma dressing.

23. When internal organs are damaged due to trauma, the contents will spill and come into contact with the _____ and produce a reaction of severe pain.
    a. periosteum
    b. peritoneum
    c. adrenal glands
    d. oblique muscle

24. An adult male who received blunt trauma to his abdomen when he lost control of his bike is lying on his back. He is very still while holding his legs drawn up. He is complaining of severe pain and will not allow you to move his legs. What is this patient doing?
    a. guarding
    b. refusing treatment
    c. bleeding to death
    d. compressing his intestines

25. When caring for a patient with abdominal trauma, the EMT must be alert for airway compromise that can be caused by:
    a. shock.
    b. vomiting.
    c. distension.
    d. herniation.

Chapter 26 Answer Form

	A	B	C	D			A	B	C	D
1.	❏	❏	❏	❏		14.	❏	❏	❏	❏
2.	❏	❏	❏	❏		15.	❏	❏	❏	❏
3.	❏	❏	❏	❏		16.	❏	❏	❏	❏
4.	❏	❏	❏	❏		17.	❏	❏	❏	❏
5.	❏	❏	❏	❏		18.	❏	❏	❏	❏
6.	❏	❏	❏	❏		19.	❏	❏	❏	❏
7.	❏	❏	❏	❏		20.	❏	❏	❏	❏
8.	❏	❏	❏	❏		21.	❏	❏	❏	❏
9.	❏	❏	❏	❏		22.	❏	❏	❏	❏
10.	❏	❏	❏	❏		23.	❏	❏	❏	❏
11.	❏	❏	❏	❏		24.	❏	❏	❏	❏
12.	❏	❏	❏	❏		25.	❏	❏	❏	❏
13.	❏	❏	❏	❏						

27

Trauma to the Head, Neck, and Spine

1. The peripheral nervous system includes which of the following structures?
   a. brain stem
   b. cerebrospinal fluid
   c. brain and spinal cord
   d. 31 pairs of spinal nerves

2. The division of the nervous system that is composed of the brain and spinal cord is the _____ nervous system.
   a. central
   b. peripheral
   c. automatic
   d. autonomic

3. The regulation of activities such as maintaining heart rate and blood pressure is under the control of the _____ nervous system.
   a. central
   b. peripheral
   c. automatic
   d. autonomic

4. _____ cushion(s) and protect(s) the brain and spinal cord from outside impact.
   a. Receptors
   b. Motor nerves
   c. Sensory nerves
   d. Cerebrospinal fluid

5. While playing softball, an outfielder was struck in the head with a ball. In addition to complaining of a headache, the player is having vision disturbances. Which part of the brain has been affected?
   a. frontal
   b. parietal
   c. occipital
   d. temporal

6. The brain is connected to the spinal cord by which of the following structures?
   a. meninges
   b. brain stem
   c. cerebellum
   d. hypothalamus

7. The _____ originate(s) in the spinal cord and lead(s) to the arms, legs, and the trunk of the body.
   a. dura mater
   b. spinal nerves
   c. cranial nerves
   d. accessory nerves

8. The spinal canal is located in an opening in the:
   a. vertebrae.
   b. fontanelle.
   c. mastoid process.
   d. foramen magnum.

9. The main nerve trunk connecting the body to the brain is the:
   a. meninges.
   b. spinal cord.
   c. spinal nerves.
   d. cranial nerves.

10. Traumatic injury to the head can cause bleeding in the brain, which raises the intracranial pressure and:
    a. causes spinal shock.
    b. causes infection.
    c. cuts off the spinal cord.
    d. shifts the brain within the skull.

11. The MOI is one of the most important factors in the assessment and treatment of an injured patient, because:
    a. even patients who have experienced minor MOIs will develop deficits later.
    b. a significant MOI will always cause some form of neurological problem for the patient.
    c. the potential for significant injury is recognized from the MOI, rather than the presence or absence of symptoms.
    d. the MOI is the absolute deciding factor in determining the need for spinal immobilization.

12. Filling the voids when splinting the spine will:
    a. minimize the pain from any new injury.
    b. prevent increased pain from preexisting back injuries.
    c. make the patient more comfortable on a long backboard.
    d. prevent the development of pain associated with lying on a backboard for a long time.

13. The patient with a suspected spinal injury is immobilized in a neutral position because:
    a. this position reduces stability.
    b. it is the most perpetual position for the spinal column.
    c. this position allows maximum comfort for the patient.
    d. this position allows the most space for the spinal cord within the spinal canal.

14. The primary goal in caring for a potential spinal injury is to:
    a. apply a rigid collar.
    b. prevent further injury.
    c. increase lung expansion.
    d. maintain a neutral position.

15. Which of the following signs or symptoms is an indication of a potential spinal injury?
    a. poorly localized cervical pain
    b. stable cervical spinous processes
    c. no deficit or loss of distal pulse, motor function, and/or sensation in one or more extremities
    d. lateral neck and shoulder pain with active movement

16. At the scene of a motor vehicle collision, you are assessing a backseat passenger with a complaint of low back pain. She is 80 years old, has a history of hypertension, and has arthritis for which she takes medications. When you assess distal pulses, motor function, and sensation in her upper extremities, she has a very weak grip, especially with the right hand. You suspect that this:
    a. is a symptom of stroke and now you will up-triage her.
    b. may be due to the arthritis and ask her if this is normal for her.
    c. weakness is a result of spinal injury, so you immobilize her to a long backboard.
    d. requires splinting the right extremity, as it may be a possible fracture or dislocation.

17. The patient you are assessing has a questionable MOI and denies neck or back pain. Before making a decision about immobilization, you:
    a. call medical control for direction.
    b. ask her if she has ever been immobilized in the past.
    c. assess for spinal tenderness by palpating each spinous process.
    d. ask her if she has a fear of being restricted with limited movement.

18. The husband of a 38-year-old woman called EMS because his wife slipped going downstairs in their home. She is alert, lying at the bottom of the stairs, and tells you that she slipped near the top and slid down on her back. She has pain in her tailbone, and when you palpate her back, there is tenderness next to but not on the lumbar spine. Treatment considerations for this patient are:
    a. to not immobilize if no deficits are noted in the distal pulses, motor function, and sensation.
    b. to immobilize her to a long backboard for a potential spinal injury.
    c. to not immobilize, because there is only tenderness and no local pain.
    d. to not immobilize, because the spinal cord does not reach as far as the tailbone.

19. Neighbors of an elderly man called EMS because they saw him fall approximately 5 feet off a ladder in his yard. They tell you that he did not lose consciousness and that they kept him lying down while waiting for you to arrive. The patient appears confused, but denies any injuries or pain in the neck, back, or extremities. When you decide that immobilization is appropriate, which of the following factors is not an indication of a spinal injury?
    a. pain with movement of the back
    b. tenderness when the spine is palpated
    c. the MOI, age of the patient, and confused mental status
    d. denial of any injuries or pain in the neck, back, or extremities

20. The victim of an assault was beaten with a bat on the head, face, and back. She is alert and has bleeding from the nose and facial injuries. As you begin to immobilize her, you consider how to keep her airway clear from all the blood that is draining from her injuries. You will manage her airway by:
    a. holding a jaw-thrust maneuver and suctioning continuously.
    b. holding a jaw-thrust maneuver and suctioning her as needed.
    c. tilting the backboard to assist with drainage and suctioning frequently.
    d. having the patient hold the suction catheter and instructing her to use it as needed.

21. Dispatch has sent you to a local department store for a fall. When you arrive, you find a crowd at the bottom of an escalator and an elderly woman lying on the ground. She has multiple skin tears and is complaining of neck and back pain. When you attempt to move her head into a neutral position, she cries out in pain. In the next attempt to stabilize her, you:
    a. do nothing and call for ALS to assist.
    b. splint her neck in the position it was found.
    c. ask her to relax and attempt a neutral position again.
    d. ask a couple of bystanders to help you move her into a neutral position using traction.

22. You are helping to teach a new EMT course, and the skill you are teaching is C-spine stabilization. You demonstrate to the students how to place the head in a neutral position and maintain stabilization until:

a. the cervical collar is securely fastened.

b. the MOI is determined to be insignificant.

c. the patient is properly secured to an immobilization device.

d. distal pulses, motor function, and sensation are assessed after immobilization.

23. A motorcyclist with a passenger had a crash. The passenger is sitting on the ground leaning against a tree, holding her helmet in her lap as you approach her. She is crying and says that she cannot feel her legs. The next step you take is to:

a. give her a hug.

b. ask the patient to lie down.

c. place a cervical collar on her neck.

d. ask the patient not to move her head.

24. Which of the following is not an indication for the use of a cervical spine immobilization device?

a. patient who is unconscious for no apparent reason

b. normal vital signs with an isolated extremity injury

c. patient appears intoxicated and the MOI is questionable

d. underage patient with a questionable MOI, who will not fit securely on a long backboard

25. A 17-year-old female was a driver in the second car of a five-car chain collision. When you arrive, she is standing next to her vehicle talking on her cell phone and crying to someone that her neck hurts. She sits in her vehicle as you approach and perform a primary assessment. You find that she is stable, but needs transport for evaluation of a potential spinal injury. You decide to:

a. apply a short-board device.

b. perform a rapid extrication onto a long backboard.

c. wait for her mother to arrive because she is 17 years old.

d. have the patient stand and perform a standing takedown immobilization.

26. The decision to apply a cervical collar is based on the:

a. MOI only.

b. chief complaint.

c. signs and symptoms.

d. MOI, signs, and symptoms.

27. A victim of an assault was strangled, and has finger and thumb impression marks on his neck. He is alert and complaining of neck pain in a strained voice. His lung sounds are clear and his vital signs are stable. As you begin to immobilize him, he tells you that he is having difficulty breathing. You suspect:

a. injury to C-4 and C-5.

b. swelling of his tongue.

c. swelling of his airway tissues.

d. bleeding of his airway tissues.

28. A child was knocked unconscious at a Little League game by a ball that struck him in the temporal skull area. When you first arrived, he was awake, but now he is becoming unconscious again. The patient is at risk for:

a. dental trauma.

b. vision disturbances.

c. vomiting and aspiration.

d. hemorrhage from an avulsion.

29. After securing an unconscious patient with a head injury to a spinal immobilization device, primary management for the patient includes ensuring:

a. that hypoxia is prevented.

b. that the patient is hyperventilated.

c. adequate distal motor function.

d. that the blood pressure stays over 110 systolic.

30. The crew chief has asked you to immobilize a stable infant who is still in her car seat. The collision was a significant MOI. The child begins to cry when your partner manually stabilizes her head. You now begin to immobilize her by:

a. fitting a pillow around her head and taping it down.

b. using a rolled towel and securing it around her neck.

c. taping the head in place with nothing around the neck.

d. doing nothing until the child stops crying, to prevent further agitation.

31. The driver of a vehicle that was involved in a low-speed collision is complaining of neck and low-backpain. After your primary assessment, you find him stable and call for help to immobilize him, because he weighs more than 400 pounds. You check to see if he will fit into your short spinal immobilization device by:

a. asking him his height.

b. sizing the device to the patient.

c. wrapping a 9-foot strap around him to see if it will close.

d. asking him to take a deep breath and hold it while you measure his waist.

32. As the second ambulance to arrive at the scene of a motor vehicle collision, you are directed to immobilize a 6-year-old child with a complaint of neck pain. A first responder is holding spinal stabilization on the patient in the second-row seat of a minivan. You size up a cervical spine immobilization device for the child patient by:
    a. considering the patient's age.
    b. considering the patient's level of distress.
    c. considering the patient's weight and height.
    d. making the adult-size device fit by securing it tighter.

33. You are working with an ALS crew to immobilize a patient who was injured in an industrial accident. The patient is unstable with a head injury, and the crew is ready to roll the patient onto the long backboard. Which responder makes the count to begin the roll?
    a. the most senior responder
    b. the responder stabilizing the head
    c. the responder with the highest level of training
    d. the responder who has established a rapport with the patient

34. The rider of an all-terrain vehicle is lying on the ground with his helmet on; he fell off the vehicle while traveling up a hill. His chief complaint is neck pain and his vital signs are stable. You have decided to leave the helmet in place and are ready to roll him onto a long backboard. The proper sequence of steps to take next is:
    a. roll on the count of three; secure to the long backboard; and assess distal pulses, motor function, and sensation.
    b. roll on the count of three; assess distal pulses, motor function, and sensation; and secure to the long backboard.
    c. assess distal pulses, motor function, and sensation; roll on the count of three; and secure to the long backboard.
    d. assess distal pulses, motor function, and sensation; roll on the count of three; secure to the long backboard; and reassess pulses, motor function, and sensation.

35. A crew of three is going to logroll a patient onto a long backboard because of a suspected spine injury. One member stabilizes the head and the other two members take a position on the patient's side and prepare to roll by taking hold of the patient's:
    a. hip and legs.
    b. shoulder and hip.
    c. stomach and legs.
    d. shoulder and legs.

36. "Bone to board" is a phrase used to describe:
    a. the proper method of securing a patient to a long backboard.
    b. the extrication of a vehicle occupant onto a short-board device.
    c. immobilizing a nontraumatic back pain patient with no cervical tenderness.
    d. those areas of the body that become tender after lying on a long backboard.

37. Your crew is immobilizing an adult patient to a long backboard because of a possible cervical injury following a fall. Now you need to strap him in tightly because you are going to carry him downstairs. The body part(s) you secure last is(are) the:
    a. hips.
    b. head.
    c. chest.
    d. lower legs.

38. The proper method of securing a patient to a long backboard is to strap the patient firmly to the board with the straps over the:
    a. upper chest, hips, and legs.
    b. head, abdomen, and ankles.
    c. lower chest, hips, and ankles.
    d. shoulders, abdomen, and thighs.

39. Which of the following hazards would preclude the EMT from using a short spine board on a stable patient with a potential spine injury?
    a. broken glass from the driver's door
    b. powder residue from a deployed airbag
    c. the use of power tools to extricate the patient
    d. smoke coming from the engine compartment

40. Dispatch has sent you to a motor vehicle collision for one patient with back pain. When you arrive, you determine that there was no collision; however, the driver was taking his wife to the hospital for spasms in her back. He pulled over when she nearly passed out from severe pain. Now she is awake and cannot move. Which of the following immobilization devices or techniques is most appropriate for removing this patient from the vehicle?
    a. long backboard
    b. rapid extrication
    c. short spine board
    d. standing takedown

41. The front-seat passenger in a Jeep was injured when the vehicle was rear-ended. She has pain in the right shoulder that radiates into her neck. Both of her knees have abrasions. You complete a primary assessment, find her to be in stable condition, and place a cervical collar on her. Which of the following immobilization devices or techniques is appropriate for removing this patient from the vehicle?
    a. long backboard
    b. rapid extrication
    c. short spine board
    d. standing takedown

42. Which of the following statements is most accurate about the use of a short spine board to immobilize a patient with a potential spine injury?
    a. Only stable patients should be secured to a short spine board.
    b. The short spine board must be secured to a long backboard before the patient is transported.
    c. A properly secured short spine board is more painful for a patient than a long backboard.
    d. A patient who is secured properly to a short spine board need not be secured to a long backboard.

43. You are assisting your partner to immobilize a young adult to a short spine board within a motor vehicle. With a cervical collar in place, you keep the patient in a neutral position and prepare to move him forward. Next, your partner:
    a. assesses distal pulses, motor function, and sensation.
    b. secures the torso straps and then the head.
    c. secures the head and then the torso straps.
    d. places the short spine board between the patient and the seat.

44. When you are using a short spine board device to immobilize a patient who has a potential cervical injury, the patient's head is manually stabilized until the:
    a. torso straps are secure.
    b. patient's torso and head are secured to the device.
    c. short spine board is secured to the long backboard.
    d. short spine board is set in place between the patient and the seat.

45. A vehicle is off the road and appears to have rolled before coming to a stop. The driver is belted in but unconscious when you gain access to the vehicle. When you touch him, he responds by moaning. His breathing is shallow and his pulse is fast and weak. Which of the following immobilization devices or techniques will you use for this patient?
    a. rapid extrication
    b. short spine board
    c. standing takedown
    d. Kendrick Extrication Device (K.E.D.)

46. Which of the following is not an indication for the use of rapid extrication?
    a. hypotensive patient
    b. trauma arrest patient
    c. heavy rainstorm in the dark
    d. spilled gas under the car

47. Rapid extrication is a special rescue removal procedure used to promptly extricate a patient from a vehicle wreck. The first step is to manually stabilize the patient's head. The piece(s) of equipment needed is(are):
    a. straps.
    b. head blocks.
    c. a long backboard.
    d. a rigid cervical collar.

48. Once the rescuers are in place with the proper equipment, the rapid extrication technique is used to remove an unstable patient from the vehicle in a manner:
    a. that takes less than 30 seconds.
    b. with the least risk of cervical movement.
    c. with the least risk of injury for the rescuers.
    d. that does not make the patient uncomfortable.

49. Performing a rapid extrication with the least possible extension, flexion, or rotation of the patient's spinal column requires:
    a. a minimum of two rescuers.
    b. rescuers who have practiced the rapid extrication technique.
    c. the patient to be unconscious and in critical condition.
    d. a short-board device, straps, tape, and a long backboard.

50. Two skaters collided hard during a hockey game and one did not get up. The skater who is down is the goalie, and he is complaining of neck pain and a loss of sensation in his legs. When you and your partner attempt to place his head in a neutral position, prior to removing his helmet, he complains of increased pain. Which immobilization technique is appropriate for this patient?
    a. Immobilize him in the position found, with his helmet on.
    b. Immobilize him in the position found, with his helmet off.
    c. Make another attempt to bring his C-spine into a neutral position.
    d. Cut away his uniform and the straps prior to removing his helmet and placing a cervical collar.

51. A football player was knocked unconscious at a scrimmage. When you arrive at his side, he is awake and lying on the ground with a coach holding manual stabilization of his head. The patient is in uniform and still has his helmet on. He is confused, has an open airway, and has adequate breathing and pulse. Distal pulses, motor function, and sensation are good in all extremities. Which immobilization technique is appropriate for this patient?
    a. Immobilize him to a long backboard with his helmet on.
    b. Remove his helmet and immobilize him to a long backboard.
    c. Remove his helmet and shoulder pads before immobilizing him.
    d. Apply a collar with the helmet in place and immobilize him to a long backboard.

52. A football helmet that has a _____ can easily be removed to access the airway, without removing the helmet from the player.
    a. shield
    b. jaw pad
    c. chin strap
    d. face guard

53. Which of the following sports utilizes helmets that may have a feature called a jaw pad, which must be removed before the helmet is removed?
    a. bicycling
    b. football
    c. motorcycling
    d. auto racing

54. Many _____ helmets are described as full-faced because of the rigid portion of the helmet that extends fully around the chin.
    a. skiing
    b. football
    c. baseball
    d. lacrosse

55. When removing the helmet of a football player who is also wearing protective shoulder pads and needs to be immobilized to a long backboard, the EMT:
    a. will need the help of the football coach or trainer.
    b. is taking a great risk and may cause further damage.
    c. first applies a cervical collar before removing the helmet.
    d. will need to pad behind the head to avoid hyperextension of the neck.

56. Many types of sports helmets can be left on the patient even if the patient needs to be immobilized. The reason for this is:
    a. the type of material they are made of.
    b. the helmets fit snugly to the head, making it easy to immobilize.
    c. the helmet manufacturers recommend leaving the helmet in place.
    d. that many of these helmets have special attachment points for immobilization.

57. When removing a full-faced helmet from a supine patient who has a possible spinal injury, the EMT should:
    a. cut all the straps before removing the helmet.
    b. use the same method as with an open-faced helmet.
    c. insert one hand inside over the face to avoid mashing the nose.
    d. tilt the helmet slightly, without moving the neck, to avoid mashing the nose.

58. You are dispatched to a motorcycle collision. You arrive to find the rider, face down, off the side of the road in the grass. He is unconscious with shallow breathing, blood is draining from his mouth, and he has a weak distal pulse. Your partner holds C-spine stabilization as you remove the helmet and together you roll him on his back. The next appropriate step is to:
    a. suction the airway.
    b. place a cervical collar on the patient.
    c. secure the patient to a long backboard.
    d. obtain vital signs and complete a secondary assessment.

59. After removing a helmet from a patient who has a suspected spinal injury, the EMT should continue to maintain cervical stabilization by:
    a. padding beneath the patient's head and the surface he is lying on.
    b. performing a jaw-thrust maneuver and supporting the patient's mandible as needed.
    c. holding manual stabilization of the head until the patient is fully secured to a long backboard.
    d. placing one hand on each side of the patient's head until a cervical collar is applied to the patient.

60. When removing a helmet from an unconscious patient, the EMT stabilizing the head will place one hand on each side of the helmet and:
    a. instruct the patient to open her mouth.
    b. instruct the helper to apply the cervical collar.
    c. support the patient's mandible with the EMT's fingers.
    d. do nothing until the helper has applied the cervical collar.

61. When a person sustains a traumatic brain injury that produces a rise in intracranial pressure, the usual response is:
    a. paralysis below the waist.
    b. an elevated blood pressure.
    c. a significant drop in blood pressure.
    d. paralysis from the neck down to the feet.

62. One major difference between stabilizing a patient's head with and without a helmet is:
    a. hand placement.
    b. when to apply the cervical collar.
    c. when to assess and reassess distal pulses, motor function, and sensation.
    d. when to secure the head to the long backboard.

63. You are transporting a patient who is immobilized to a long backboard. She complains of nausea and suddenly vomits. Which straps do you unfasten so that you can roll the patient on her side, while still maintaining spinal immobilization?
    a. none of the straps should be unfastened
    b. the strap holding the cervical collar in place
    c. the stretcher straps holding the long backboard in place
    d. the straps securing the patient to the long backboard

64. When a trauma patient has a known or suspected cervical spine injury, the entire spine is immobilized using a long backboard because this:
    a. is the most comfortable position for the patient.
    b. is the safest way to transport a trauma patient.
    c. position helps to reduce excess pressure on the spinal cord.
    d. position will prevent any further injury to the patient.

65. The rationale for using a short spine immobilization device when moving a patient from the sitting to the supine position is to protect and immobilize the entire spine immediately and:
    a. to build trust and confidence with the patient.
    b. to keep the patient from talking on the cell phone.
    c. to prevent the patient from going into spinal shock.
    d. continuously until the patient is secured to the long backboard.

66. The short spine board device is used to immobilize and:
    a. secure the patient's entire body before the patient is moved.
    b. effectively prevent any further pain for the patient.
    c. extricate patients who are found seated in an automobile.
    d. rapidly correct any misalignment of the spine resulting from the collision.

67. In which of the following patients might the use of rapid extrication make the difference between life and death?
    a. decompensated shock
    b. impaled object in the eye
    c. penetrating injury to the arm
    d. open fracture of the lower leg

68. The use of the rapid extrication technique on a patient who is stable may:
    a. cause nausea for the patient.
    b. increase the risk of further spinal injury.
    c. cause increased pressure on the abdomen.
    d. allow the patient to better follow your instructions during the move.

69. On the site at a construction project, a worker was struck in the head by a falling object. The object struck his hard hat and left a dent. The patient is alert, ambulatory, and denies any injury, but when you palpate his cervical spine he has tenderness. You decide to immobilize and transport him for evaluation. What method do you use?
    a. Immobilize the patient with the hard hat on.
    b. Remove the hard hat and perform a standing takedown.
    c. Remove the hard hat and instruct the patient to sit down on the long backboard.
    d. Any of these above methods is appropriate.

70. Which of the following is an indication for leaving a helmet on a patient?
    a. Removal will not cause further injury.
    b. There is adequate head movement within the helmet.
    c. There is no face shield that flips up to allow access to the face.
    d. Proper immobilization can be accomplished with the helmet on.

Chapter 27 Answer Form

	A	B	C	D		A	B	C	D
1.	❑	❑	❑	❑	32.	❑	❑	❑	❑
2.	❑	❑	❑	❑	33.	❑	❑	❑	❑
3.	❑	❑	❑	❑	34.	❑	❑	❑	❑
4.	❑	❑	❑	❑	35.	❑	❑	❑	❑
5.	❑	❑	❑	❑	36.	❑	❑	❑	❑
6.	❑	❑	❑	❑	37.	❑	❑	❑	❑
7.	❑	❑	❑	❑	38.	❑	❑	❑	❑
8.	❑	❑	❑	❑	39.	❑	❑	❑	❑
9.	❑	❑	❑	❑	40.	❑	❑	❑	❑
10.	❑	❑	❑	❑	41.	❑	❑	❑	❑
11.	❑	❑	❑	❑	42.	❑	❑	❑	❑
12.	❑	❑	❑	❑	43.	❑	❑	❑	❑
13.	❑	❑	❑	❑	44.	❑	❑	❑	❑
14.	❑	❑	❑	❑	45.	❑	❑	❑	❑
15.	❑	❑	❑	❑	46.	❑	❑	❑	❑
16.	❑	❑	❑	❑	47.	❑	❑	❑	❑
17.	❑	❑	❑	❑	48.	❑	❑	❑	❑
18.	❑	❑	❑	❑	49.	❑	❑	❑	❑
19.	❑	❑	❑	❑	50.	❑	❑	❑	❑
20.	❑	❑	❑	❑	51.	❑	❑	❑	❑
21.	❑	❑	❑	❑	52.	❑	❑	❑	❑
22.	❑	❑	❑	❑	53.	❑	❑	❑	❑
23.	❑	❑	❑	❑	54.	❑	❑	❑	❑
24.	❑	❑	❑	❑	55.	❑	❑	❑	❑
25.	❑	❑	❑	❑	56.	❑	❑	❑	❑
26.	❑	❑	❑	❑	57.	❑	❑	❑	❑
27.	❑	❑	❑	❑	58.	❑	❑	❑	❑
28.	❑	❑	❑	❑	59.	❑	❑	❑	❑
29.	❑	❑	❑	❑	60.	❑	❑	❑	❑
30.	❑	❑	❑	❑	61.	❑	❑	❑	❑
31.	❑	❑	❑	❑	62.	❑	❑	❑	❑

	A	B	C	D		A	B	C	D
63.	❑	❑	❑	❑	67.	❑	❑	❑	❑
64.	❑	❑	❑	❑	68.	❑	❑	❑	❑
65.	❑	❑	❑	❑	69.	❑	❑	❑	❑
66.	❑	❑	❑	❑	70.	❑	❑	❑	❑

CHAPTER

28

Multisystem Trauma

1. An unconscious male was removed from the driver's seat of a motor vehicle and placed on a long backboard by the fire department as your ambulance approached the scene of a high-speed collision. He is rapidly immobilized and placed in your ambulance. The patient remains unconscious, is breathing slow and shallow, and has no external bleeding, but his right ankle is deformed. His vital signs are respirations 12 and regular, pulse rate is 140 and regular, BP 90/50, and his skin is pale, dry, and cool. What type of injuries do you suspect at this point?

   a. head injury and ankle fracture
   b. chest and abdominal trauma
   c. head injury and internal bleeding
   d. spinal shock and chest trauma

2. (Continuing with the previous question) You insert an oral airway and administer high-flow oxygen; his lung sounds are clear. What action is appropriate at this point?

   a. Begin rapid transport to the nearest hospital.
   b. Begin routine transport to the nearest hospital.
   c. Begin rapid transport to the nearest trauma center.
   d. Do not transport, request air-medical transport, complete a secondary assessment, and assist ventilations.

3. A person who has sustained a significant electrical shock is typically immobilized by EMS personnel because of the potential for head injury caused by:

   a. the exit wound.
   b. trauma from falling.
   c. the entrance wound.
   d. loss of reflex control.

4. The victim of a gunshot wound was shot in the abdomen. He is alert, weak, and losing a lot of blood. When you roll him to inspect his back, you find an exit wound. You find no pain or deformity upon palpation of his neck and spine. You quickly place a trauma dressing on the exit wound and fully immobilize him to a long backboard because:

   a. he has the MOI for a spinal injury.
   b. this is the easiest way to move him.
   c. bleeding is best controlled when lying supine.
   d. he will be easy to restrain if he becomes agitated or combative

5. While returning from the hospital, you and your partner witness a serious motor vehicle collision at a busy intersection. The driver of one vehicle is slumped on the wheel so that the horn is continuously blowing. You park the ambulance as your partner notifies dispatch. The other two drivers are out of their vehicles and deny having any injuries, but as you approach the last driver it is quickly apparent that he is unconscious, and his breathing is inadequate with snoring respirations. The next step you take is to:

   a. begin a rapid extrication.
   b. suction his airway and apply a cervical collar.
   c. apply a cervical collar and begin ventilations with a bag mask device.
   d. lift his head into a neutral position and perform a jaw thrust.

6. Dispatch has sent you to the scene of a motor vehicle collision with a motorcycle. When you arrive, the first ambulance on scene directs you to go to a rider who is lying in the road with an EMT holding manual stabilization of his C-spine. The rider is conscious, alert, and appears to have an open fracture of the left femur. His airway is clear and he denies difficulty breathing or chest pain. After you complete a rapid trauma exam, you begin to apply a traction splint and then the patient loses consciousness. What steps do you take next?

   a. Remove his helmet and assess his airway and breathing.
   b. Assess his airway and breathing and then remove the helmet.
   c. Assess his ABCs and remove the helmet if you need to manage the airway.
   d. Remove his helmet, apply a cervical collar, and roll him onto a long backboard.

7. It is 03:30 when a call comes in for a motor vehicle collision with multiple patients. When you arrive, the fire department is on scene assessing three patients from a vehicle that struck a tree. One person is out of the vehicle and appears to have minor injuries. The driver is confused but denies injury, and the backseat passenger is in respiratory arrest. The tree on one side of the vehicle and the driver are blocking access to the backseat passenger. Rapid extrication is needed for:

   a. both patients still in the vehicle.
   b. just the backseat occupant.
   c. none of the occupants of this vehicle.
   d. just the driver, to gain access to the backseat occupant.

8. You and your partner are removing a helmet from a supine patient who has a possible head injury and difficulty breathing. While you stabilize the patient's head, using both hands, your partner should:

   a. secure a cervical collar on the patient.
   b. cut all the straps before removing the helmet.
   c. use two hands to stretch the sides of the helmet by pulling outward.
   d. place one hand under the neck and support the head in the occipital region.

9. Your ambulance has a special assignment to stand by at the Funny Car auto races that are in town for the night. While you are standing by, track officials wave you out to the driver of a vehicle that rolled on the track. He is still in the vehicle, which is upright, but he has been knocked out. Blood is dripping down his face, so you decide to remove his helmet to assess him. For this patient, it is appropriate to:

   a. not remove the helmet.
   b. remove the helmet with the patient in the vehicle.
   c. rapidly extricate him and then remove the helmet.
   d. wait until the patient is in the ambulance and then remove the helmet.

10. A 12-year-old male rode his bike through an intersection without stopping and struck a vehicle. His helmet came off when he hit the vehicle. He has been unconscious since the collision and when you do your primary assessment he begins to move. His jaw clenches, his arms and legs extend straight and stiffen, and his hands and feet flex. What is happening with this patient?

   a. He is seizing.
   b. His brain is herniating.
   c. He is going into cardiac arrest.
   d. He is becoming paralyzed.

11. (Continuing with the previous question) What is the priority in managing this patient?

   a. obtaining vital signs
   b. maintaining an airway
   c. administering high-flow oxygen
   d. completing a secondary assessment

12. A Pop Warner football player was knocked out during a tackle and upon wakening is complaining of cervical neck pain that radiates in the shoulder. The patient must be immobilized to a long backboard, but he has nausea and is at risk for vomiting. Ideally, the helmet and shoulder pads should be:

   a. removed by the coach or parent.
   b. removed by you and your partner.
   c. removed by the athletic trainer on scene.
   d. left in place until arriving at the hospital.

13. The two primary factors for the extent of traumatic injury a patient may be subjected to are anatomic structures that are involved and:

   a. the patient's age.
   b. the patient's past medical history.
   c. the time of day the injury occurred.
   d. amount of energy exchanged to the body.

14. Which of the following multisystem trauma patients should be transported to the nearest hospital, even if it is not a trauma center?

   a. traumatic cardiac arrest
   b. head injury and unstable pelvis
   c. critical burns on the face, head, arms, and legs
   d. pregnant patient involved in a high-speed crash

15. When a bullet is fired into the abdomen, the energy forces are transferred to the tissues, causing them to move apart. This is called:

   a. cavitation.
   b. barotraumas.
   c. the third collision.
   d. conservation of energy.

16. The patient you are assessing fell from a second-story window. Which of the following features of the mechanism of injury is most important?

   a. height of the fall
   b. the body's point of initial impact
   c. the combination of forces involved
   d. the type of surface the patient landed on

17. As a general rule, the exit hole from a gunshot wound is larger that the entrance because of:

   a. cavitation.
   b. dissection.
   c. the proximity of the shooter.
   d. the position of the patient when hit.

18. The EMT can make a significant impact on the life or death of a multisystem trauma patient by:

    a. minimizing scene time.
    b. taking the appropriate standard precautions.
    c. transporting the patient to the nearest hospital.
    d. stabilizing the patient on the scene prior to transport.

19. While on the scene where there is a traumatic injury, the most important information for the EMT to obtain is the:

    a. mechanism of injury.
    b. patient's organ donor status.
    c. patient's severity of pain.
    d. patient's past medical history.

20. Which of the following multiple trauma situations is an indication for the use of air-medical transport?

    a. extremely combative patient
    b. limited access to a remote area
    c. patient with injuries due to barotrauma
    d. weather too severe for ground transport

21. You are sizing up the scene of a motor vehicle collision of a multisystem trauma patient whose vehicle was first rear-ended, then struck another vehicle in the front. What type of force(s) has this patient experienced in her mechanism of injury?

    a. penetrating
    b. rapid acceleration
    c. rapid deceleration
    d. rapid acceleration and deceleration

22. The "golden hour" for the trauma victim begins:

    a. when the first EMT arrives at the scene.
    b. immediately after the injury is sustained.
    c. when the ambulance leaves the scene.
    d. immediately upon arriving at the emergency department.

23. An unrestrained driver involved in a crash in an intersection bent the steering wheel. He is conscious and is bleeding from the nose, has two missing front teeth, has a large bruise on his sternum and abdomen, open wound on both lower legs, and a deformed right ankle. Which of these injuries is most critical?

    a. chest
    b. abdomen
    c. the upper airway
    d. extremities

24. You have responded to a call for a fall. A 20-year-old female was thrown from a horse while riding inside a barn. She is having difficulty breathing, is bleeding from the right side of her chest, and has an open femur fracture with severe angulation. A witness reports there was no loss of consciousness. What assessment step should be performed first?

    a. listen to lung sounds
    b. obtain a blood pressure
    c. determine the amount of blood lost
    d. complete a secondary assessment

25. Trauma patients who have sustained pulmonary contusions will often have other severe chest and _____ injuries, so the EMT must assume that multiple associated injuries are present.

    a. head
    b. neck
    c. abdominal
    d. spinal cord

Chapter 28 Answer Form

	A	B	C	D		A	B	C	D
1.	❏	❏	❏	❏	14.	❏	❏	❏	❏
2.	❏	❏	❏	❏	15.	❏	❏	❏	❏
3.	❏	❏	❏	❏	16.	❏	❏	❏	❏
4.	❏	❏	❏	❏	17.	❏	❏	❏	❏
5.	❏	❏	❏	❏	18.	❏	❏	❏	❏
6.	❏	❏	❏	❏	19.	❏	❏	❏	❏
7.	❏	❏	❏	❏	20.	❏	❏	❏	❏
8.	❏	❏	❏	❏	21.	❏	❏	❏	❏
9.	❏	❏	❏	❏	22.	❏	❏	❏	❏
10.	❏	❏	❏	❏	23.	❏	❏	❏	❏
11.	❏	❏	❏	❏	24.	❏	❏	❏	❏
12.	❏	❏	❏	❏	25.	❏	❏	❏	❏
13.	❏	❏	❏	❏					

CHAPTER

29

Environmental Emergencies

1. It is a hot day and you see a sun worshipper tanning in the park. She is spraying a water mister to keep cool. What method of cooling is she enjoying?
   a. radiation
   b. convection
   c. conduction
   d. evaporation

2. You are trying to cool a patient who is suffering from heat exposure. By allowing a fan to blow over the patient, you are cooling him by which method?
   a. radiation
   b. convection
   c. conduction
   d. evaporation

3. You have been called to care for a person found lying outside in the snow. You find the patient, who is cold and shivering. This patient has lost a significant amount of body heat in a short time, primarily by means of:
   a. radiation.
   b. conduction.
   c. convection.
   d. evaporation.

4. You have just discovered a person who has been exposed to the cold for a prolonged period of time and has frostbite on multiple toes. Which signs and symptoms can you expect to find?
   a. The toes will appear white and feel numb.
   b. The toes will look shriveled, but have normal color.
   c. The toes will feel cold, look red, and the patient will have severe pain.
   d. The toes will appear black and blue and the patient will have severe pain.

5. For a victim of sudden exposure to extremely cold temperatures, such as falling through the ice into freezing water, decreased coordination and motor function are _____ findings.
   a. early
   b. very late
   c. unreliable
   d. nonassociated

6. For a victim of prolonged cold exposure, which of the following signs indicates that the condition is critical?
   a. frost nip
   b. urinary incontinence
   c. decreased mental status
   d. decreased fine motor function

7. A 60-year-old male went to get the newspaper and fell in his driveway between high snow banks. He lay there for nearly an hour before being discovered. He is alert, cold, wet, and appears to have a severely deformed open fracture of his ankle. Choose the management steps in the appropriate order.
   a. Move him out of the cold, splint the ankle, administer high-flow oxygen, and transport rapidly.
   b. Check ABCs, splint the ankle, move the patient into the ambulance, remove his wet clothing, and provide warmth.
   c. Check ABCs, remove the wet clothing, splint the ankle and control any bleeding, and move the patient out of the cold and provide warmth.
   d. Control any bleeding, splint the ankle and elevate the leg, administer high-flow oxygen, move the patient into the ambulance, and transport.

8. You are dispatched for an elderly patient who has fallen. Upon arrival, you find a conscious and confused woman who may have been on the floor for more than 18 hours. She is incontinent of urine and is complaining of being really cold. The first priority after managing the ABCs is to:
   a. stop ongoing heat loss.
   b. provide warm, humidified oxygen.
   c. cover the patient with a blanket and begin transport in a warm ambulance.
   d. call medical control for an order to assist with oral high-concentration glucose.

9. Two men who were out snowshoeing became lost for a few hours, then found their way out of the woods. EMS was called because one had developed frostbite on the toes of his left foot. Management of the extremity includes:

   a. beginning to warm the extremity while keeping it elevated.
   b. splinting the extremity and keeping it from further cold exposure.
   c. keeping the extremity from warming until the patient reaches the hospital.
   d. placing the foot in tepid water for 5 minutes, and then splinting the extremity.

10. The EM can best recognize dehydration associated with prolonged exposure to heat by the patient's:

   a. sweaty skin.
   b. inability to sweat.
   c. past medical history.
   d. signs and symptoms.

11. A healthy person with a mild to moderate heat exposure might be expected to have which of the following signs and symptoms?

   a. shock
   b. weak pulse
   c. altered mental status
   d. nausea and vomiting

12. Which of the following signs and symptoms of heat exposure are most severe?

   a. confusion or dizziness
   b. any compromise to the ABCs
   c. muscle twitching and sweating
   d. increased body temperature and intense thirst

13. You have been dispatched to a vehicle that is stopped in a parking lot, for a 2-year-old child who is having seizures. When you arrive, the parents tell you that the child's eyes rolled back into his head, he began to seize, and appeared to have stopped breathing. They also state that this has never happened before. The child appears to be sleeping and is slowly waking. He is bundled up in a snowsuit, which is appropriate for the weather. What are your next management steps?

   a. Remove some of the clothing, provide oxygen, and transport the child in his car seat.
   b. Let the mother hold the child with an oxygen mask on the child's face and transport them together.
   c. Pour cool water over the child's head, provide oxygen, and transport him immobilized on a short board.
   d. Let the mother hold the child outside of the vehicle in the cold to lower his temperature, and then transport the child on a stretcher.

14. Your crew is standing by at an outdoor soccer tournament on a very warm afternoon. The humidity is high and the players have been participating in multiple games. A player has collapsed, apparently from the heat. He is conscious but not alert. You begin to treat him by giving him high-flow oxygen by non-rebreather mask, and then:

   a. remove his clothing.
   b. blow a fan on him and mist him with water.
   c. put him into your air-conditioned ambulance as soon as possible.
   d. all of the above.

15. If rapid cooling is not begun for the victim of a severe heat disorder, _____ may result.

   a. hypertension
   b. hypoglycemia
   c. congestive heart failure
   d. permanent brain damage

16. A group of water skiers were on the lake practicing when one went down in the water. He was initially unconscious when pulled from the water and awoke in the boat as he was brought to the dock. When you arrive, he is awake but does not recall what happened. What should you do next?

   a. Consider that the patient may be hyperthermic.
   b. Attempt to obtain a SpO2 and blood glucose reading.
   c. Consider that the patient may have a heart condition.
   d. Take spinal precautions and prepare to fully immobilize the patient.

17. Two boaters were tossed into the water when their canoe overturned. Both had personal floatation devices on, but one could not swim, and it took them nearly 2 hours to get to shore. The nonswimmer was acting confused, so EMS was called. The patient appears cyanotic and is cold to the touch. Vital signs are: respiration 16, adequate; pulse 68, regular; BP 100/50. What do you suspect is the primary problem at this point?

   a. shock
   b. hypoxia
   c. hypothermia
   d. near-drowning

18. You are dispatched to the local marina for a sick person. Upon arrival, you find the patient complaining of motion sickness, headache, and aches in the neck and shoulders. She denies difficulty breathing or chest pain. The patient is a new employee of a dive shop and she did not dive today, but she did two dives yesterday. How should you manage this patient?

    a. Be prepared for this patient to go into respiratory arrest.
    b. Consider that this patient needs decompression therapy.
    c. She has no life-threatening injuries, so refer her to her own physician.
    d. Consider this to be a decompression emergency only if she dove below 33 feet.

19. Which of the following statements regarding near-drowning is most accurate?

    a. Kidney failure is common following a near-drowning episode.
    b. Aspiration of either salt water or fresh water results in hypoxia.
    c. The EMT must treat every victim of near-drowning for hypothermia.
    d. All victims of near-drowning should be placed in Trendelenburg position, to allow drainage of the lungs.

20. In the primary assessment of a victim of near-drowning, the patient may appear normal. In the reassessment, however, the EMT should expect signs and symptoms of problems related to:

    a. infection.
    b. breathing.
    c. decompression sickness.
    d. bleeding in the brain.

21. Which of the following factors is typically not associated with victims of near-drowning?

    a. alcohol
    b. frostbite
    c. spinal injury
    d. hypothermia

22. During a domestic dispute, one patient sustained human bites on the back and upper left arm. There are no other injuries and the patient denies any other symptoms. This patient should be transported for evaluation:

    a. only if she is over 60 years of age.
    b. only if she is less than 16 years of age.
    c. only if the biter has not been vaccinated for tetanus.
    d. if the bites have broken through the skin and are bleeding.

23. A victim of snakebite is alert and shows you two fang marks on his left calf. The bite occurred 20 minutes ago. He is not sure what type of snake it was, but remembers that it was brown. Emergency medical care for this type of injury includes supporting the ABCs and:

    a. elevating and icing the extremity.
    b. cleaning the wound using suction.
    c. applying a tourniquet above the injury site.
    d. splinting the extremity and keeping the patient still.

24. The patient you are assessing was bitten multiple times on the lower arms and hands in an attack by an unfamiliar dog. She complains of severe pain at the injury sites and is bleeding from the wounds. Emergency medical care for this patient begins with:

    a. pain management.
    b. wrapping and splinting the arms and hands.
    c. determining if the dog has a collar and tags.
    d. determining when the patient's last tetanus shot was.

25. You are assessing a 72-year-old male who is on the sidelines of a soccer field. He has been sitting in the sun for a couple of hours watching his grandson play in a soccer tournament. His clothing is wet with perspiration, he is pale, and his skin temperature feels normal. He is complaining of dizziness when he attempts to stand up. Which of the following conditions do you suspect he is experiencing?

    a. heat stroke
    b. heat cramps
    c. heat exhaustion
    d. exertional heat stress

26. The formation of nitrogen bubbles in the blood or tissues, associated with diving, is known as:

    a. the bends.
    b. nitrogen narcosis.
    c. hyperbaric sickness.
    d. recompression sickness.

27. People who _____ are at an increased risk of experiencing a heat exhaustion emergency when exposed to warm conditions for lengthy periods.

    a. work outside
    b. take diuretics
    c. exercise routinely
    d. drink alcohol excessively

28. _____ is the formation of ice crystals within the tissues as a result of prolonged exposure to cold temperatures.

    a. Frostnip
    b. Frostbite
    c. Air embolism
    d. Decompression illness

29. Which of the following conditions is not a predisposing factor for hypothermia?

a. child less than 1 year old
b. an elderly person who is living alone
c. a female in the third trimester of pregnancy
d. a person who is intoxicated with alcohol

30. For a victim of a sting from a marine life form, the general approach to emergency care includes:

a. transport for evaluation.
b. splinting and/or elevating the affected area.
c. assisting with an epinephrine auto-injector.
d. applying ice to reduce the pain and swelling.

31. EMS was called for a 12-year-old female who was having a seizure in the pool. Another child described the patient as having lost consciousness. A parent was nearby when the seizure began and quickly pulled the patient from the pool. Your general impression is that of a conscious patient with an open airway who is coughing. Underneath the blanket she is wrapped in, you can see that her skin is pink, warm, and still wet. She is alert to your voice and responds appropriately. Her lung sounds are clear. You administer oxygen and obtain vital signs. She has no history of seizures, takes no medicine, and has no allergies. What action is appropriate?

a. Suspect possible trauma and perform a secondary assessment.
b. Call medical control to consult about possible hypothermia.
c. Perform a secondary assessment due to possible hypothermia associated with submersion.
d. Finish obtaining vital signs and continue to observe the patient for a few more minutes before making a transportation decision.

32. (Continuing with the preceding question) There was no apparent traumatic MOI. After talking to the patient and the other child, you discover that the seizure activity began when they were swimming underwater and competing to see who could hold their breath the longest. The patient appears well and is moving all extremities. Vital signs are: respiratory rate 20, with good effort; pulse 84, strong and regular; BP 118/74; SpO2 100 percent. The patient's father is convinced that she did not swallow any water and says he will follow up with the child's own pediatrician for the possible seizure activity. He is willing to sign your patient refusal paperwork, but you try to convince him to have the patient seen in the ED because:

a. the seizure activity could be a new onset of epilepsy.
b. the patient may attempt to go back into the water and could have another seizure.
c. serious complications, including death, can occur many hours after a submersion.
d. you believe the father is making an irrational decision that could be considered child neglect.

33. Your ambulance is dispatched for a 54-year-old male who has abdominal pain. When you arrive at his residence, he is alert and in distress from severe muscle spasms in the abdomen. He says that he has never experienced anything like this before and denies difficulty breathing, chest pain, or loss of consciousness. His wife asks you to look at his hand and says that he was in the attic earlier and was bitten by an insect, perhaps a spider. She wants to know if the muscle spasms are related to the bite. The area of the bite is red and swollen and the patient states that there is a dull ache. Which of the following insect bites or stings could produce these symptoms?

a. tick
b. fire ant
c. black widow spider
d. brown recluse spider

34. (Continuing with the preceding question) You quickly obtain a SAMPLE history and focused physical exam. The cramping did begin after the bite. The patient is taking medications for hypertension and high cholesterol, he has no known allergies, and his last meal was lunch (soup and ham sandwich). His vital signs are: respiratory rate 22, nonlabored; pulse 90, weak and irregular; BP 100/50. The patient's abdomen is rigid and now he is feeling weak. Select the appropriate management steps for the patient.

a. Treat for shock and provide wound care for the hand.
b. Apply ice to the area of the bite and perform a secondary assessment.
c. Pour vinegar over the area of the bite to denature the toxin or sprinkle meat tenderizer over the area.
d. Place a tourniquet above the area of the bite, splint the extremity, and transport the patient to the nearest trauma center.

35. Dispatch has sent your crew to the city park for a possible alcohol overdose. The police are on the scene with a male in his fifties, who smells of alcohol and urine. His pants are wet and he is shivering uncontrollably, even though the ambient temperature is nearly 70°F. The police tell you that they got reports that the patient has been lying in the bushes for hours. The patient is able to answer your questions and understands where he is and what is happening. He denies any injury, but is hungry. This patient's mental status and body shivering indicate that:

a. his body is trying to generate heat.
b. his core body temperature is below 90°F.
c. his core body temperature is critically low.
d. he has suffered chronic exposure to mild temperatures.

Chapter 29 Answer Form

	A	B	C	D			A	B	C	D
1.	❏	❏	❏	❏		19.	❏	❏	❏	❏
2.	❏	❏	❏	❏		20.	❏	❏	❏	❏
3.	❏	❏	❏	❏		21.	❏	❏	❏	❏
4.	❏	❏	❏	❏		22.	❏	❏	❏	❏
5.	❏	❏	❏	❏		23.	❏	❏	❏	❏
6.	❏	❏	❏	❏		24.	❏	❏	❏	❏
7.	❏	❏	❏	❏		25.	❏	❏	❏	❏
8.	❏	❏	❏	❏		26.	❏	❏	❏	❏
9.	❏	❏	❏	❏		27.	❏	❏	❏	❏
10.	❏	❏	❏	❏		28.	❏	❏	❏	❏
11.	❏	❏	❏	❏		29.	❏	❏	❏	❏
12.	❏	❏	❏	❏		30.	❏	❏	❏	❏
13.	❏	❏	❏	❏		31.	❏	❏	❏	❏
14.	❏	❏	❏	❏		32.	❏	❏	❏	❏
15.	❏	❏	❏	❏		33.	❏	❏	❏	❏
16.	❏	❏	❏	❏		34.	❏	❏	❏	❏
17.	❏	❏	❏	❏		35.	❏	❏	❏	❏
18.	❏	❏	❏	❏						

SECTION

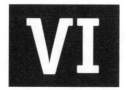

SPECIAL POPULATIONS

CHAPTER 30

Obstetric and Gynecologic Emergencies

1. The umbilical cord consists of:
   a. a muscular tube.
   b. one artery and two veins.
   c. one vein and two arteries.
   d. a self-contained feeding system.

2. *Afterbirth* is a lay term for which of the following organs or components of childbirth?
   a. uterus
   b. placenta
   c. amniotic fluid
   d. umbilical cord

3. Physical assessment of a contraction is best palpated:
   a. over the umbilicus.
   b. over the symphysis pubis.
   c. on the fundus (top) of the uterus.
   d. on the cervix (bottom) of the uterus.

4. The contents of an obstetric kit are:
   a. sterile.
   b. clean, but not sterilized.
   c. enough to care for two babies.
   d. only for use by a trained and certified EMT.

5. You have just finished immobilizing the driver of a vehicle that was involved in a MVC. She is complaining of neck and low-back pain and she is pregnant, in her 38th week. When you put her into the ambulance, she becomes unconscious. What step do you take next?
   a. Elevate her legs.
   b. Administer high-flow oxygen.
   c. Check for breathing and a pulse.
   d. Tilt the backboard slightly up to the left side.

6. A pregnant 32-year-old patient, in the third trimester, is complaining of severe abdominal pain, which began suddenly. She denies any vaginal bleeding or discharge. When you palpate her abdomen, you find that the uterus is rigid. What life-threatening condition do you suspect?
   a. preeclampsia
   b. placenta previa
   c. abruptio placenta
   d. ectopic pregnancy

7. You respond to a call for pregnancy with vaginal bleeding and discover a 24-year-old female in her third trimester of pregnancy. She is frightened and tells you that suddenly she began having heavy vaginal bleeding. She denies any pain or traumatic injury and reports that the bleeding has not stopped. What life-threatening condition do you suspect?
   a. placenta previa
   b. premature labor
   c. abruptio placenta
   d. ectopic pregnancy

8. During the transport of a woman in active labor, the patient tells you that the baby is coming. You examine her and find the baby crowning. The hospital is 10 minutes away, so now you:
   a. stop the ambulance and assist with the delivery.
   b. continue transport and assist with the delivery en route.
   c. continue transport and tell the mother to close her legs until you arrive.
   d. continue transport and instruct the mother not to push with contractions.

9. Prior to transporting a woman in active labor, you assessed her for crowning and saw none. During transport, the contractions become stronger and closer together. Which of the following signs is an indication of an imminent delivery?
   a. severe back pain
   b. abdominal cramping
   c. the patient feels an urge to move her bowels
   d. the patient has been leaking clear fluid for several hours

10. You have responded to a residence for a young woman in labor. She called EMS because she has no other way of getting to the hospital. Her contractions are strong, regular, occur every 5 minutes, and last for 30 seconds. You should:
    a. transport the patient.
    b. request a second ambulance.
    c. prepare the mother for delivery.
    d. instruct the mother to close her thighs together.

11. Your unit has been called to transfer a high-risk pregnant patient woman to the hospital for admission. The staff reports that the patient is 25 weeks pregnant and is experiencing Braxton Hicks contractions. Her vital signs are stable. Management of this patient includes:

    a. declining transport and calling an ALS ambulance.
    b. position of comfort, high-flow oxygen, and rapid transport.
    c. supportive care, position of comfort, and routine transport.
    d. having a staff member ride along on the transport.

12. EMS has been called for a woman who is having seizures. Upon arrival, you confirm that there was a brief seizure and find a pregnant female who is conscious, confused, and complaining of severe headache. She is 36 weeks along in gestation and is being treated for hypertension. Your primary assessment findings, together with the patient's history, indicate that the patient is experiencing:

    a. eclampsia, a life-threatening condition.
    b. preeclampsia, a life-threatening condition.
    c. eclampsia, a non-life-threatening condition.
    d. preeclampsia, a non-life-threatening condition.

13. (Continuing with the preceding question) After completing a focused physical exam, you find swelling in the patient's face, hands, lower legs, and feet. Her vital signs are: pulse 110, regular; respiration 20, regular; BP 186/100; skin is flushed, warm, and dry. Management of this patient should include:

    a. high-flow oxygen, calling for ALS, and rapid transport.
    b. high-flow oxygen, position of comfort, and rapid transport.
    c. notifying her physician's office and offering to transport her there.
    d. low-flow oxygen, position of comfort, and routine transport.

14. During emergency childbirth, which of the following factors should the EMT be alert for as a possible cause of an airway problem?

    a. nausea and vomiting
    b. the patient biting her tongue during a contraction
    c. the patient holding her breath during a contraction
    d. the patient putting her face into a pillow to scream

15. When preparing the mother for delivery in emergency childbirth, the EMT should:

    a. use only absolutely sterile equipment.
    b. allow the mother to go to the toilet before she delivers.
    c. allow the husband or friend to be present during delivery.
    d. allow only one other person to be present during delivery.

16. Once you have determined that birth is imminent, you will need to prepare the mother for delivery by:

    a. asking her to empty her bladder.
    b. letting her take a position of comfort.
    c. administering high-concentration oxygen.
    d. positioning her on her back on the stretcher.

17. Management of the third stage of delivery includes:

    a. watching for the baby's head to push through the vaginal opening.
    b. frequently assessing the patient for signs of hypertension and eclampsia.
    c. waiting to begin transport, but calling the ED to advise of the current status.
    d. coaching the patient to deliver the placenta and assessing for signs of shock.

18. Immediately after the baby's head is delivered, the next step in assisting with a delivery is to:

    a. prepare to deliver the upper shoulder.
    b. prepare to deliver the lower shoulder.
    c. check for the cord around the baby's neck.
    d. wipe the head off so that it is not so slippery.

19. A woman in active labor is crowning and pushing with contractions. She tells you that the baby is coming. She is in the delivery position and you that see the baby's head emerging. The next step is to:

    a. wipe the baby's head and assess for meconium.
    b. use a sterile dressing to prepare to catch the baby.
    c. take a suction bulb in one hand and get ready to suction.
    d. place your hand on the baby's head to prevent an explosive delivery.

20. The priority in the care of the baby as the head delivers is:

    a. suctioning the airway.
    b. assessing the skin color, temperature, and condition.
    c. wiping the eyes clear of fluid with a sterile pad.
    d. not to stimulate the infant to breathe until it is delivered.

21. The steps in suctioning the baby during delivery begin with:

    a. suctioning the nose, then the mouth after the baby is delivered.
    b. using a bulb syringe to rapidly evacuate the mouth, nose, and ears.
    c. keeping the baby's head in a slightly downward position for drainage.
    d. suctioning the mouth, then the nose once the baby's head is delivered.

22. The most common presentation of the baby's head from the vaginal opening is:

    a. face up.
    b. face down.
    c. turned to the left side.
    d. turned to the right side.

23. When assisting with an emergency childbirth, the EMT should clamp and cut the cord:
    a. when a prolapsed cord is present.
    b. only after the baby has been delivered.
    c. only after the placenta has been delivered.
    d. when it cannot be unwrapped from around the neck.

24. After clamping and cutting the umbilical cord, you observe that the end of the cord attached to the baby is leaking blood. You should manage this by:
    a. pinching the stump of the cord until it stops bleeding.
    b. carefully placing a second clamp proximal to the first.
    c. elevating the cord and placing an ice pack on the stump.
    d. keeping the cord warm and letting the natural clotting process stop the bleeding.

25. When the placenta is delivered and a portion is visibly missing, the EMT can expect:
    a. significant vaginal bleeding to follow.
    b. the remaining portion to deliver within minutes.
    c. the remaining portion to deliver within the hour.
    d. no problems during the time it takes to finish transport.

26. When assisting the mother to deliver the placenta, the EMT should expect:
    a. that the cord can easily become entangled in the placenta.
    b. no bleeding following expulsion of the placenta.
    c. significant bleeding following expulsion of the placenta.
    d. contractions that are painful and similar to those occurring with delivery of the baby.

27. When delivery of the placenta occurs in the prehospital setting, the EMT is required to bring the placenta to the hospital for which of the following reasons?
    a. proper disposal
    b. blood typing
    c. stem cell research
    d. inspection of completeness

28. A home delivery for the third child of a woman in her late twenties was assisted by a midwife. The delivery of the baby and placenta was reported as uncomplicated, but the mother has heavy vaginal bleeding and transport to the hospital is requested. Care for this patient includes:
    a. considering the possibility of delivery of a second baby.
    b. treating for shock, calling for ALS, and rapid transport.
    c. calling for ALS and treating for shock until the paramedics arrive.
    d. treating the patient and notifying child protective services about the home delivery.

29. Following delivery, the EMT may have to manage a rip in the skin and bleeding from the mother in the area known as the:
    a. anus.
    b. pubis.
    c. placenta.
    d. perineum.

30. After assisting the mother with an uncomplicated emergency delivery, management of the mother should be focused on:
    a. rapid transport and treatment for shock.
    b. letting the mother hold the baby if she is capable.
    c. performing uterine massage to reduce pain and bleeding.
    d. supportive care, comfort, and reassessment for signs of shock.

31. After 30 seconds of drying, warming, suctioning, and stimulation, a newborn baby is not responding well. The heart rate is slow and breathing is inadequate. The next step in resuscitation is to:
    a. start chest compressions.
    b. retilt the head and suction again.
    c. check the umbilical cord for bleeding.
    d. administer oxygen and prepare to assist ventilations.

32. Stimulating a newborn baby to breathe can be accomplished by any of the following methods, *except*:
    a. rubbing the baby's back.
    b. clicking the bottom of the feet.
    c. drying the baby with clean, dry towels.
    d. holding the baby upside down to allow fluids to drain.

33. Within 1 minute of delivery of a newborn, if the heart rate is less than _____ beats per minute and is not increasing with stimulation and oxygenation, the EMT should begin chest compressions.
    a. 90
    b. 80
    c. 70
    d. 60

34. For the baby that presents with the buttocks first in the mother's vaginal opening, the EMT should first:
    a. place the mother on her back with legs elevated and transport quickly.
    b. place the mother on her side with both legs closed and transport quickly.
    c. place her gloved fingers into the vagina to keep the baby's airway open.
    d. support the buttocks and legs as the baby delivers, to prevent injury to the baby's neck.

35. A frightened young mother-to-be has called EMS because her water broke and she is having contractions. When you assess her for crowning, you see about 6 inches of the umbilical cord hanging out of the vaginal opening and no baby. At this point you should:
   a. do nothing, as this is a typical finding.
   b. quickly prepare for delivery, as birth is imminent.
   c. keep the mother still while you wait for ALS to arrive.
   d. consider this a true emergency and begin rapid transport.

36. Which of the following abnormal deliveries should not be attempted in the prehospital setting?
   a. twins or triplets
   b. premature baby
   c. limb presentation
   d. breech presentation

37. Twins that are born from the same placenta will always be:
   a. premature.
   b. the same size.
   c. the same gender.
   d. one of each gender.

38. The size of each twin baby will be different at birth, yet the EMT can expect both twins to be _____ single babies.
   a. larger than
   b. smaller than
   c. the same size as
   d. premature compared to

39. The procedure for assisting with delivery of twins is _____ that for single babies, and the EMT can typically expect the first baby to appear _____.
   a. different from, feet first
   b. different from, head first
   c. the same as for, feet first
   d. the same as for, head first

40. The danger associated with the presence of meconium in amniotic fluid is:
   a. that the baby will be difficult to stimulate or resuscitate.
   b. that the baby has likely suffered irreversible brain damage.
   c. that the immature lungs cannot tolerate aggressive suctioning.
   d. aspiration of meconium, leading to respiratory distress syndrome.

41. When meconium is present during the delivery, the EMT should suction the baby:
   a. as soon as the head appears.
   b. immediately after the baby is delivered.
   c. only after the umbilical cord is clamped.
   d. after the umbilical cord is clamped and cut.

42. Meconium staining in the amniotic fluid is a sign of:
   a. a traumatic labor.
   b. a premature infant.
   c. imminent cardiac arrest.
   d. fetal distress during the pregnancy.

43. A baby that is born prematurely is at increased risk for:
   a. hypercarbia.
   b. hypothermia.
   c. hyperglycemia.
   d. hyperventilation syndrome.

44. The EMT can recognize a premature infant because the baby:
   a. weighs less than 5.5 pounds.
   b. is born before 39 weeks' gestation.
   c. has a darker skin color than a full-tern baby.
   d. has a lighter skin color than a full-term baby.

45. You are assessing a 56-year-old female who has severe abdominal pain. She tells you that she has a history of hypertension and had a hysterectomy 4 years ago. She looks pale, is tachycardic, and her blood pressure is 110/50. Management of this patient should begin with:
   a. calling ALS for pain management.
   b. an examination for vaginal bleeding.
   c. high-flow oxygen and treatment for shock.
   d. attention to the ABCs and suspicion of an ectopic pregnancy.

46. Abdominal pain, low-back pain, fever, nausea, and abnormal vaginal discharge are signs and symptoms associated with:
   a. kidney stones.
   b. ectopic pregnancy.
   c. urinary tract infection.
   d. sexually transmitted disease.

47. A 21-year-old female is complaining of abdominal pain with cramping in the left-lower quadrant. She denies being pregnant and has no vaginal discharge. Which condition should be suspected first?
   a. appendicitis
   b. kidney stone
   c. sexual trauma
   d. ectopic pregnancy

48. Which of the following can cause irregular fetal development when the mother is taking it or is exposed to it?
   a. calcium
   b. folic acid
   c. vitamin A
   d. vitamin C

49. If a pregnant woman sustains an injury that results in shock, her body will engage a self-protective mechanism that:
    a. masks signs of shock in the baby.
    b. delays the normal signs of shock in the baby.
    c. directs blood from the baby to keep the mother alive.
    d. directs blood from the mother to keep the baby alive.

50. A serious motor vehicle collision has resulted in the cardiac arrest of a woman in her thirties who appears to be in the third trimester of pregnancy. CPR has been started and she will be ready for transport quickly. The fetus's chance of survival in this case:
    a. is near-zero.
    b. depends on the quality of prenatal care.
    c. is better if the bag of waters has not ruptured.
    d. depends on aggressive resuscitation of the mother.

51. The normal term of gestation (pregnancy) is _____ weeks.
    a. 36 to 40
    b. 38 to 42
    c. 40 to 44
    d. 42 to 46

52. The _____ is actually fetal membranes which are commonly called the "bag of waters."
    a. embryo
    b. placenta
    c. amniotic sac
    d. amniotic fluid

53. _____ is an inflammation of the mucous membrane that lines the uterus, which is caused by bacterial infection or sexually transmitted diseases.
    a. Cystitis
    b. Estrogen
    c. Endometritis
    d. Progesterone

54. The most common sexually transmitted disease for both men and women is:
    a. chlamydia.
    b. gonorrhea.
    c. hepatitis.
    d. syphilis.

55. For the victim of a sexual assault, the EMT must assess and manage any life-threatening conditions first, then:
    a. clean superficial wounds.
    b. provide emotional support.
    c. preserve evidence of the crime.
    d. report the crime to the police.

56. The primary complication of uncontrolled vaginal bleeding is:
    a. infection.
    b. infertility.
    c. tissue scaring.
    d. shock and death.

57. A 23-year-old female in the ladies room at her work place. Coworkers called EMS because she is in severe pain which came on suddenly. The patient is pale and in obvious pain. She complains of abdominal cramping that began 15 minutes ago. She has no vaginal discharge and denies being pregnant. What condition do you suspect is present?
    a. ruptured ovarian cyst
    b. ectopic pregnancy
    c. urinary tract infection
    d. kidney stone

58. (Continuing with the previous question) The patient is nauseous and her vital signs are: respiratory rate 22 and panting due to the pain, pulse rate 118 and regular, and BP 98/54. What action should be taken next?
    a. Call for ALS.
    b. Begin rapid transport.
    c. Prepare for the patient to vomit.
    d. Keep the patient calm and warm.

59. _____ is an example of a secondary injury resulting from a sexual assault.
    a. Rectal tearing
    b. Bruising on the thighs
    c. Sexually transmitted disease
    d. Lacerations to the external genitalia

60. An 18-year-old female is complaining of having a fever since yesterday and today has nausea and menstrual cramps that are more painful than she has ever had. What condition do you suspect?
    a. trauma
    b. sexual assault
    c. urinary tract infection
    d. pelvic inflammatory disease

Chapter 30 Answer Form

	A	B	C	D			A	B	C	D
1.	❏	❏	❏	❏		31.	❏	❏	❏	❏
2.	❏	❏	❏	❏		32.	❏	❏	❏	❏
3.	❏	❏	❏	❏		33.	❏	❏	❏	❏
4.	❏	❏	❏	❏		34.	❏	❏	❏	❏
5.	❏	❏	❏	❏		35.	❏	❏	❏	❏
6.	❏	❏	❏	❏		36.	❏	❏	❏	❏
7.	❏	❏	❏	❏		37.	❏	❏	❏	❏
8.	❏	❏	❏	❏		38.	❏	❏	❏	❏
9.	❏	❏	❏	❏		39.	❏	❏	❏	❏
10.	❏	❏	❏	❏		40.	❏	❏	❏	❏
11.	❏	❏	❏	❏		41.	❏	❏	❏	❏
12.	❏	❏	❏	❏		42.	❏	❏	❏	❏
13.	❏	❏	❏	❏		43.	❏	❏	❏	❏
14.	❏	❏	❏	❏		44.	❏	❏	❏	❏
15.	❏	❏	❏	❏		45.	❏	❏	❏	❏
16.	❏	❏	❏	❏		46.	❏	❏	❏	❏
17.	❏	❏	❏	❏		47.	❏	❏	❏	❏
18.	❏	❏	❏	❏		48.	❏	❏	❏	❏
19.	❏	❏	❏	❏		49.	❏	❏	❏	❏
20.	❏	❏	❏	❏		50.	❏	❏	❏	❏
21.	❏	❏	❏	❏		51.	❏	❏	❏	❏
22.	❏	❏	❏	❏		52.	❏	❏	❏	❏
23.	❏	❏	❏	❏		53.	❏	❏	❏	❏
24.	❏	❏	❏	❏		54.	❏	❏	❏	❏
25.	❏	❏	❏	❏		55.	❏	❏	❏	❏
26.	❏	❏	❏	❏		56.	❏	❏	❏	❏
27.	❏	❏	❏	❏		57.	❏	❏	❏	❏
28.	❏	❏	❏	❏		58.	❏	❏	❏	❏
29.	❏	❏	❏	❏		59.	❏	❏	❏	❏
30.	❏	❏	❏	❏		60.	❏	❏	❏	❏

CHAPTER

31

Pediatric Emergencies

1. At 1 and 5 minutes after birth, the EMT assesses and scores the newborn's:
   a. birth weight and length.
   b. eye opening, verbal, and motor response.
   c. appearance, pulse, grimace, activity, and reflex.
   d. blood pressure, pulse, oxymetry, and blood glucose.

2. You and your partner are assisting with the delivery of a premature baby. You have assessed the infant after 1 minute and have determined that the baby's heart rate is 58 beats per minute even after you have warmed, dried, stimulated, and provided blow-by oxygen. What action should you perform next?
   a. Start CPR.
   b. Suction for meconium.
   c. Repeat the assessment.
   d. Assist ventilations with a bag mask device.

3. When meconium is present in amniotic fluid during childbirth it is:
   a. a sign of fetal distress.
   b. completely normal.
   c. a sign of birth defect.
   d. a life-threatening condition.

4. _____ is(are) a sign of neonatal respiratory distress.
   a. Belching
   b. Hiccups
   c. Sternal retractions
   d. Belly breathing

5. After resuscitating a neonate that was having respiratory distress, the EMT must stabilize the baby by:
   a. keeping the baby warm and providing oxygen.
   b. allowing the mother to attempt to nurse the baby.
   c. assessing the heart rate and blood pressure every 5 minutes.
   d. preventing seizures.

6. _____ is the leading cause of death in children.
   a. Asthma
   b. Poisoning
   c. Overdose
   d. Trauma

7. The unexpected death of an infant from an unexplained etiology is:
   a. called Reye's syndrome.
   b. common in children of Asian descent.
   c. called sudden infant death syndrome.
   d. rare in infants less than 6 months old.

8. The respiratory system of the infant is different from that of an older child or an adult in that the:
   a. lung tissue is less fragile.
   b. lung capacity is increased.
   c. accessory muscles are immature and fatigue easily.
   d. chest wall is more rigid, causing diaphragmatic breathing.

9. _____ is a sign of respiratory distress that is observed in children, but rarely seen in adults.
   a. Grunting
   b. Coughing
   c. Choking
   d. Wheezing

10. Which of the following signs of respiratory distress indicates the most severe distress in a child?
    a. grunting and crying
    b. stridor and coughing
    c. wheezing and sneezing
    d. slow and gasping breaths

11. The most prominent indicator that a child is progressing from respiratory distress to respiratory failure is:
    a. changing skin color.
    b. increasing respiratory rate.
    c. use of accessory muscles.
    d. decreasing level of consciousness.

12. The small airways of the pediatric patient are prone to obstructions from:
    a. secretions.
    b. dry air.
    c. humidified air.
    d. stuffed animals.

13. When a child 1 to 3 years of age has a sudden onset of respiratory distress or stridor, the EMT should first suspect:

    a. croup.
    b. epiglottitis.
    c. secretions.
    d. an aspirated foreign body.

14. A respiratory emergency that presents with great difficulty exhaling and may occur in any pediatric age group, is:

    a. croup.
    b. asthma.
    c. epiglottitis.
    d. pneumonia.

15. You are helping to teach a CPR class, and your station is foreign body airway obstruction in the unresponsive child with no injuries. When you teach your students to open the airway, you demonstrate the:

    a. jaw-thrust maneuver.
    b. cross-finger technique.
    c. tongue jaw-lift maneuver.
    d. head-tilt chin-lift maneuver.

16. While on duty, you stop for lunch at a fast-food restaurant. As you enter, you hear a woman cry for help and see a crowd gathering around a child who appears to be unconscious in his mother's arms. When you approach and ask what happened, the mother tells you that her 6-year-old son was choking on a mouthful of French fries before he passed out. The next step you take is to:

    a. perform a finger sweep.
    b. attempt to ventilate the child.
    c. position the child supine on the floor.
    d. reposition the head and chin and attempt to ventilate.

17. (Continuing with the preceding question) You are unable to ventilate the child, because of the obstruction, so you perform abdominal thrusts and attempt to ventilate again. You do this several times without success as your partner notifies dispatch and requests ALS to the scene. What steps do you take next?

    a. Continue with abdominal thrusts.
    b. Attempt back blows and chest thrusts.
    c. Check for a pulse; if no pulse is present, begin CPR.
    d. Perform a finger sweep, reposition the head, and attempt to ventilate.

18. It is time to recertify in CPR, and you are practicing foreign body airway obstruction on an infant mannequin. After you confirm that the infant cannot make a sound or breathe and is not moving, the next step you take is to perform:

    a. a tongue-jaw lift.
    b. a finger sweep.
    c. five back blows.
    d. five chest thrusts.

19. You have been dispatched for an asthma attack. Your initial impression of the 5-year-old male patient is severe respiratory distress. The child looks pale and exhausted and is working hard to breathe. You calmly give him oxygen and get ready to assist his ventilations and ask your partner to call:

    a. the child's pediatrician to get confirmation of a history of asthma.
    b. medical control for an order to assist with a bronchodilator treatment.
    c. medical control for an order to assist with an anti-inflammatory treatment.
    d. the child's pediatrician to determine if this type of event has happened before.

20. A first-time mother of a 10-week-old infant calls EMS because her baby is not acting right. The baby appears to be struggling to breathe and the mother states that the baby did not want to drink her bottle. You assess the baby and find that her nose is congested with mucus, and you hear congestion in her breathing. The next step you take is to suction the:

    a. nose with a bulb syringe.
    b. mouth with a bulb syringe.
    c. nose with a rigid-tip catheter.
    d. mouth with a rigid-tip catheter.

21. The parents of a 3-year-old boy called EMS because the boy awoke crying, scared, and complaining that he cannot breathe. The boy is alert, tugging at his neck, and crying when you approach. His skin is very warm and pale. You suspect that he has croup when you hear his barking cough. The primary approach to the management of this patient is:

    a. to avoid alarming or agitating the child.
    b. rapid transport, oxygen, and call for ALS.
    c. to assist ventilation with a bag mask device and call for ALS.
    d. to allow one of the parents to help you assist ventilations.

22. A 2-year-old has been sick for 24 hours with diarrhea and vomiting. Her airway is clear and breath sounds are adequate, but the respiration rate is fast. Her brachial pulse is 150 and regular. Skin CTC is pale, warm, and dry, and capillary refill is 5 seconds. You suspect:

    a. sepsis.
    b. bronchiolitis.
    c. compensated shock
    d. decompensated shock.

23. A 6-month-old infant was treated and discharged from the hospital 3 days ago for dehydration. Since she has been home, she has not fed well and is fussy. The mother took her temperature and found that it is 101°F. The infant has nasal flaring and grunting, and she is working hard to breathe. Skin is cyanotic, warm, and dry. The child has signs and symptoms of:
    a. respiratory failure.
    b. respiratory distress.
    c. compensated shock.
    d. decompensated shock.

24. You arrive at a day care center for a seizure call. The patient is 18 months old and is sleepy. The airway is clear, breathing is adequate, and the skin is warm and moist. The caregiver reports seeing the child have a seizure that lasted approximately a minute. There is no history of seizures with this patient, but the child was given acetaminophen for a fever this morning. You suspect a febrile seizure and
    a. dehydration.
    b. adequate perfusion.
    c. compensated hypoperfusion.
    d. decompensated hypoperfusion.

25. Which of the following is an indirect measure of end-organ perfusion?
    a. urine output
    b. capillary refill
    c. mental status
    d. distal versus proximal pulses

26. One of your partners is assessing the vital signs of a sick baby while you obtain a history from the mother. What piece of information does she provide to you that suggests the baby may have inadequate end-organ perfusion?
    a. The baby was born premature.
    b. The baby is using fewer diapers than normal.
    c. The baby has been crying and fussing for hours.
    d. The last temperature taken on the baby was 101.1°F.

27. When assessing the perfusion in a child, which of the following findings suggests that cardiac output is less than adequate?
    a. systolic BP of 90 mm Hg
    b. pink mucous membranes
    c. capillary refill less than 2 seconds
    d. cool extremities in a warm setting

28. The EMT who is assessing and treating a very sick child can reduce the chance of cardiac arrest and significantly increase the chance of recovery by:
    a. providing rapid transport to the nearest hospital.
    b. recognizing respiratory distress and treating it appropriately.
    c. recognizing the signs of child abuse and reporting it appropriately.
    d. obtaining a focused history from the parent prior to transporting the patient.

29. Which of the following is the primary cause of cardiac arrest in children?
    a. suicide
    b. toxic ingestion
    c. infection/sepsis
    d. respiratory arrest

30. The mother of a 10-day-old infant calls 9-1-1 because the baby is unresponsive after a possible seizure. En route to the call, you consider the most common possible causes of seizure in babies and recall that a seizure caused by _____ is often the most straightforward to manage in the prehospital setting.
    a. fever
    b. toxic ingestion
    c. congenital defect
    d. trauma from childbirth

31. You are assessing an 11-year-old child who is postictal from his first seizure. The child is sleepy, breathing slowly and shallowly, and is hot and moist to the touch. The caregiver states that the child stayed home from school today because of a fever, aches, and pains. You suspect the cause of the seizure is:
    a. trauma.
    b. epilepsy.
    c. infection.
    d. brain tumor.

32. The causes of seizures vary for each age group, but the one cause that remains common in all pediatric age groups is:
    a. trauma.
    b. congenital.
    c. drug related.
    d. alcohol related.

33. The family of a special-needs child calls EMS because their 4-year-old is in status epilepticus and his anti seizure medication is not working today. The patient is seizing in his bed when you arrive. Special care steps for this patient include:
    a. no transport, calling ALS, and suction while waiting.
    b. suction, high-flow oxygen, and rapid transport.
    c. high-flow oxygen and calling the pediatrician for specific instructions.
    d. high-flow oxygen, cooling, and bringing the caregiver with you to the ED.

34. The school nurse called EMS because a student with a history of epilepsy experienced seizures in class. When you arrive, the 8-year-old female is alert and resting. The nurse tells you that the patient may have missed taking her anti seizure medication and that it has happened before. The parents have been notified and will meet you at the hospital. The next step in the care of this patient is:

    a. supportive care with attention to the airway.
    b. removal of any excess clothing to keep the child from overheating.
    c. searching the patient for a MedicAlert™ tag identifying her as an epileptic.
    d. to call medical control and ask for permission to assist the patient in taking her anti seizure medication.

35. The parents of a 24-month-old are very upset and describe seeing their baby have a seizure that lasted for approximately 2 minutes. They said that the baby stopped breathing. Your primary assessment shows that the child is sleepy, but is breathing adequately. The child has been sick with cold symptoms since last night. The next step in the care of the child is to:

    a. insert an OPA.
    b. remove the child's clothing.
    c. administer high-flow oxygen.
    d. administer acetaminophen for the fever.

36. Because of their disproportionate sizes, the _____ are injured more frequently in children than in adults.

    a. chest and abdomen
    b. head and abdomen
    c. head, face, and neck
    d. airway and abdomen

37. An infant who experiences a fall from a height of three times her own is more likely to suffer a/an _____ injury than a child or adult falling from a proportionate height.

    a. head
    b. chest
    c. extremity
    d. abdominal

38. Children are at high risk for injury to internal organs of the chest in a traumatic event, because:

    a. of the lack of use of child restraints in motor vehicles.
    b. of the improper use of child restraints in motor vehicles.
    c. their developing bones are not as strong as mature bones.
    d. injury from child abuse is more prevalent in the chest area.

39. The use of an OPA in an unconscious infant with traumatic injury is:

    a. never recommended.
    b. the same method of insertion as for an adult.
    c. appropriate in the absence of a gag reflex.
    d. appropriate in the presence of a gag reflex.

40. A 6-year-old was knocked off his bike by a vehicle that was backing up. The child was wearing a helmet, which was removed by a parent. Spinal stabilization is being maintained. The child is unconscious, has labored breathing, and his abdomen appears to be distended. Which management step do you begin first?

    a. Assist ventilations.
    b. Perform a detailed physical exam.
    c. Immobilize to a long backboard.
    d. Remove his clothing and perform a rapid trauma exam.

41. A family of five traveling in a minivan was involved in a high-speed rollover collision. You have been assigned to assess the youngest member of the family, who is a 2-year-old still in the car seat. The child appears to be stable and has no distress, but the MOI is significant enough to warrant transport for evaluation. You will transport the patient:

    a. immobilized in the car seat.
    b. immobilized to a short spine board.
    c. in the car seat without immobilization.
    d. on your stretcher with no immobilization.

42. Which of the following findings is not associated with signs of sexual abuse of a child?

    a. hearing or speech deficit
    b. difficulty walking or sitting
    c. anxious child who avoids eye contact
    d. child who is uncooperative with certain aspects of an assessment

43. A baby with mouth and gum lacerations may suggest abuse with an MOI of:

    a. improper nourishment.
    b. shaken baby syndrome.
    c. a bottle being shoved too hard, repeatedly, into the mouth.
    d. chewing on an electrical cord in the absence of parental supervision.

44. You are documenting findings related to a possible child abuse situation. Which of the following observations would be inappropriate to document?

    a. evidence of alcohol use
    b. your opinion about the caretaker's character
    c. family members giving different accounts of the MOI
    d. an MOI that does not fit the situation found on scene

45. When managing a pediatric patient who may be a victim of child abuse, EMTs should report their findings to the:
    a. ED staff.
    b. caregiver or parent.
    c. national registry for victims of abuse.
    d. relative who is not living with the patient.

46. When documenting a call that involves suspected child abuse, the EMT is the ideal health care provider to:
    a. identify appropriate interaction with the caregiver or parent.
    b. provide information about the family's past medical history.
    c. provide information about the condition of the child's home environment.
    d. notify the parent or care giver in writing of his/her suspicions.

47. Which of the following statements is most correct regarding child abuse?
    a. Child abuse is a crime.
    b. Not every EMT is required to report suspected child abuse.
    c. When abuse is suspected, the primary assessment of the child is modified.
    d. Some form of alcohol or drug use is always associated with child abuse.

48. You and your partner have arrived at the hospital with a 10-year-old male who is your partner's cousin. The patient was the victim of a near-drowning and is still unresponsive upon arrival at the ED. Before you go back into service, you should first:
    a. get a probable diagnosis from the ED physician.
    b. talk about the call with your partner and assess his reaction.
    c. notify your supervisor to take your partner out of service for the day.
    d. notify your supervisor about the relation of the patient to your partner.

49. Which of the following statements about the need for debriefing following a difficult infant or child emergency call is most correct?
    a. Some EMTs do not need an organized debriefing session.
    b. EMTs should talk about the call with the medical director.
    c. EMTs always talk about the call with the other crew members as soon as possible.
    d. All EMTs need an organized debriefing session.

50. After arriving at the ED with a 4-month-old who is in cardiac arrest, you give report and begin documenting the call. After being at the hospital for a while, the initial feedback from the staff is that SIDS may be the cause of death. You and your crew are feeling upset about the call. What is one of the most effective things you can do first to help debrief this call?
    a. Talk to your crew.
    b. Talk to the parents.
    c. Go home for the remainder of the shift.
    d. Go back to work to take your mind off this call.

51. Which of the following statements is most correct about the special considerations for taking pediatric vital signs?
    a. Most adult emergency medical equipment will fit pediatric patients.
    b. The EMT should memorize the normal BP values for each age group.
    c. An adult BP cuff can be used to obtain an accurate BP on a young child.
    d. The EMT should use a reference for vital sign values instead of memorization.

52. To rapidly determine the severity of an illness or injury of a pediatric patient, the EMT must:
    a. keep the child from crying.
    b. approach the patient the same way as he would an adult.
    c. perform an age-appropriate primary and secondary assessment.
    d. consider the use of immobilization for the uncooperative infant or young child.

53. In which age group should the EMT begin to involve the child in the history-taking process?
    a. toddler
    b. preschool
    c. grade school
    d. adolescent

54. You have been dispatched for a cardiac arrest call. The patient is an 8-month-old infant who was last seen awake in the middle of the night. At 7:00 a.m., the infant was found blue, warm, apneic, and pulseless. The family is crying and you find it difficult to obtain any additional information. CPR is begun and you attend to the feelings of the family by:
    a. removing the child to the ambulance.
    b. reinforcing that the treatment of the child is your first priority.
    c. telling them that you need them to give you the child's medical history.
    d. explaining that nothing can be done for the child at this time.

55. You are splinting the arm of a 5-year-old girl who has a painful, swollen, and deformed wrist. The father is very anxious and is asking a lot of questions. While you splint the arm, you:

a. are thinking that this is a possible act of child abuse.

b. honestly explain the procedure and keep him informed.

c. ask him to step out of the room, as he is upsetting the child.

d. stop what you are doing and ask him to let you care for the child without interruption.

56. A mother called EMS when her 3-year-old daughter fell off the couch and cut her scalp on the coffee table. When you get there, the mother is crying and tells you that it is all her fault, because she was out of the room when the child fell and injured her head. You quickly see that the injury is superficial, with bleeding that has already stopped. The mother is still really upset, so you:

a. allow her to assist you in the treatment.

b. call the police to investigate the incident.

c. consider that she may be guilty of neglect.

d. reassure her that the bleeding is controlled and permit her to observe.

57. It would not be uncommon for an EMT who is a parent to _____ caring for an ill or injured pediatric patient.

a. burn out after

b. feel nothing at all while

c. feel emotional stress while

d. avoid whenever possible

58. Remaining calm and reassuring the parents of a sick or injured child will:

a. support the child's environmental needs.

b. help to establish trust with both the parents and the patient.

c. reinforce the parents' perceived loss of control of the situation.

d. help the EMT understand his own emotional response to the call.

59. When managing a complex pediatric call, each of the following considerations is paramount, *except*:

a. avoiding overwhelming the patient.

b. having the correctly sized equipment ready and available.

c. the need to examine the patient while the child is in the parent's arms.

d. assigning a crew member to inform and deal with the parents or caregiver.

60. When assessing and interviewing a teenager in the presence of her parents, the EMT should:

a. not take sides in disputes with the parents.

b. consider using a Broslow tape or other pediatric reference.

c. ask the parents to leave while the patient is being examined.

d. approach this patient exactly the same way as he would an adult.

61. Which cause of cardiac arrest is more common in adults than children or infants?

a. trauma

b. toxic ingestion

c. airway obstruction

d. myocardial infarction

62. At 22:30, your crew is dispatched on a call for a 4-year-old male who is having difficulty breathing. At the residence, a nervous father flags you down and brings you inside to his son, who is crying in high-pitched, squeaking sounds. The father says the boy woke up crying and stated that he could not breathe. The boy has been sick with a viral infection and cold symptoms for several days. There is no history of asthma or other respiratory disease, although this happened once before about a year ago. They had to call the ambulance then, too. The boy is tugging at his throat and nasal flaring is prominent. In addition to administering oxygen, what is going to be a key approach to the management plan for this patient?

a. providing aggressive ventilation assistance using a bag mask device

b. transporting the child safely strapped into his own car seat

c. inspecting the inside of the patient's mouth and throat if possible

d. letting the patient stay in a position of comfort with minimal disturbance

63. (Continuing with the preceding question) Your partner, with the help of the father, administers oxygen to the patient. You obtain vital signs carefully, without upsetting the child. It is cool outside and you have the father cover the child with a blanket and proceed to the ambulance. The transport time is short and the patient improves significantly on the ride in. What do you suspect is the cause of the respiratory distress?

a. croup

b. epiglottitis

c. bronchiolitis

d. new onset of asthma

64. A mother of a 4-month-old infant calls EMS because her child is sick. The mother reports that the child has been fussy, has not been feeding well, and has been vomiting. She laid the infant down for a nap and now is unable to arouse her. The patient does not appear to respond to your touch. The airway is open, she has a rapid respiratory rate, her skin is pale and dry, her extremities are cool, she has no peripheral pulses, and capillary refill time is 6 seconds. What do these signs indicate?

    a. hypoperfusion
    b. physical abuse
    c. respiratory failure
    d. respiratory distress

65. (Continuing with the preceding question) You call dispatch and request an ALS intercept. Next, you administer high-flow oxygen and prepare the patient for transport. What additional care will you provide until ALS can meet you?

    a. Hyperventilate with an infant-sized bag mask device.
    b. Suction the patient, elevate her legs, and attach the AED.
    c. Administer oxygen, provide warmth, and begin rapid transport.
    d. Apply hot packs to the extremities, cover the head, and begin rapid transport.

Chapter 31 Answer Form

	A	B	C	D		A	B	C	D
1.	❏	❏	❏	❏	34.	❏	❏	❏	❏
2.	❏	❏	❏	❏	35.	❏	❏	❏	❏
3.	❏	❏	❏	❏	36.	❏	❏	❏	❏
4.	❏	❏	❏	❏	37.	❏	❏	❏	❏
5.	❏	❏	❏	❏	38.	❏	❏	❏	❏
6.	❏	❏	❏	❏	39.	❏	❏	❏	❏
7.	❏	❏	❏	❏	40.	❏	❏	❏	❏
8.	❏	❏	❏	❏	41.	❏	❏	❏	❏
9.	❏	❏	❏	❏	42.	❏	❏	❏	❏
10.	❏	❏	❏	❏	43.	❏	❏	❏	❏
11.	❏	❏	❏	❏	44.	❏	❏	❏	❏
12.	❏	❏	❏	❏	45.	❏	❏	❏	❏
13.	❏	❏	❏	❏	46.	❏	❏	❏	❏
14.	❏	❏	❏	❏	47.	❏	❏	❏	❏
15.	❏	❏	❏	❏	48.	❏	❏	❏	❏
16.	❏	❏	❏	❏	49.	❏	❏	❏	❏
17.	❏	❏	❏	❏	50.	❏	❏	❏	❏
18.	❏	❏	❏	❏	51.	❏	❏	❏	❏
19.	❏	❏	❏	❏	52.	❏	❏	❏	❏
20.	❏	❏	❏	❏	53.	❏	❏	❏	❏
21.	❏	❏	❏	❏	54.	❏	❏	❏	❏
22.	❏	❏	❏	❏	55.	❏	❏	❏	❏
23.	❏	❏	❏	❏	56.	❏	❏	❏	❏
24.	❏	❏	❏	❏	57.	❏	❏	❏	❏
25.	❏	❏	❏	❏	58.	❏	❏	❏	❏
26.	❏	❏	❏	❏	59.	❏	❏	❏	❏
27.	❏	❏	❏	❏	60.	❏	❏	❏	❏
28.	❏	❏	❏	❏	61.	❏	❏	❏	❏
29.	❏	❏	❏	❏	62.	❏	❏	❏	❏
30.	❏	❏	❏	❏	63.	❏	❏	❏	❏
31.	❏	❏	❏	❏	64.	❏	❏	❏	❏
32.	❏	❏	❏	❏	65.	❏	❏	❏	❏
33.	❏	❏	❏	❏					

CHAPTER

32

Geriatric Emergencies

1. In late adulthood, the heart is less able to respond to exercise because the:
   a. muscle is less elastic.
   b. muscle is more elastic.
   c. heart rate becomes too slow.
   d. muscle becomes too large.

2. Aging affects the blood vessels, causing the walls to thicken which results in:
   a. increased blood pressure.
   b. decreased blood pressure.
   c. increased blood flow to organs.
   d. decreased cardiac workload.

3. The elderly patient will often have subtle signs such as weakness or shortness of breath when experiencing an acute coronary problem. One reason this occurs is:
   a. decreased heart muscle.
   b. diminished pain perception.
   c. decreased hormone production.
   d. because of non-acute confusion.

4. Changes in the respiratory system in late adulthood lead to:
   a. increased mucous production.
   b. overactive respiratory drive.
   c. a generalized decrease in lung capacity.
   d. increased diffusion of gases through the alveoli.

5. Older persons often have _____ due to decreasing muscle mass and weakening bone structure in the chest wall.
   a. lung cancer
   b. small rib fractures
   c. non-healing rib fractures
   d. an ineffective cough reflex

6. A 72-year-old male has difficulty breathing today. He was well yesterday when he returned home from the hospital where he was treated for a respiratory infection. He slept well, but this morning he is short of breath when he walks. He is a smoker and during the day his dyspnea has been worsening. His skin is very warm, dry, and pale. His lung sounds are diminished on the left lower side. Respiratory rate is 24 and shallow, pulse rate is 66 and regular, and BP is 146/86. What do you suspect is his problem today?
   a. pneumonia
   b. pulmonary embolism
   c. exacerbation of emphysema
   d. exacerbation of chronic bronchitis

7. (Continuing with the previous question) What information could best help you strengthen your differential diagnosis?
   a. a body temperature reading
   b. a pulse oximetry reading
   c. the presence or absence of a productive cough
   d. the number of cigarettes that the patient has smoked since returning home

8. The family of a 68-year-old female who is confined to bed due to severe complications from a stroke has requested transport from your ambulance service. The patient is to be taken to the emergency room for evaluation of a possible respiratory infection. During the move to your stretcher, you see she has open wounds on her knees, ankles, and elbows. What is the most likely cause of these open wounds?
   a. physical abuse
   b. emotional neglect
   c. severe infection
   d. prolonged periods of immobilization

9. Elderly patients can have a poor response to their prescribed medications due to:
   a. osteoporosis.
   b. bowel obstructions.
   c. a decline in kidney function.
   d. excessive hormone production.

10. _____ is one of the major changes in the endocrine system function during late adulthood.
    a. Diminished vision
    b. Increased pain perception
    c. Increased insulin production
    d. Decreased insulin production

11. _____ is a chronic and progressive neurological condition that robs memory and intellect and is the most common form of dementia.
    a. Diabetes
    b. Depression
    c. Alzheimer's disease
    d. Transient ischemic attack

12. Dementia can be caused by trauma, metabolic disorders, organic damage, or:
    a. heredity.
    b. obesity.
    c. menopause.
    d. the presence of a tumor.

13. Any older person that relies on others can become a victim of abuse, with the most common abuser(s) being the:
    a. spouse.
    b. children.
    c. roommate.
    d. health care provider.

14. _____ is(are) the most common form of elder abuse perpetrated by family members.
    a. Burns
    b. Neglect
    c. Bruises
    d. Broken bones

15. When the EMT performs the physical exam on an elderly patient, he must proceed gently so as not to:
    a. displace any clothing.
    b. cause any additional injury.
    c. increase the patient's blood pressure.
    d. force the patient to receive unwanted care.

16. After hip fractures, the most common complication associated with osteoporosis in the elderly patient is:
    a. obesity.
    b. rib fractures.
    c. spinal fractures.
    d. pulmonary embolism.

17. You are attempting to interview an elderly resident in a nursing home when it becomes obvious that he cannot hear you. What action should you take to improve communication with the patient?
    a. Ask the staff to help you.
    b. Make eye contact and shout at the patient.
    c. Locate the patient's hearing aids and help insert them.
    d. Write down your questions and formulate them with yes or no answers.

18. An elderly patient with a head injury is more likely to have a poorer outcome than a younger adult because:
    a. the skull becomes thinner with age and cracks more easily.
    b. the brain softens with age and is susceptible to bruising.
    c. the brain shrinks with age and is more susceptible to injury.
    d. preexisting illnesses make it difficult for the older patient to heal.

19. You have been dispatched for a "fall." When you arrive you find a 76-year-old female on the floor unable to get up. She is alert and oriented, denies any injury or illness, and states she fell because she tripped over her slipper. You and your crew help her up and assess her. Her vital signs are unremarkable, but she has multiple bruises of various ages on her arms and legs. She tells you that the medication she is taking causes the bruising. Which of the following classifications of medications would cause the bruising?
    a. stool softener
    b. blood thinner
    c. antihypertensive
    d. diuretic

20. (Continuing with the previous question) The patient also has a bump on the back of her. She denies losing consciousness, has no headache, and does not want to go to the hospital again. You give her an ice pack for the bump and:
    a. allow her to refuse medical attention.
    b. insist that she has no option other than to go to the hospital.
    c. help her call a friend or relative to stay with her for a while.
    d. attempt to convince her to go to the emergency department for evaluation.

21. When an elderly patient appears to be hypothermic and there is no obvious environmental explanation, the EMT should assume that the patient has _____ until proven otherwise.
    a. a severe infection
    b. low blood sugar
    c. a thyroid problem
    d. a medication reaction

22. When an elderly patient has a new and sudden onset of confusion, the EMT should administer high-flow oxygen and assess for:
    a. dementia.
    b. Alzheimer's
    c. low blood sugar.
    d. medication overdose.

23. An 83-year-old male fell out of bed and has neck and back pain after falling. The patient has severe curvature of the spine, which is normal for him. In an effort to avoid injuring the patient further, the EMT should apply a cervical collar and _____ prior to transporting the patient for evaluation.
    a. skip the backboard immobilization
    b. place the patient flat on a long backboard
    c. immobilize the patient to a short backboard
    d. carefully pad and pack all voids around the patient immobilized on a long backboard

24. An elderly patient who is ill or injured may not exhibit signs and symptoms of shock that you would see in a younger adult because of:
    a. hardening of the arteries.
    b. diminished perception of pain.
    c. the medications they are taking.
    d. excessive hormone production.

25. _____ is a disease associated only in the late adult patient.
    a. COPD
    b. Cancer
    c. Arthritis
    d. Dementia

Chapter 32 Answer Form

	A	B	C	D
1.	❑	❑	❑	❑
2.	❑	❑	❑	❑
3.	❑	❑	❑	❑
4.	❑	❑	❑	❑
5.	❑	❑	❑	❑
6.	❑	❑	❑	❑
7.	❑	❑	❑	❑
8.	❑	❑	❑	❑
9.	❑	❑	❑	❑
10.	❑	❑	❑	❑
11.	❑	❑	❑	❑
12.	❑	❑	❑	❑
13.	❑	❑	❑	❑

	A	B	C	D
14.	❑	❑	❑	❑
15.	❑	❑	❑	❑
16.	❑	❑	❑	❑
17.	❑	❑	❑	❑
18.	❑	❑	❑	❑
19.	❑	❑	❑	❑
20.	❑	❑	❑	❑
21.	❑	❑	❑	❑
22.	❑	❑	❑	❑
23.	❑	❑	❑	❑
24.	❑	❑	❑	❑
25.	❑	❑	❑	❑

CHAPTER 33

Emergencies of Patients with Special Challenges

1. Which of the following clues should lead the EMT to suspect that a patient is a victim of abuse?
   a. The patient has very poor hygiene.
   b. The patient has injuries that do not match the story given.
   c. The patient is unable to tell how his injury occurred.
   d. The patient is unwilling to provide a past medical history.

2. When a caregiver fails to properly care for the basic needs of another, that caregiver is:
   a. guilty of neglect.
   b. guilty of malfeasance.
   c. failing to communicate.
   d. not always responsible for his actions.

3. When caring for a victim of domestic violence, the EMT will have a heightened awareness of scene safety, appreciate various patterns of abuse, treat the patient, complete documentation requirements, and:
   a. preserve evidence.
   b. provide full disclosure.
   c. consult medical control.
   d. complete mandatory reporting.

4. Transport has been requested for a dehydrated home-care patient with a dialysis shunt in his left arm. The patient is nonverbal and restricted to a bed due to a stroke from several years ago. The patient does not appear to be in distress and vital signs are stable. During your secondary exam, you find that the patient has a red streak going up his arm, originating at the site of the shunt. The skin at the site is very warm to the touch and the patient indicates discomfort when you touch them there. What do you suspect is the problem with the patient's left arm?
   a. infection
   b. defective shunt
   c. physical abuse or neglect
   d. it is normal for this patient

5. You and your crew have responded to a call for cardiac arrest. When you arrive, a family member who is visibly upset tells you that she found her mother unresponsive in bed and that she believes she is dead. Her mother has been terminally ill and they are working with hospice. When you assess the patient, you find obvious signs that the patient died several hours earlier. What action should be taken next?
   a. Begin CPR until ALS arrives and takes charge of the call.
   b. Contact hospice to confirm what the daughter has told you is correct.
   c. Ask the family if the patient has a "Do Not Resuscitate Order."
   d. Provide comfort care to the family while you wait for the police to arrive.

6. The EMT is assessing a child who she suspects is a victim of potential child abuse. The EMT should:
   a. confront the parent about her suspicions.
   b. get a detailed description of the mechanism of injury.
   c. report assessment findings to the emergency department nurse.
   d. notify the dispatcher to have police meet the ambulance at the hospital.

7. Which of the following is an example of child neglect?
   a. unusual burns
   b. signs of malnourishment
   c. multiple bruises of various ages
   d. injuries that do not match the mechanism of injury

8. High-risk factors found to be a common denominator in many child abuse situations include:
   a. female toddlers.
   b. children in affluent families.
   c. a medical or physical disability.
   d. children in the care of grandparents.

9. When caring for patients with cultural backgrounds that differ from your own, a very important concept to keep in mind is that:
   a. patients with cultural differences have special needs.
   b. cultural differences will limit the EMT's ability to care for the patient.
   c. language barriers will never complicate assessment or care.
   d. culture-related preferences may conflict with the EMT's learned medical practice.

10. When assessing a patient who is significantly obese with large arms, the EMT should use a larger-than-normal-sized blood pressure cuff to avoid:
    a. embarrassing the patient.
    b. causing the patient unnecessary pain.
    c. obtaining a falsely elevated pressure reading.
    d. obtaining a falsely lowered pressure reading.

11. When moving and transporting a very large person, the EMT should use special "bariatric" equipment when the:
    a. transport is more than 10 miles.
    b. transport will take longer than 30 minutes.
    c. patient requests to be transported sitting upright.
    d. patient's weight exceeds the maximum load capacity of the stretcher.

12. An EMT at some point may encounter parents of children who use a(n) _____ monitor, a device that detects changes in chest or abdominal movement and heart rate.
    a. apnea
    b. cardiac
    c. oximetry
    d. end-tidal

13. You and your crew have been assigned to a call at an assisted living facility with limited information. When you arrive at the patient's room, there is a strong odor of stool and the staff tells you that the patient needs transport to the emergency department to have his ostomy repaired because the bags will not attach properly. During your assessment of the patient, you look at the ostomy located on the patient's:
    a. flank.
    b. rectum.
    c. abdomen.
    d. chest wall.

14. EMS is likely to be called for the patient on a ventilator at home when:
    a. there is a power failure.
    b. the patient requires suctioning.
    c. the patient requires a breathing treatment.
    d. the decision has been made to discontinue use.

15. In which of the following situations might the family, caring for a patient at home with an airway device, call EMS to assist them?
    a. replacing tubing
    b. obstructed tubing
    c. apnea monitor alarm
    d. changing a patient's position

16. _____ provide palliative and support services under medical supervision for the terminally ill patient.
    a. HMOs
    b. Hospice programs
    c. Nursing facilities
    d. Church organizations

17. A major component of _____ is the work toward the relief of pain and suffering for the chronically ill patient.
    a. acute care
    b. support services
    c. palliative care
    d. health management organizations

18. When a person living at home has a tracheostomy tube, one reason he may need to call EMS for assistance related to the tube is that the:
    a. inner tube has become clogged.
    b. outer tube needs to be changed.
    c. patient needs a treatment of humidified oxygen.
    d. patient no longer needs the adjunct and needs help removing it.

19. When it becomes necessary to suction the patient with a tracheostomy tube, the EMT must:
    a. call ALS.
    b. suction using non-sterile gloves.
    c. suction using disposable sterile gloves.
    d. hyperventilate between attempts of suctioning.

20. As many as one in four infants with Down syndrome are born with:
    a. diabetes.
    b. hearing deficit.
    c. vision impairment.
    d. a congenital heart defect.

21. A developmental disability refers to an impaired or insufficient development of the brain, resulting in an inability to:
    a. concentrate.
    b. communicate.
    c. learn at the usual rate.
    d. mature into adulthood.

22. When caring for a child with autism spectrum disorder (ASD), the EMT should:
    a. talk directly to the child and allow extra time for answers.
    b. avoid upsetting the child by talking directly to the parents or caregivers.
    c. assume that when the child is overwhelmed he or she will become violent.
    d. always use the same approach when assessing and interviewing the child.

23. A patient with autism who has a significant injury or illness:
    a. may not exhibit normal pain response.
    b. will not allow a stranger to physically assess them.
    c. can only be cared for by someone they are familiar with.
    d. must be transported to a hospital equipped for developmentally delayed patients.

24. Caring for homeless patients can be challenging because the patient often
    a. has poor hygiene.
    b. is mentally ill and uncooperative.
    c. numerous concurrent health problems.
    d. chooses hospitals that will not accept patients who cannot pay.

25. You have responded to a scene with police already present. The police tell you that the person they are talking to is homeless, they are familiar with her, and she is not a threat. She has been sick and today is too weak to move. The patient is dressed in multiple layers of clothing, is pale, and is coughing. The immediate concern for you at this point is:
    a. getting consent from the patient.
    b. exposure to an infectious cough.
    c. that the patient cannot pay for medical care.
    d. that the patient is a victim of physical abuse.

Chapter 33 Answer Form

	A	B	C	D			A	B	C	D
1.	❏	❏	❏	❏		14.	❏	❏	❏	❏
2.	❏	❏	❏	❏		15.	❏	❏	❏	❏
3.	❏	❏	❏	❏		16.	❏	❏	❏	❏
4.	❏	❏	❏	❏		17.	❏	❏	❏	❏
5.	❏	❏	❏	❏		18.	❏	❏	❏	❏
6.	❏	❏	❏	❏		19.	❏	❏	❏	❏
7.	❏	❏	❏	❏		20.	❏	❏	❏	❏
8.	❏	❏	❏	❏		21.	❏	❏	❏	❏
9.	❏	❏	❏	❏		22.	❏	❏	❏	❏
10.	❏	❏	❏	❏		23.	❏	❏	❏	❏
11.	❏	❏	❏	❏		24.	❏	❏	❏	❏
12.	❏	❏	❏	❏		25.	❏	❏	❏	❏
13.	❏	❏	❏	❏						

SECTION

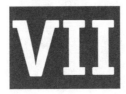

VII

OPERATIONS

CHAPTER

34

EMS Operations

1. It is your turn to perform the daily check of the extrication equipment located on your agency's emergency vehicle. As you go through the equipment, which of the following items appear out of place?
   a. ropes
   b. penlight
   c. Stokes rescue basket
   d. socket set with sockets

2. The Occupational Safety and Health Administration (OSHA) or the state equivalent of OHSA requires each EMS service to have an exposure control plan that specifies:
   a. cleaning requirements.
   b. when to open air vents in the ambulance.
   c. how to transport communicable patients.
   d. what type of mask to place on a patient with tuberculosis.

3. In the daily inspection of your vehicle mechanical systems, which of the following items is not a component of that inspection?
   a. oil level
   b. fuel level
   c. brake test
   d. stretcher mount

4. Replacing equipment on the ambulance and completing an inventory of equipment are tasks typically performed in each of the following phases of an ambulance call, *except*:
   a. at the scene.
   b. at the hospital.
   c. during the daily shift inspection.
   d. in the station after the call.

5. During which phase of an ambulance call would the EMT typically obtain permission to treat a patient?
   a. at the scene
   b. after the call
   c. at the hospital
   d. en route to the scene

6. When responding to the scene of a motor vehicle collision (MVC), the EMT should consider which of the following guidelines first?
   a. Use lights and siren only if the need exists.
   b. Notify the hospital with necessary patient information.
   c. Know the type of equipment needed and where it is stored.
   d. Listen for a status report from a first responder on the scene.

7. According to vehicle and traffic regulations, emergency vehicles may use lights and sirens to respond:
   a. to a drill.
   b. when returning from a call.
   c. to a medical emergency.
   d. during driver training on the road.

8. While you are transporting a patient, your ambulance is struck by another vehicle at an intersection. The driver of the ambulance must:
   a. continue to the ED if the patient is critical or unstable.
   b. continue, but she must notify the police through the dispatcher.
   c. stop to assess damage, render aid, and exchange information.
   d. stop to assess damage; if there is none, she can continue.

9. You are responding to a high-priority call on a divided highway. The motorist in front of you is not yielding the right of way. The proper action to take now is to:
   a. follow the vehicle while using excessive siren tones.
   b. wait for a safe location to pass the vehicle on the left.
   c. flash your high beams continuously until the driver moves to the right.
   d. edge up to the vehicle's rear bumper so he can better see your lights.

10. Your ambulance is transporting a high-priority patient to the ED when you notice that a family member is driving right behind your ambulance with his flashers on. The family member has just followed your ambulance through an intersection with a red light. What action is appropriate at this point?

a. Continue driving and do nothing about the family member.

b. Turn off your lights and siren and continue to the hospital in a safe manner.

c. Continue driving and notify your dispatcher about the illegal driving actions of the family member.

d. Stop the ambulance and talk to the family member and discourage him from using the ambulance as an escort.

11. You and your partner have just completed an emergency vehicle operator course (EVOC). Having completed this course means that you both have:

a. taken extra effort to ensure safe driving practices.

b. authorization to drive all types of emergency vehicles.

c. special immunity from lawsuits resulting from motor vehicle collisions involving your emergency vehicle.

d. learned all the vehicle and transportation laws associated with the operation of emergency vehicles.

12. According to most state laws, whenever the driver of an ambulance exercises privileges during an emergency response, that driver:

a. is not held to a higher standard in the eyes of the law.

b. assumes the burden of driving with due regard for others.

c. is not responsible if someone is injured because of his driving.

d. is personally immune from any lawsuit resulting from an ambulance crash.

13. While driving the ambulance to a low-priority call, an animal runs out in the road directly in your path. Which of the following actions is appropriate for this situation?

a. Turn on your siren to encourage the animal to move.

b. Adjust your speed and employ evasive maneuvers.

c. Decelerate suddenly while swerving to avoid the animal.

d. Flash your headlights several times to encourage the animal to move.

14. The first priority of the ambulance operator is to:

a. operate the vehicle safely.

b. transport the patient to the ED.

c. rapidly transport the patient and crew to the hospital.

d. learn all the vehicle and transportation laws in her state.

15. A request for an escort should be considered:

a. only if the escort is a police car.

b. very rarely, because it is so dangerous.

c. only if the escort is another ambulance.

d. if you are unable to locate the patient's location.

16. When two emergency vehicles are responding to high-priority calls and are within view of each other:

a. one operator should shut off the siren.

b. both operators should shut off the sirens.

c. the operators should use different siren modes.

d. one operator should use the horn instead of the siren.

17. Part of the EMT's driving responsibilities is exercising due regard for the safety of others. An example of this is:

a. allowing other motorists enough time to clear a path.

b. deciding which priority to use to transport the patient to the ED.

c. conserving fuel and reducing vehicle wear by using slow start-up and stopping procedures.

d. notifying the dispatcher that your patient needs alternative transportation if the ambulance breaks down.

18. "A reasonable and careful person performing similar duties and under the same circumstances would act in the same manner" is an accepted definition of:

a. due regard.

b. emergency privileges.

c. OSHA regulation 1910.

d. Good Samaritan privileges.

19. The shift supervisor has asked you to train a new EMT. To start, you review with the new EMT what information is essential to respond to a call. You include all the pertinent factors for these procedures and place the highest emphasis on:

a. arriving safely.

b. address information.

c. nature of illness or injury.

d. responder mode using lights and sirens.

20. The time between the receipt of a call by the dispatcher and the time the call is given to the unit to respond is called the:

a. queue time.

b. public access time.

c. system-ready phase.

d. prearrival instruction phase.

21. Dispatch has given you a call for an unconscious patient in a large motel. You are told that the caller is someone who is calling for the patient, but is not in direct contact with the patient. This type of call is a _____ party caller.

a. first-

b. second-

c. third-

d. fourth-

22. The enhanced 9-1-1 system helps to decrease response time to an emergency call by:
    a. providing GPS displays of the caller's location.
    b. identifying the caller's voice and level of distress.
    c. providing instant callback capability in case a caller hangs up too fast.
    d. providing instructions for emergency care until the ambulance arrives.

23. During the early part of your shift, the dispatcher notifies you that there is a problem with the _____. This problem means that portable radios will not be powerful enough to reach the base station from some locations.
    a. repeater
    b. telemetry
    c. simplex system
    d. multiple system

24. While taking a shower, a very large lady fell in the tub and was unable to get out on her own. Her only injury is a possible ankle sprain. With the help of additional crew members, you are able to get her out of the tub. The house is a bungalow with little space to move around. Which of the following devices would be most appropriate to use to move her out of the house?
    a. Reeves
    b. stretcher
    c. stair chair
    d. Stokes rescue basket

25. (Continuing with the preceding question) During the move out of the house, the patient complained of severe pain in her ankle. After you get outside and before you can load her into the ambulance, she says that she feels like she is going to pass out—and then she does. Now which device is the most appropriate to move the patient with?
    a. Reeves
    b. stretcher
    c. stair chair
    d. long backboard

26. You are assessing a 48-year-old morbidly obese female who injured herself when she tripped and fell. She is lying on the floor on her side and refuses to roll onto her back because of the increased pain when she moves. After completing a secondary assessment, you determine that she has a possible hip fracture or dislocation and decide to move her to the ambulance by using a:
    a. stretcher.
    b. stair chair.
    c. long backboard and stretcher.
    d. traction splint, long backboard, and stretcher.

27. (Continuing with the preceding question) You have discovered the patient lying on the floor on her side with a possible hip fracture or dislocation. The device you have chosen to move the patient to the ambulance with:
    a. will serve as a splint for the possible fracture or dislocation.
    b. is appropriate because no additional splinting is required with this type of injury.
    c. is appropriate, but the patient will need to be splinted with another device once she is inside the ambulance.
    d. is appropriate because the patient will be splinted and can be moved right into the ambulance without any additional equipment.

28. An elderly patient with moderate respiratory distress due to congestive heart failure lives in a small apartment on the first floor. She is sitting on the couch in the living room near the front door. A stretcher will not fit into the apartment, so you choose to move her out to the ambulance by:
    a. stair chair.
    b. laying her in a Reeves stretcher.
    c. carrying her on your long backboard.
    d. having her walk outside and sit on the stretcher outside.

29. Noting the official transfer of a patient to a nurse or physician on your patient care report:
    a. protects you from litigation.
    b. helps document that you did not abandon the patient.
    c. ensures that the patient's personal belongings will not get lost.
    d. guarantees a quick turnaround so you can get back into service.

30. The timely completion of a patient care report (PCR), using accurate and complete information with no misspelled words, will:
    a. impress the ED staff.
    b. impede the continuity of patient care.
    c. provide professional data for evaluation of quality of care.
    d. ensure that the EMT will never be involved in litigation.

31. The typical patient care report (PCR) includes information that will be used for which of the following functions?
    a. administrative recordkeeping
    b. legal tool to protect the patient
    c. personnel assignment record
    d. equipment maintenance record

32. The steps taken to prepare your ambulance for the next response are:
   a. required by OSHA.
   b. key to the safety and health of you and your crew.
   c. necessary for the safety and health of your patient.
   d. vital for the safety and health of you, your crew, and the patient.

33. Once a patient is transferred to the hospital and paperwork is completed, the crew should prepare as quickly as possible for the next response by:
   a. quickly getting back to the station to restock and clean the vehicle.
   b. cleaning and restocking the ambulance before notifying the dispatcher of availability.
   c. notifying the dispatcher of availability, making a list of restock items, and returning to the station.
   d. checking the fuel, washing the ambulance, and notifying the dispatcher of availability.

34. The patient you just transferred to the ED vomited in your ambulance during the transport. There is a spill on the floor and the ambulance smells bad. You take which steps to clean and disinfect this type of mess?
   a. Use a disposable towel first, then use soap and water and let it air-dry.
   b. Open all the doors, don gloves, use a disposable towel first, and then wipe the surface with a germicidal solution and air-dry.
   c. Document the spill, notify dispatch that you are out of service, and begin sterilization procedures.
   d. Turn on the ambulance and let the AC and vents run, don gloves and wipe the surface with germicidal solution, then close all the doors and spray a deodorizer inside.

35. During the last call, you had an infectious exposure. Which of the following steps is necessary only on *high-exposure* calls before returning to service?
   a. Wash the area of contact thoroughly.
   b. Change your entire uniform, including socks and shoes.
   c. Document the situation in which the exposure occurred.
   d. Describe the actions taken to reduce chances of infection.

36. Which of the following steps is out of place for the completion of a call and return to service?
   a. washing your hands
   b. verifying proper immunization boosters
   c. giving a verbal report on the patient
   d. transferring the patient's personal belongings

37. It is your turn to clean the equipment used on the last call and return it to the ambulance. The long backboard that was used has blood on it, so you get it ready to go back into service by:
   a. cleaning it with soap and water.
   b. sterilizing it while at the hospital.
   c. disinfecting it with a germicidal cleaner.
   d. hosing it down with water and wiping it with a disposable towel.

38. The product you are using to clean equipment after a call states on the label that it will kill most bacteria, some viruses, and some fungi, but not *Mycobacterium tuberculosis* or bacterial spores. This level of cleaning is:
   a. sterilization.
   b. low-level disinfection.
   c. high-level disinfection.
   d. intermediate-level disinfection.

39. _____ is a process that kills all forms of microbial life on medical instruments.
   a. Cleaning
   b. Sterilization
   c. High-level disinfection
   d. Intermediate-level disinfection

40. The process of removing dirt from the surface of an object using soap and water is called:
   a. cleaning.
   b. sanitizing.
   c. sterilization.
   d. disinfection.

41. The cleanup of a blood spill on the floor of the ambulance begins with removing moist blood with a paper towel, followed by a:
   a. high-level disinfection with hot water.
   b. soap-and-water mopping and air-drying.
   c. towel wipe down with a sanitizer and AC drying.
   d. wipe down with a spray disinfectant and air-drying.

42. When using a plastic spray bottle of concentrated household bleach as a disinfectant for cleaning, the usual recommended dilution in water is:
   a. 1:1.
   b. 1:10.
   c. 1:100.
   d. 1:1000.

43. During cleanup and restock after a call, you have reusable equipment that must be decontaminated from urine and vomit. You should place those items in a _____ bag.
   a. red
   b. clear
   c. yellow
   d. orange

44. Proper verbal report of patient information, upon arrival at the ED, is necessary to:
    a. get a patient properly registered.
    b. rapidly locate a specialty physician.
    c. have a bed ready for the patient upon arrival at the ED.
    d. help prevent any confusion that may potentially be harmful to the patient.

45. The patient information included in the typical radio report to the ED:
    a. is a courtesy and not mandatory.
    b. helps prepare the ED for the patient's arrival.
    c. enables the patient to prepare for arrival at the ED.
    d. allows other EMS agencies to be aware of busy hospitals.

46. Basic ambulance maintenance, such as oil and filter changes, are typically the responsibility of the:
    a. EMT.
    b. junior EMS responder.
    c. senior EMS responder.
    d. agency's vehicle mechanic.

47. The primary purpose of completing a daily ambulance checklist is to:
    a. have the unit prepared to respond to a call.
    b. prevent or reduce the risk of lawsuits.
    c. help the crew learn the location of the medical equipment.
    d. help the crew learn the location of the nonmedical equipment.

48. Air medical transport has been requested to the scene of a serious MVC with multiple patients. The head-on collision occurred on a high-speed road at night. Both drivers and one passenger are dead. A front-seat passenger in his early twenties has a head injury with altered mental status. One passenger who was ejected is in cardiac arrest, with CPR in progress. There is a toddler in a car seat who appears uninjured and a 10-year-old with a possible fractured forearm and ankle. Which patient has the highest priority for air medical transport?
    a. toddler
    b. cardiac arrest
    c. head injury with AMS
    d. 10-year-old with extremity injuries

49. (Continuing with the preceding question) A landing zone is being set up in a field 50 yards from the collision. Command has been notified that the helicopter is small, that it can take one patient, and that the ETA is 5 minutes. This aircraft will require a landing zone that is:
    a. 50×50 feet.
    b. 60×60 feet.
    c. 60×60 yards.
    d. 100×100 feet.

50. You and your partner have been assigned to do a long-distance transport of a stable patient who requires constant oxygen by non-rebreather mask at 10 lpm. The transport will take 2 hours. The onboard oxygen tank is an M cylinder with 1,500 psi.

    Using the following formula, estimate the time in minutes you have available with the current onboard tank.

    $$\frac{1.56 \times 1500}{10 \,(1pm)} \text{(cylinder constant for an M tank)}$$

    a. 96 minutes
    b. 234 minutes
    c. 960 minutes
    d. 2,340 minutes

Chapter 34 Answer Form

	A	B	C	D		A	B	C	D
1.	❏	❏	❏	❏	26.	❏	❏	❏	❏
2.	❏	❏	❏	❏	27.	❏	❏	❏	❏
3.	❏	❏	❏	❏	28.	❏	❏	❏	❏
4.	❏	❏	❏	❏	29.	❏	❏	❏	❏
5.	❏	❏	❏	❏	30.	❏	❏	❏	❏
6.	❏	❏	❏	❏	31.	❏	❏	❏	❏
7.	❏	❏	❏	❏	32.	❏	❏	❏	❏
8.	❏	❏	❏	❏	33.	❏	❏	❏	❏
9.	❏	❏	❏	❏	34.	❏	❏	❏	❏
10.	❏	❏	❏	❏	35.	❏	❏	❏	❏
11.	❏	❏	❏	❏	36.	❏	❏	❏	❏
12.	❏	❏	❏	❏	37.	❏	❏	❏	❏
13.	❏	❏	❏	❏	38.	❏	❏	❏	❏
14.	❏	❏	❏	❏	39.	❏	❏	❏	❏
15.	❏	❏	❏	❏	40.	❏	❏	❏	❏
16.	❏	❏	❏	❏	41.	❏	❏	❏	❏
17.	❏	❏	❏	❏	42.	❏	❏	❏	❏
18.	❏	❏	❏	❏	43.	❏	❏	❏	❏
19.	❏	❏	❏	❏	44.	❏	❏	❏	❏
20.	❏	❏	❏	❏	45.	❏	❏	❏	❏
21.	❏	❏	❏	❏	46.	❏	❏	❏	❏
22.	❏	❏	❏	❏	47.	❏	❏	❏	❏
23.	❏	❏	❏	❏	48.	❏	❏	❏	❏
24.	❏	❏	❏	❏	49.	❏	❏	❏	❏
25.	❏	❏	❏	❏	50.	❏	❏	❏	❏

CHAPTER

35

Highway Safety and Vehicle Extrication

1. Extrication is a process in which actions are taken to free a patient trapped in a:
   a. tunnel vision.
   b. vehicle.
   c. swimming pool.
   d. bathtub.

2. The purpose of extrication is to:
   a. ensure the safety of the rescuer and the patient.
   b. remove a patient from entrapment without causing further injury.
   c. develop specialized teams with skills for different types of rescues.
   d. have an effective preplan that includes specific equipment for various rescues.

3. _____ is a rescue term associated with the removal of parts or debris from around a patient in an effort to free that patient from a vehicle compartment or structure.
   a. Recovery
   b. Hazard control
   c. Disentanglement
   d. Rapid extrication

4. With the proper training and equipment, the EMT may not participate in which phase of a rescue?
   a. size-up and hazard control
   b. gaining access to the patient
   c. disentanglement and patient packaging
   d. providing ALS care to the patient

5. In a rescue operation, the next step after gaining access to a patient is:
   a. disentanglement.
   b. patient packaging.
   c. body recovery and stabilization.
   d. medical assessment and treatment.

6. Rescue awareness for the EMT means that she has enough knowledge to:
   a. recognize when a patient is stable or unstable.
   b. recognize when it is not safe to gain access to a patient.
   c. gain access to a patient for treatment purposes in any circumstance.
   d. gain access to a patient for assessment purposes in any circumstance.

7. For EMS personnel working at the scene of a highway rescue operation, the _____ is(are) the greatest hazard.
   a. traffic
   b. crowds
   c. fire hazards
   d. broken glass

8. When the EMT arrives at the scene of a highway rescue operation and stages the ambulance, he should adjust the emergency lights so that:
   a. they are all shut off.
   b. they are all turned on.
   c. only minimal warning lights are on.
   d. the alternating head lights are on.

9. When using flares at the scene of a motor vehicle collision, the flares should:
   a. not be directly exposed to traffic.
   b. only be placed by law enforcement personnel.
   c. not be used when the road is wet or has snow cover.
   d. direct the flow of traffic away from emergency workers

10. The phase of extrication that includes estimating the severity of injuries and the patient transport needs is the _____ phase.
    a. scene size-up
    b. transportation
    c. disentanglement
    d. medical treatment

11. For the EMTs who must make a rescue from a vehicle that has gone off the road and into tall grass, an additional safety concern that they must be aware of is that the:
    a. vehicle may be difficult to locate.
    b. potential for a fire hazard is increased.
    c. patient(s) may wander from the scene.
    d. potential for an electrical hazard is greater.

12. The final component or phase of an extrication for the EMT is the:
    a. overhaul.
    b. cleanup.
    c. transportation.
    d. patient packaging.

13. An often overlooked hazard for EMS personnel at the scene of a motor vehicle crash is an energy-absorbing bumper because:
    a. they have the potential to explode.
    b. they can leak a highly flammable fluid.
    c. if loaded, it can release unexpectedly.
    d. the true damage to the vehicle may be hidden.

14. A potential danger for the EMT working at the scene of a motor vehicle collision that involves a vehicle with an alternative fuel source is:
    a. that the battery cannot be disconnected.
    b. not being able to turn off the vehicle.
    c. not being able to stabilize the vehicle.
    d. that the engine is too quiet to hear, if it is running.

15. Your partner has gained access to the driver of a motor vehicle, who is trapped with his legs pinned, and is stabilizing the patient's cervical spine. The rescue crew with the fire department is about to break the glass in the door before prying the door off with a power tool. What item can you give your partner to protect the patient from the glass?
    a. a short backboard
    b. a disposable blanket
    c. an aluminized fire blanket
    d. any of these items will work

16. You and your crew have arrived at the scene of a car crash. The vehicle is off the road on an embankment on its side and the occupants are crying out for help. The first action to take is to:
    a. stabilize the vehicle.
    b. gain access to the patients.
    c. disentangle any patient that is trapped.
    d. extricate any patients that cannot get out on their own.

17. Once a vehicle is determined to be in a stable position, the first attempt to gain access to a patient in that vehicle should be to:
    a. locate an unlocked door.
    b. force open the door nearest to the patient.
    c. force open the door farthest from the patient.
    d. locate an unlocked door farthest from the patient.

18. Once you have determined that the scene is safe, and the vehicle with a crushed driver-side door and a trapped patient is stabilized, you should first attempt to gain access to the patient by:
    a. trying to open the door.
    b. breaking the glass on the passenger door.
    c. breaking the glass farthest from the patient.
    d. directing the patient to roll down the window.

19. When the EMT is attempting to gain access to a patient through the doors of a vehicle that was involved in a collision, she should first try all doors. If she cannot gain access through a door, then she should try gaining access:
    a. by forcing open the trunk or rear hatch.
    b. by breaking the windshield with a pry bar.
    c. through the window nearest to the patient.
    d. through the window furthest from the patient.

20. The driver of a vehicle that was involved in a collision in an intersection is uninjured but unable to open her door. It is an older vehicle, and all the doors are manually locked from the inside. You ask her to try to roll down a window so that you can get inside to stay with her until the fire department can get her out. This type of access is:
    a. noninvasive.
    b. simple access.
    c. complex access.
    d. disentanglement.

21. The fire department is attempting to gain access into a motor vehicle that has extensive damage. None of the doors will open easily, and the firefighters have broken the glass in the rear window to allow access to the patient. This type of entry into the vehicle is referred to as:
    a. simple access.
    b. horizontal entry.
    c. complex access.
    d. disentanglement.

22. Arriving at the scene of a motor vehicle collision, you see a car on its hood. The fire department has stabilized the vehicle with cribbing and now it is safe to attempt to gain access to the patient. The rear driver-side door opens enough for you to climb in. This type of access is referred to as:
    a. simple access.
    b. complex access.
    c. disentanglement.
    d. upside-down entry.

23. Which of the following factors would significantly change the treatment of a patient involved in a rescue effort, making treatment different from that of any other patient?
    a. the patient's past medical history
    b. lengthy time before access to the patient
    c. any past experience the patient may have had with a rescue
    d. the amount of psychological support needed for the patient

24. The potentially greatest hazard for the EMT working at the scene of a collision is:
    a. the traffic.
    b. fire or explosion.
    c. glass and sharp metal edges.
    d. exposure to leaking fluids such as fuel and oil.

25. The roof supports of an automobile are identified as A, B, C, or D posts. Which post supports the roof at the windshield?
    a. A
    b. B
    c. C
    d. D

Chapter 35 Answer Form

	A	B	C	D			A	B	C	D
1.	❏	❏	❏	❏		14.	❏	❏	❏	❏
2.	❏	❏	❏	❏		15.	❏	❏	❏	❏
3.	❏	❏	❏	❏		16.	❏	❏	❏	❏
4.	❏	❏	❏	❏		17.	❏	❏	❏	❏
5.	❏	❏	❏	❏		18.	❏	❏	❏	❏
6.	❏	❏	❏	❏		19.	❏	❏	❏	❏
7.	❏	❏	❏	❏		20.	❏	❏	❏	❏
8.	❏	❏	❏	❏		21.	❏	❏	❏	❏
9.	❏	❏	❏	❏		22.	❏	❏	❏	❏
10.	❏	❏	❏	❏		23.	❏	❏	❏	❏
11.	❏	❏	❏	❏		24.	❏	❏	❏	❏
12.	❏	❏	❏	❏		25.	❏	❏	❏	❏
13.	❏	❏	❏	❏						

Hazardous Materials, Multiple Casualty Incidents, and Incident Management

1. The amount of responsibility an EMT typically has at the scene of a hazmat incident is determined by:

   a. dispatch.

   b. the most experienced EMS provider on the scene.

   c. the local hazmat plan and level of hazmat training the EMT has.

   d. how many patients are involved and the type of chemical involved.

2. Of the following tasks, which must the EMT do first upon arrival at a scene with a potential hazmat?

   a. Perform triage.

   b. Complete a scene size-up.

   c. Establish a decon corridor.

   d. Assume the role of safety officer.

3. The role of the EMT as the first to arrive at the scene of a hazmat incident is to:

   a. determine what type of hazmat specialist will be needed.

   b. keep herself and the crew from being exposed or injured.

   c. identify the chemical substance involved using the NFPA 704 placard system.

   d. determine the type of decontamination procedure that will be needed.

4. Ensuring bystander safety at the scene of an multiple casualty incident (MCI) is the primary responsibility of the:

   a. police.

   b. safety officer.

   c. incident commander.

   d. senior EMT or paramedic.

5. Establishing safety zones should be completed _____ a hazmat operation.

   a. in the later phase of

   b. in the early phase of

   c. in the cleanup phase of

   d. after a hazmat specialist arrives at

6. To keep bystanders safe at or near a hazmat operation, the EMT should first:

   a. establish safety zones.

   b. call for the police to assist.

   c. call for the fire department to assist.

   d. assign the task to the safety officer.

7. You believe that a product with a flammability hazard is present at the scene. Your partner goes to the ambulance and brings back a hazmat resource guide, which states that a flammability hazard may have any of the following warnings, *except*:

   a. may be fatal if inhaled.

   b. may cause fire or explosion.

   c. may ignite other combustible materials.

   d. may be ignited by heat, sparks, or flames.

8. After responding to a low-priority call for a sick person, you quickly discover that there are two others in the residence with the same symptoms as the patient, but to a lesser degree. All three have headache, nausea, and dizziness and you suspect possible inhalation poisoning. The next action you take is to:

   a. establish safety zones.

   b. get everyone out of the residence.

   c. open all the windows in the residence.

   d. attempt to identify the poisonous substance.

9. On the scene of a call for a sick person, you suspect that there is a hazard in the basement. The patient had been working down there for an hour when he developed a cough, watery eyes, and nausea. You are upstairs and do not have any resources immediately available to help with information about the substance he was working with. At this point you:

   a. search the residence for the MSDS.

   b. interrogate the patient and family members.

   c. call dispatch and request a hazmat response.

   d. go into the basement to find the packaging label for the substance.

10. When approaching the scene of a hazmat incident, the ambulance needs to stay clear of all spills, vapors, fumes, and smoke. This is usually achieved by:

   a. parking at least 500 feet from the scene.
   b. parking behind the largest fire apparatus.
   c. approaching and parking downwind of the scene.
   d. approaching and parking upwind and uphill of the scene, if possible.

11. As an EMT trained to the hazmat awareness level, your duties are to:

   a. recognize a hazmat and carry out basic confinement.
   b. recognize a hazmat, back off, and call for the appropriate help.
   c. select and don appropriate PPE, then carry out basic control and containment.
   d. establish incident command and assign duties to incoming rescue personnel.

12. Dispatch has put out a call for a 30-year-old male with possible exposure to a hazardous material. Before you arrive at the scene, an updated report from dispatch informs you that the material was liquid chlorine and that it was splashed in the patient's face. When you arrive, as you perform a scene size-up your first priority is to:

   a. determine the need for additional resources.
   b. avoid any exposure to yourself and your crew.
   c. assess for any risks of primary or secondary contamination of the patient.
   d. assess for any risks of primary or secondary contamination of other responders.

13. When arriving at the scene of a hazmat incident in progress, the ambulance should report and stage in the _____ zone.

   a. hot
   b. cold
   c. warm
   d. control

14. You are assisting in the decontamination of a patient who accidentally splashed diesel fuel on his head, face, chest, and extremities. The first step you took was to instruct the patient to remove his clothing and then pour water on himself. This step is referred to as _____ decontamination.

   a. self-
   b. gross
   c. tertiary
   d. secondary

15. During a hazmat incident, a treatment sector (group) is established so that EMS can:

   a. dress and actively monitor the teams working in the hot zone.
   b. monitor the hazmat team before and after entry into the hot zone.
   c. determine what type of decontamination is appropriate for the incident.
   d. directly report any irregularities on the part of the hazmat team to the incident commander.

16. _____ is the process of removing hazardous materials from exposed persons and equipment at a hazmat incident.

   a. Corrosion
   b. Extrication
   c. Degradation
   d. Decontamination

17. An early-morning fire in an apartment complex has 36 residents out on the street watching their homes being destroyed. Many of the residents were asleep when the fire started, and nearly half of them are coughing or complaining of a burning sensation in the throat. Until proven otherwise, EMS should suspect that:

   a. there may still be residents in the building.
   b. one of the residents is most likely an arsonist.
   c. there is a possibility of carbon monoxide poisoning in all the victims of this fire.
   d. many of these victims may have seizures within an hour.

18. Your unit was dispatched to stand by at a tire fire in a junkyard. You have been staged a quarter-mile away. From there you can see that the fire is significant and that black smoke is rising in extremely large clouds. With residential housing surrounding three sides of the junkyard, which of the following environmental factors could create an immediate hazard for these residents?

   a. rain
   b. snow
   c. lightning
   d. wind direction

19. Dispatch sends you down to Pier 3 for an injured worker. When you arrive, you discover that the victim is pinned by a piece of iron and a second person was injured while attempting to free the first victim. This incident is now a(n):

   a. hazmat.
   b. confined space rescue.
   c. multiple casualty incident (MCI).
   d. extrication with two patients on scene.

20. It is 23:00 hours and you are responding to a private residence for an alcohol overdose. Police are on the scene when you arrive; they advise you that there was a party with teenage drinking. As you size up the scene, it is apparent that several teenagers are highly intoxicated. You immediately advise dispatch to send two additional ambulances and declare this to be a(n):

    a. rescue operation.
    b. EMS sector (branch).
    c. multiple casualty incident (MCI).
    d. prolonged and involved incident involving minors.

21. At 07:00 hours, it is a foggy morning and you are dispatched to a motor vehicle collision. When you arrive and complete a scene size-up, you find a bus on its side with the unresponsive driver still inside, but no additional passengers. A second vehicle is involved, and there are four occupants with various complaints of injury. This incident is a:

    a. hazmat incident.
    b. confined space rescue.
    c. complicated extrication.
    d. multiple casualty incident (MCI).

22. The EMT who establishes command at a large incident will determine how many sector (group) functions to establish based on:

    a. the level of his training.
    b. how many sector (group) vests are available.
    c. the number of patients each hospital can accept.
    d. the complexity of the incident and the number of staff.

23. As the first ambulance to arrive at the scene of an extrication involving a hazardous material, you complete a scene size-up, notify dispatch, and begin any possible hazard control. The EMT's approach to hazard control should be limited to:

    a. creating a safe perimeter.
    b. attempting to contain the substance involved.
    c. keeping reporters away from the danger zone.
    d. rapidly getting any victims who can walk out of the area.

24. Your assignment at the scene of a multiple casualty incident is to oversee the treatment of patients who have been triaged. This assignment is designated:

    a. treatment officer.
    b. medical command.
    c. staging sector (group).
    d. treatment sector (group).

25. When you have more than one patient to manage, you need to determine which one is more severely injured or ill. This is referred to as:

    a. triage.
    b. patient identification.
    c. rapid physical examination.
    d. patient discovery and classification.

26. As the second ambulance arriving on scene at a large office building, which has begun evacuation of its employees because of an unusual odor, you are assigned the detail of triage tagging. This phase is important because:

    a. it helps to eliminate the need to repeatedly reassess each patient.
    b. using triage tags eliminates the need for nonemergency treatment.
    c. using triage tags eliminates the need for rapid emergency treatment.
    d. the first ambulance to arrive is too busy with other assignments on the scene.

27. Typically, the only treatment completed on a patient in the triage stage of a multiple casualty incident is:

    a. splinting for children.
    b. CPR for a cardiac arrest.
    c. opening a patient's airway.
    d. none; no treatment is done during the triage stage.

28. Under the incident command system, the _____ section is responsible for coordinating services and materials, such as the communications unit, medical unit, or food unit, for major incidents.

    a. logistics
    b. planning
    c. operations
    d. command

29. The role of the EMT in a disaster operation is to:

    a. follow the national disaster plan.
    b. provide medical and psychological support to those who need it.
    c. get involved in the preplanning and training for disaster operations.
    d. acknowledge Homeland Security (HLS) efforts and work with HLS teams.

30. The EMT can better understand what his role may be in disaster operations by:

    a. becoming involved in preplanning and training.
    b. realizing that there is really no way to prepare for major disasters.
    c. obtaining the highest level of medical training affordable.
    d. talking to as many people as possible who have been in disasters.

31. An incident has become large enough to require the resources of agencies outside of the community. Communication among all the resources will:

    a. work best when plain English only is used.
    b. be designated by the incident commander.
    c. use the common "disaster system" terminology.
    d. use the code system of the originating jurisdiction.

32. Before a disaster that could involve numerous victims occurs, many communities preplan and train for various possibilities. These plans use a tool called _____, which manages personnel and resources during a multiple casualty incident.
    a. Homeland Security (HLS)
    b. incident management system (IMS)
    c. disaster and rescue operations (DRO)
    d. environmental disaster management (EDM)

33. The larger a multiple casualty incident (MCI) is, the more functional components may be required. With enough resources, the incident commander can utilize up to four components, which include:
    a. fire, police, media, and mutual aid.
    b. treatment, transport, logistics, and finance.
    c. operations, planning, logistics, and finance.
    d. operations, logistics, treatment, and transport.

34. Many emergency departments will _____ before they accept a hazmat patient, even when that patient was decontaminated at the scene.
    a. contact the hazmat team specialist
    b. ask you to decontaminate the patient again
    c. take the patient through their own decontamination procedures
    d. have the local fire department respond to inspect a patient for contamination

35. To prevent unnecessary contamination of EMS equipment at the scene of a hazmat incident, the EMT should:
    a. use only disposable items.
    b. use only the equipment of the hazmat team.
    c. stage equipment in the cold zone of an operation.
    d. not use any equipment until the patients have been decontaminated.

36. To help prevent contamination of the ambulance by a patient who has been exposed to a hazardous material, during the decontamination phase the:
    a. patient's clothing must be removed in the hot or warm zones.
    b. trained hazmat personnel will give the patient special instructions.
    c. EMT will follow special instructions given by the trained hazmat chief.
    d. patient will be wrapped in a special sealed blanket and an oxygen mask applied.

37. As a proactive EMT, you have been reviewing the local MCI plan. Now you want to learn more about the areas in your community where hazardous materials are stored in large quantities and the location of possible sites for an incident. Therefore, you:
    a. research at the local library.
    b. contact the local or state office of OSHA.
    c. get all the information from research online.
    d. go to the local fire department for the information.

38. The role of EMS command within the incident command system at a large incident is to:
    a. train and lead volunteers.
    b. be involved in planning and education.
    c. work cooperatively with other emergency commanders.
    d. circle the perimeter to observe all aspects of the incident.

39. _____ is the cooperation of multiple agencies working at one major incident, such as fire or train derailment.
    a. Unified command
    b. Singular command
    c. Incident command
    d. Multiple casualty incident

40. At the scene of a multiple casualty incident, the consolidated action plan is typically developed at the:
    a. dispatch center.
    b. unified command post.
    c. singular command post.
    d. first arriving emergency vehicle.

41. EMS and fire are dispatched for a fire alarm at a dance club. When you arrive, there is a crowd standing outside the building and the police and fire departments are on the scene. The club manager reports that a spotlight over the stage started smoking and set off the fire alarm; the crowd panicked and a few customers were injured while exiting the building. You grab your triage tags and begin to get a count of the number of patients, and you start sorting them to determine which ones will need immediate emergency care. After an initial triage, which of the following patients can be considered a P-3, green, or categorized with minor injuries?
    a. a 23-year-old female having an asthma attack from smoke inhalation
    b. a 43-year-old female complaining of headache, nausea, and vomiting
    c. a 44-year-old female with a nosebleed and a possible fractured nose
    d. a 28-year-old male with a swollen and deformed ankle and abrasions on both hands

42. (Continuing with the preceding question) Which patient is most in need of immediate emergency care?
    a. a 23-year-old female having an asthma attack from smoke inhalation
    b. a 43-year-old female complaining of headache, nausea, and vomiting
    c. a 44-year-old female with a nosebleed and a possible fractured nose
    d. a 28-year-old male with a swollen and deformed ankle and abrasions on both hands

43. Your unit has been dispatched to a local produce farm for a patient who has abdominal pain. Two hours after beginning work today, a 19-year-old male began complaining of severe abdominal cramps and nausea, and he has a new skin irritation with redness and itching on both arms and his neck. Shortly after arriving, you discover that there are multiple patients on the scene, with similar symptoms, who are all going to require transport for evaluation. Three more patients are complaining of headache, eye irritation, sore throat, nausea, and dizziness. What is the next action to take?

a. Triage and tag each patient, then request the appropriate number of ambulances.
b. Notify dispatch that you are declaring an MCI with a hazmat exposure.
c. Avoid any contamination of yourself and your crew by retreating to the ambulance to wait for additional resources.
d. Avoid any further possible contamination by identifying a decontamination area, and begin washing the patients.

44. A medical emergency that creates a number of patients and places excessive demands on personnel and available equipment is referred to as a(n):

a. disaster.
b. mass-casualty incident.
c. multiple casualty incident.
d. incident management system.

45. You have been dispatched with the fire department for two people stuck in an elevator. When you arrive, you learn that the power is out because of an electrical fire in the building. There is a smoke condition and the building is being evacuated. What can you do to protect the two victims in the elevator?

a. Tape a sheet over the outside of the elevator door.
b. Stay by the elevator and provide supportive instructions.
c. Stand by until the fire department has extricated the victims.
d. Attempt to pass oxygen tubing through the floor of the elevator.

46. _____ is the type of terrain that can become dangerous, because of difficult footing, when carrying a patient in a basket.

a. Low angle
b. High angle
c. Short angle
d. Vertical rescue

47. A teenager is stranded on a large rock in fast-running water approximately 25 feet from the shore. A special rescue team has been called and you are awaiting its arrival. What can you do until the rescue team arrives?

a. There is really nothing to do at this point.
b. Attempt to throw a rope out to the victim.
c. Throw a personal flotation device (PFD) to the victim.
d. Attempt to rescue the victim while wearing a personal flotation device (PFD).

48. Ropes, an exposure suit, and a personal flotation device (PFD) are the equipment needed for which type of rescue?

a. low angle
b. ice or water
c. confined space
d. hazardous materials

49. Confined spaces are deceiving and can present a great threat to a rescuer because:

a. these spaces may contain very little oxygen.
b. employees infrequently work in and around them.
c. OSHA requires a work-site permit to work in them.
d. many EMTs are too large to gain access to them.

50. Plenty of resources have been dispatched to a motel fire, but your ambulance is the first unit to arrive. Flames and smoke are visible, and you quickly identify two victims at a third-floor window who are trapped by the fire. You should attempt a rescue only when:

a. the victims are children, elderly, or disabled.
b. the victims will perish before the fire department arrives.
c. you are trained to do so and have the proper equipment.
d. you should never attempt such a rescue, as it is the job of the fire department.

Chapter 36 Answer Form

	A	B	C	D			A	B	C	D
1.	❑	❑	❑	❑		26.	❑	❑	❑	❑
2.	❑	❑	❑	❑		27.	❑	❑	❑	❑
3.	❑	❑	❑	❑		28.	❑	❑	❑	❑
4.	❑	❑	❑	❑		29.	❑	❑	❑	❑
5.	❑	❑	❑	❑		30.	❑	❑	❑	❑
6.	❑	❑	❑	❑		31.	❑	❑	❑	❑
7.	❑	❑	❑	❑		32.	❑	❑	❑	❑
8.	❑	❑	❑	❑		33.	❑	❑	❑	❑
9.	❑	❑	❑	❑		34.	❑	❑	❑	❑
10.	❑	❑	❑	❑		35.	❑	❑	❑	❑
11.	❑	❑	❑	❑		36.	❑	❑	❑	❑
12.	❑	❑	❑	❑		37.	❑	❑	❑	❑
13.	❑	❑	❑	❑		38.	❑	❑	❑	❑
14.	❑	❑	❑	❑		39.	❑	❑	❑	❑
15.	❑	❑	❑	❑		40.	❑	❑	❑	❑
16.	❑	❑	❑	❑		41.	❑	❑	❑	❑
17.	❑	❑	❑	❑		42.	❑	❑	❑	❑
18.	❑	❑	❑	❑		43.	❑	❑	❑	❑
19.	❑	❑	❑	❑		44.	❑	❑	❑	❑
20.	❑	❑	❑	❑		45.	❑	❑	❑	❑
21.	❑	❑	❑	❑		46.	❑	❑	❑	❑
22.	❑	❑	❑	❑		47.	❑	❑	❑	❑
23.	❑	❑	❑	❑		48.	❑	❑	❑	❑
24.	❑	❑	❑	❑		49.	❑	❑	❑	❑
25.	❑	❑	❑	❑		50.	❑	❑	❑	❑

CHAPTER

37

EMS Response to Terrorism

1. Which of the following clues should the EMT recognize as a potential terrorism event?
   a. a patient experiencing seizures in a supermarket
   b. a motor vehicle collision with a vehicle containing incendiary items
   c. a traveler at a bus station or airport who is pulling luggage on wheels
   d. an unconscious patient who appears to have fallen from a significant height

2. Classification of biological agents that may be used at a terrorism incident include:
   a. viral agents, bacterial agents, and toxins.
   b. nerve agents, blister agents, and blood agents.
   c. choking agents, tear gas, and pepper spray.
   d. alpha and beta particles.

3. In which of the following situations should the EMT recognize the signs where chemical, biological, radiological, nuclear, or explosive (CBRNE) materials have been used?
   a. an alarm drop in an assisted living facility
   b. an abandoned city building that homeless people are using as shelter
   c. two unconscious patients with no minimal or no signs of trauma
   d. a mass gathering of young adults at a RAVE party who suddenly disperse

4. Patient(s) exhibiting acute signs and symptoms of salivation, lacrimation, urination, defecation, GI upset, emesis, or muscle twitching (SLUDGEM) have had exposure to:
   a. radiation.
   b. explosives.
   c. a nerve agent.
   d. a blister agent.

5. Once the EMT has credible information of the presence of CBRNE, his next action is to:
   a. evacuate the area.
   b. establish EMS command.
   c. notify neighboring communities of the threat.
   d. attempt to identify signs of specific agent exposure.

6. When an incident is suspected as possible terrorism, it is essential that the EMT knows:
   a. how to enter an unstable situation.
   b. how to stabilize a toxic atmosphere.
   c. how to mitigate all the hazards at the scene.
   d. when it is or is not safe to gain access to patients.

7. When the EMT recognizes that the scene she is working in is an incident of terrorism and a crime scene, in addition to safety and patient care she will need to:
   a. take a few days off from work.
   b. take notes on what she has seen.
   c. organize a posttraumatic stress debriefing.
   d. complete a posttraumatic stress debriefing.

8. Upon arriving at an incident involving a weapon of mass destruction (WMD), the EMT's role includes:
   a. establishing command and performing a scene size-up.
   b. reporting to command and then to an assigned sector (group).
   c. providing the initial scene report to dispatch and requesting additional resources.
   d. identifying yourself and your level of training to the transportation sector officer.

9. The purpose of a "dirty bomb" is to spread _____ in the area of the explosion to frighten people and to make buildings and land unusable for a long period of time.
   a. nerve agents
   b. nuclear material
   c. radioactive material
   d. biological agents

10. One of the easiest ways an EMT can protect himself from radiation exposure at an incident is to:
    a. hand wash frequently.
    b. decon as soon as possible.
    c. decrease the distance from the radiation source.
    d. decrease the amount of time spent near the source.

11. Acute radiation sickness (ARC) is most likely to occur from:
    a. chest x-rays.
    b. a dirty bomb explosion.
    c. radiation therapy to treat cancer.
    d. a single brief exposure to beta particles.

12. The immediate signs and symptoms of acute radiation sickness (ARS) include:
    a. seizures.
    b. internal bleeding.
    c. nausea and vomiting.
    d. destruction of bone marrow.

13. Other than _____ agents, inhalation is the primary route of exposure for chemical agents.
    a. nerve
    b. blister
    c. choking
    d. irritating

14. Patients with chemical exposure need decontamination and the first action to take is to:
    a. have the patient remove his clothing.
    b. gather and isolate all the patients into one area.
    c. flush the patient with soap and water from a hose.
    d. perform a primary and secondary assessment.

15. Agents such as tear gas and pepper spray are designed to:
    a. cause pulmonary edema.
    b. temporarily incapacitate.
    c. cause confusion and hallucinations.
    d. cause peripheral nervous system dysfunction.

16. The symptoms associated with an exposure to biological agents used as weapons appear within:
    a. seconds.
    b. minutes.
    c. an hour.
    d. hours to days.

17. A primary safety concern for emergency responders at the scene of an explosive incident is:
    a. the fallout from the debris.
    b. an exposure to bleeding patients.
    c. the potential for a secondary device.
    d. an unsecured perimeter.

18. Explosive devices can be designed to spread:
    a. propaganda.
    b. bloodborne pathogens.
    c. fear and panic.
    d. chemical and biological agents.

19. Your ambulance is the first to arrive at the scene of an explosion. Your initial role as the EMS provider is to establish command and:
    a. survey the scene.
    b. establish a triage sector.
    c. call for additional resources.
    d. set up a treatment sector.

20. The Mark 1 Kit includes a single injector containing two antidote drugs, which is used for _____ exposure.
    a. anthrax
    b. nerve agent
    c. severe tear gas
    d. mustard gas

21. The EMTs responding to a terrorism incident involving weapons of mass destruction can use the acronym _____ to recognize types of harm posed by specific threats.
    a. OPQRST
    b. SLUDGEM
    c. TRACEM-P
    d. HAZMAT

22. _____ is an example of a toxin that has been used in terrorism incidents in the United States and worldwide.
    a. Ricin
    b. Ebola
    c. Small pox
    d. Yellow fever

23. When making the determination of what type of personal protective equipment to don at the scene of an incident of terrorism, the EMT must consider:
    a. how readily available the equipment is.
    b. that too much protection can create additional hazards.
    c. how many patients are symptomatic and asymptomatic.
    d. how many patients have wandered away from the incident.

24. Any mechanical, electrical, or chemical device used intentionally to initiate combustion and start a fire is:
    a. an incendiary device.
    b. not illegal to possess.
    c. legal to own, but not sell or transfer.
    d. never a hazard when handled by trained professionals.

25. A bomb was remotely detonated on a city bus carrying a dozen civilians. Five of the civilians survived the blast and had the chief complaint of severe difficulty breathing and were coughing up blood. What is the most likely problem with the survivors?
    a. blunt force trauma
    b. smoke inhalation
    c. blast lung injury
    d. upper airway burns

Chapter 37 Answer Form

	A	B	C	D			A	B	C	D
1.	❑	❑	❑	❑		14.	❑	❑	❑	❑
2.	❑	❑	❑	❑		15.	❑	❑	❑	❑
3.	❑	❑	❑	❑		16.	❑	❑	❑	❑
4.	❑	❑	❑	❑		17.	❑	❑	❑	❑
5.	❑	❑	❑	❑		18.	❑	❑	❑	❑
6.	❑	❑	❑	❑		19.	❑	❑	❑	❑
7.	❑	❑	❑	❑		20.	❑	❑	❑	❑
8.	❑	❑	❑	❑		21.	❑	❑	❑	❑
9.	❑	❑	❑	❑		22.	❑	❑	❑	❑
10.	❑	❑	❑	❑		23.	❑	❑	❑	❑
11.	❑	❑	❑	❑		24.	❑	❑	❑	❑
12.	❑	❑	❑	❑		25.	❑	❑	❑	❑
13.	❑	❑	❑	❑						

Appendix A:
Answer Key with Rationales

Chapter 1: Introduction to Emergency Medical Care

1. d. An EMS system is a network of services working together to provide patient care at the scene, during transport, and until the patient is received at the emergency department (ED).

2. c. Access to EMS with a cell phone is not any faster than with a landline. In fact, in many cases cell phone use has caused significant delay with deleterious results. However, improvements are being made, such as use of modified GPS locators.

3. c. One role of the EMT is to act as a liaison between the patient and the other health care providers you interact with while taking care of a patient. The goal is to help improve or maintain a high quality of health care.

4. c. In 1978, doctor Jeff Clawson introduced EMD, a system that involves prearrival instructions and dispatch according to medical priority protocols.

5. b. EMD is emergency medical dispatch, and a dental technician is not part of ED staff. These are examples of health care professionals or allied health personnel.

6. b. In nonmedical workplace sites, the first responder is typically the first trained person to arrive at a patient's side to provide care for an acute illness or injury. Many workplaces have a nurse on site during specific hours. However, it is not as common to staff a nurse 24/7 or have the nurse leave an office to respond at the site of a workplace accident.

7. a. Additional examples of advocating for your patients are protecting their confidentiality and not allowing your personal biases to affect patient care.

8. d. A deficit in color vision would not hinder one's ability to take an EMT certifying exam, maintain emergency equipment, or keep good documentation. However, color recognition is important to the emergency vehicle operator. The operator has to be able to distinguish colors on traffic signals and signs.

9. a. Activating EMS is typically done by the public; a physician does issuing standing orders; registering with NAEMT is an option, not a responsibility.

10. c. Honesty, integrity, and sympathy are all great traits for persons employed in the field of emergency medicine (as well as for life in general), but each has a slightly different meaning.

11. c. When responding to any scene, the number one priority is your personal safety and the safety of your crew.

12. b. Personal safety includes maintaining good health. The components of good health or wellness are proper nutrition and keeping mentally and physically fit. This includes keeping immunizations up to date.

13. b. There are many primary prevention activities that the EMT can get involved with: injury prevention, playground safety, bicycle-related head injuries and the use of helmets, child passenger and motor vehicle safety, preventing falls, medication safety, recognizing signs of a stroke or heart attack, and updating vaccinations are just a few topics.

14. b. The issuance of certification or licensure based on prior training in another state is referred to as *reciprocity.*

15. d. Placing the needs of your patients as a priority, including protecting their personal belongings and information while patients are in your care, is an example of patient advocacy.

16. a. The process called *continuous quality improvement* is designed to uncover problems through the practice of reviewing and auditing and to provide solutions to those problems within an EMS system.

17. a. *Protocols* are guidelines for the management of specific patient problems.

18. a. Training is one of the areas that continuous quality improvement recognizes as a source of potential problems and an area that can be improved.

19. b. The primary role of the medical director is to ensure quality patient care.

20. c. Written protocols are also referred to as *offline* or *indirect medical control.*

21. b. *Online* or *direct medical control* is the ability to obtain real-time direction and orders.

22. c. A medical director of an EMS agency has authority over patient care, and the EMS provider in that agency is acting as a designated agent or an extension of the physician.

23. d. The PCR contains patient information and administrative information such as patient demographics, run times, and dispatch information.
24. d. Local, regional, and state authorities can authorize the policies and procedures used by an EMS system.

25. a. Staying informed about changes in patient care and keeping skills sharp is the responsibility of the individual EMT. Fortunately there are a variety of ways to obtain continuing education.

Chapter 2: Well-Being of the EMT

1. c. Stress can come from a single incident or accumulate with multiple incidents over a short or lengthy period of time. There are many ways to deal with stress and each person deals with stress using coping skills acquired in their lifetime.
2. a. Talking with crew members enables emergency personnel to vent feelings and facilitates an understanding of stressful situations.
3. a. The stress generated by involvement in trauma, death, disaster, and crime scenes can cause delayed stress reactions for the EMT. This stress commonly leads to burnout.
4. c. Many medical emergencies call for the EMT to provide supportive care for the family members on the scene or at the hospital. This is especially true when death or near-death is a likely outcome. Supportive care includes listening and answering questions as best as you can without providing false hope.
5. d. The stages of the grieving process are shock, denial, anger, bargaining, depression, and acceptance. As EMTs, you and your coworkers as well as terminal patients and their family members may experience grief from death and dying. The EMT is expected to be able to recognize the stages of grieving and allow those experiencing grief to express their feelings.
6. c. Denial is a defense mechanism. It is the inability or refusal to believe the reality of the event and is part of the normal grieving process.
7. b. When family or caretakers are inconsolable despite efforts to explain the reality of the current situation, the EMT must see this as part of the grieving process and provide some form of support. Getting the patient out of sight in the ambulance allows some people a brief opportunity to begin to realize what is happening. This is a form of support.
8. a. *Acceptance* is the realization of fate and obtaining a reasonable level of comfort with the anticipated outcome or loss.
9. c. Many terminally ill patients experience the stages of the grieving process. Until you talk to them, you will not be able to know which stage they are experiencing. The approach to take with any terminally ill patient is to make her as comfortable as possible, maintain her dignity, and show respect at all times.

10. d. Your family's unhappiness typically adds to the stress in your life. Addressing these concerns is important and should not be ignored.
11. b. Getting a call near the end of the shift and not getting out on time is the nature of this sometimes stressful business. Although it is not always possible, you should avoid scheduling anything close to the end of a shift. This is one way to avoid placing additional stress on yourself, your friends, and your family.
12. a. Participation is voluntary and confidential. For some EMTs debriefing can be very helpful to understand their feelings and reactions during and after the incident.
13. d. The stress experienced during a critical incident and the effects from the incident will be different for each EMT. The way a person handles stress is directly affected by previous exposures to stress and the coping mechanisms that person has developed.
14. c. The symptoms described are indications of excessive stress.
15. c. A crisis-induced stress reaction can produce a range of negative signs and symptoms both during and after an incident.
16. b. Self-medication may include the use of alcohol, drugs, or a combination. It may be dangerous and is not a recommended technique for reducing stress.
17. b. In this case, anger comes from frustration related to the inability to control the situation. The anger may be focused on anyone or anything. Do not take it personally or argue with the person. As long as there is no physical threat to you, allow them to express their feelings.
18. d. Physical conditioning improves brain function, metabolism, personal appearance, and self-image. The more physically fit a person is, the better equipped she is to handle stress.
19. b. The EMT must think safety first. When 9-1-1 is activated in the middle of the night, it would be normal and expected for a light to be turned on at the caller's residence. No lights could mean that the caller is blind or unable to turn the lights on, but it could also mean that a crime has occurred or is still in progress.

20. c. Think safety first. Have dispatch send the police, if they are not there already. Do not turn your back on the patient. Keep an exit open and guarded by a crew member. Be prepared to leave quickly.

21. b. An icy walkway can be managed easily with rock salt. The fire department will stabilize a vehicle that is leaking fuel, and the police are needed to handle violence and other crime scenes.

22. d. BSI is a method of protecting against disease transmission by pathogens in blood or other body fluids.

23. c. Hand washing after every patient contact and after each call is the responsibility of the individual EMT and every health care provider.

24. a. Once an exposure has been reported, it is the employer's responsibility to arrange for you to be evaluated by a health care professional as soon as possible. The agency's exposure control plan includes having this policy in writing, and it must be available for the employee to review and understand.

25. c. Hepatitis is a bloodborne pathogen and staph is transmitted by direct contact or touch.

26. d. The immunizations currently recommended for the EMT are chickenpox, hepatitis B, influenza, Lyme disease, measles, mumps, polio, rubella, tetanus, and diphtheria. After September 11, 2001, many military personnel were required to get the smallpox immunization. Smallpox immunization for the general public is available but is not strongly recommended.

27. a. For geographical locations with higher-than-average numbers of known TB cases, screening is recommended twice a year.

28. b. At a minimum, gloves should be considered for any patient contact. The more information you have about the patient, the more PPE you may find necessary.

29. b. The current recommendations for the use of PPE for bacterial meningitis with a transmission mode of oral and nasal secretions are to wear gloves and a surgical mask, followed by hand washing after patient contact.

30. b. The current recommendations for the use of PPE for whooping cough with a transmission mode of respiratory secretions and airborne droplets are to wear gloves and a surgical mask, followed by hand washing after patient contact.

31. a. The EMT's primary responsibility is personal safety. Even when working at a scene with an established safety officer, police officer, or EMS supervisor, the EMT must make her own safety the top priority.

32. d. It is one of the EMT's responsibilities to attempt to keep bystanders from becoming victims at a scene with hazards.

33. b. Preventing exposure of another ill or injured patient, yourself, or a crewmember is the reason for properly cleaning and decontaminating equipment as soon as possible.

34. d. Dressing the part of a professional is important, but many agencies have a policy on uniforms that leaves little choice. Routinely demonstrating good sense in taking protective measures against infectious disease is a great trait for a coach or mentor.

35. c. Talking about using PPE is one thing, but actually having the students put it on is better, especially during initial training.

Chapter 3: Medical, Legal, and Ethical Issues

1. c. State law identifies the actions and care that the EMT is legally permitted to perform. The specific skills and medical interventions vary from each state's "scope of practice" legislation.

2. a. When documenting, the EMT should always try to use objective language and not make judgments.

3. d. The driver of an emergency vehicle must exercise *due regard,* which means that "a reasonably careful person performing similar duties and under the same circumstances would act in the same manner."

4. a. EMT certification or licensure is granted by the state. Reciprocity can occur for certification or licensure, and is typically granted based on the type of training and/or experience the applicant has.

5. b. The DNR is signed by a patient and his physician. When a patient is not capable of signing, his legal custodian can sign for him.

6. b. Advance directives, such as a DNR or a living will, are legal documents that contain instructions on treatment and the patient's wishes and are drawn up before an event to which they would apply has occurred.

7. d. A durable power of attorney or health care proxy allows a person to designate an agent to act when the person is unable to make decisions himself.

8. c. A *living will* is a document that states the type of life-saving medical treatment a patient wants or does not want to be used in case of terminal illness, coma, or persistent vegetative state. These decisions are typically made in the hospital setting.

9. c. For patients of legal age or emancipated minors who are able to make reasoned decisions, the EMT must obtain consent to treat, either verbally (most often the case), nonverbally, or in writing. That same patient can revoke consent at any time.

10. d. There are many acceptable ways to ask for consent.

11. a. When an adult patient with severe mental disability requires life-saving treatment, implied consent is the rule. When the problem is not life-threatening,

consent must be obtained from the patient's guardian.

12. c. For patients of legal age or emancipated minors who are able to make reasoned decisions, the EMT must obtain express consent.

13. b. Implied consent, also called the *emergency doctrine,* is the type of consent that remains in effect for as long as the patient requires life-saving treatment.

14. d. The emergency doctrine, also called *implied consent,* is the type of consent that remains in effect for as long as the patient requires life-saving treatment.

15. b. Implied consent, also called the *emergency doctrine,* is the type of consent that remains in effect for as long as the patient requires life-saving treatment.

16. c. A person makes a threat or gesture of suicide to ask for help rather than die. Any patient who has expressed the intent to harm himself needs help and must be transported for a psychological evaluation.

17. a. A pediatric patient who is experiencing a life-threatening condition with no parent present is treated under implied consent.

18. d. A minor who is married, pregnant, or a parent, and living on his or her own; or who is in the armed forces, is considered emancipated and can legally give consent for or refuse care. The definition of emancipated minor varies by state. Be familiar with your state's definition of an emancipated minor.

19. a. A living will is an advance directive. It states the type of lifesaving medical treatment a patient wants or does not want to be employed in case of terminal illness, coma, or persistent vegetative state.

20. a. Consent to treat a minor must be obtained from a parent or legal guardian, unless the illness or injury is life-threatening, in which case consent is implied.

21. d. A competent adult may refuse care or any part of care. The EMT should explain the possible dangers associated with refusing, carefully document the refusal, and have the patient sign the refusal.

22. d. A minor cannot legally refuse treatment for a life-threatening injury. Treatment for a non-life-threatening injury requires the consent or refusal of a parent or legal guardian.

23. c. There are specific conditions that preclude a patient from refusing care (e.g., mentally incompetent adult, minor, an unresponsive patient, a patient with an altered mental status).

24. b. When a competent adult refuses care or transport and you feel this may cause further harm, consider trying to get a family member or friend to stay with him or transport him.

25. c. A competent adult may refuse care or any part of care. The EMT should explain the possible dangers associated with refusing, carefully document the refusal, and have the patient sign the refusal.

26. a. *Negligence* is deviation from the accepted standard of care (typically as a result of carelessness or inattentiveness).

27. c. Once a patient–provider relationship has been established, the EMT must stay with the patient until that patient can be turned over to another health care provider with an equal or higher level of training.

28. a. The EMT was assaulted. Some states or jurisdictions have made it a serious crime to assault or strike an EMS provider while he is in the course of his duties.

29. a. Transporting a patient without permission or detaining a patient without his consent or legal authority is considered false imprisonment or kidnapping. This is one of the reasons why it is so important to get consent before taking a patient to the hospital.

30. a. Touching a competent adult patient without consent may be considered assault or battery.

31. b. A duty to act is a legal responsibility to provide service to the patient. The EMT's first priority is personal safety, and he may delay action if there is a safety issue.

32. d. When you are off duty or out of your jurisdiction, your ability to practice may be limited by the lack of medical control. The safest approach when faced with a life-threatening medical emergency or injury outside your medical control region is to limit your care to lifesaving BLS treatment as a first responder.

33. b. The EMT has a responsibility at a crime scene to first and foremost protect herself and other EMS providers. Next is to provide patient care, observe and document any items moved or anything unusual at the scene, and to protect potential evidence whenever possible.

34. c. State and local laws do vary as to "duty to act." For example, in some states the EMT must stop to assist an ill or injured person even when the EMT is not on duty.

35. a. To maintain the patient–EMS provider relationship, information about the patient's history, the assessment findings, and treatment rendered must remain confidential.

36. c. The release of patient information requires written permission from the patient or the patient's legal guardian.

37. b. *Slander* is an act in which a person's character or reputation is injured by the false or malicious spoken words of another person, such as when spreading rumors.

38. b. The law in each state requires mandatory child abuse reporting. The method of reporting and to whom the suspected abuse is reported varies from state to state.

39. c. Morals relate to societal standards and ethics relate to personal standards. Covering up a medication error violates the EMT Code of Ethics and is considered record tampering and is illegal.

40. d. The EMT can identify a potential organ donor by an organ donor card, by a signature or sticker on a

driver's license indicating such, and/or by a family member providing the information.

41. c. A potential organ donor should be treated the same as any other patient requiring emergency care. In addition, the EMT should contact medical control and advise of the potential for organ donation.

42. a. A potential organ donor should be treated the same as any other patient requiring emergency care. In addition, the EMT should contact medical control and advise of the potential for organ donation.

43. a. The knot is evidence and should not be untied or even handled, if possible. The correct approach is to make a clean cut with a sharp knife at least 6 inches from the knot.

44. a. The body should be left in the position found. Many EMS and police agencies require that an EKG be obtained, and this can be done without moving the patient.

45. c. The EMT must not allow the victim to remove any clothing or bathe. If possible, the victim should not use the bathroom. The ED will use a rape kit to obtain evidence samples from the victim's body and clothing.

46. d. As with any documentation, only objective information should be included. Your suspicions are subjective and should not be included in documentation.

47. a. Mandatory reporting varies from state to state, but EMS providers usually have a requirement to make a report or personally notify a mandated reporter in cases that may involve child abuse or neglect, elder or spousal abuse, sexual assault, gunshot and stab wounds, animal bites, and communicable diseases.

48. a. Most states make it mandatory for the EMT to report violent crimes such as rape and abuse. Failure to do so may result in criminal charges and/or disciplinary action against the EMT.

49. b. Patient care comes first. Advising the ED of your suspicions right away and not waiting is appropriate, though. Documentation should include only objective information.

50. c. There is no absolute guarantee for avoiding lawsuits. EMTs however, can avoid lawsuits by always being respectful and pleasant to patients, their families, and property; providing competent patient care; and completing clear and accurate documentation.

Chapter 4: Medical Terminology and Anatomy and Physiology

1. c. In the anatomical position, the body is standing erect, facing forward, with arms down and palms facing forward.

2. a. *Plane* is the surface of an object split down the middle.

3. a. The cervical spine is comprised of 7 vertebrae: the thoracic has 12, the lumbar has 5, the sacrum has 5, and the coccyx has 3 to 5 fused.

4. b. *Bilateral* refers to two sides; *proximal* means close to; *superior* is above.

5. c. *Supine* means lying on the back; *prone* means lying face down; *lateral* means the side; *anatomical* position is standing facing forward.

6. c. The quadrants of the abdomen are named for the location on the body: upper left and right, and lower left and right.

7. c. The esophagus lies directly in the midline of the body. The stomach is in the ULQ, the heart is near the midline, and the large intestine lies in all four quadrants of the abdomen.

8. b. *Midshaft* describes the location of the middle of a long bone.

9. d. Mid-axillary describes the location under the armpit (axilla) and the vertical middle line. The two vertical lines on either side of the mid-axillary line are the anterior-axillary and posterior-axillary lines.

10. c. The cervical spine is located in the posterior (back) of the neck.

11. d. The pharynx is the cavity or space just in back of the mouth into which the nostrils, esophagus, and trachea open. The glottis is a slit-like opening between the vocal cords. The nares are the openings of the nose, and sinuses are any of several cavities in the skull.

12. a. The larynx, located in the upper part of the trachea, contains the vocal cords.

13. d. The epiglottis is a thin plate of flexible tissue that protects (covers) the airway during swallowing.

14. a. Alveoli are small sacs in the lungs. During inspiration, they fill with air; a gas exchange between oxygen and carbon dioxide then takes place within the pulmonary capillaries, and carbon dioxide is released during exhalation.

15. b. The end expiratory pressure in the lungs is negative.

16. c. The primary muscles used for breathing are the diaphragm, a sheet of muscle between the chest and abdominal cavities, and the intercostal muscles, the muscles between the ribs.

17. d. The prefix *pneumo* is used for terms relating to air, breathing, and the lungs.

18. c. During inhalation, the diaphragm and the intercostals contract. The diaphragm also moves downward.

19. d. The lungs adhere to the chest wall with a tension surface created by serous fluid, similar to the way two sheets of glass would stick together if a few drops of water were trapped between them.

20. a. The respiratory system is comprised of the organs that are responsible for gas exchange. Oxygen moves into the cells and carbon dioxide moves out.

21. d. Heart sounds are created by the opening and closing of heart valves, which occurs with contraction and relaxation of the heart muscle.

22. a. The throbbing sensation, or *pulse*, that can be felt in the arteries is caused by contraction of the heart.

23. b. Blood returns to the heart by way of the vena cava, the largest vein in the body. The superior vena cava receives blood from the upper body and the inferior vena cava receives blood from the lower body.

24. b. Blood flows into the heart by passing through the tricuspid valves, then through the pulmonary valve into the lungs, and then out of the heart by way of the bicuspid and aortic valves.

25. c. The pulmonary artery carries blood from the right ventricle to the lungs. It is the only artery that carries deoxygenated blood.

26. d. Plasma contains serum, the fluid portion of blood that contains minerals, salts, and proteins.

27. c. At birth, both ventricles are about the same size. As an infant matures, the left ventricle becomes larger and more muscular.

28. b. The coronary arteries supply the heart with blood. The pulmonary arteries supply the lungs, the carotid arteries supply the brain and head, and the superior vena cava is a vein.

29. c. The peripheral or distal circulation supplies the extremities with blood.

30. a. *Infarct* and *necrosis* both mean dead tissue.

31. d. When working properly, the pulmonic valve should prevent any backflow of blood from the pulmonary artery back into the right ventricle.

32. a. The tibial pulse is felt in the back of the lower leg. The femoral pulse can be palpated on the upper inside thigh, the dorsalis pedis on the top of the foot, and the brachial pulse on the inside upper arm.

33. a. Deoxygenated blood is returned to the heart by veins.

34. b. An *embolism* is an obstruction in a blood vessel caused by a blood clot or other substance. *Varicose* describes a swollen vein, *edema* is an abnormal accumulation of fluid, and *palpation* is touching.

35. d. Special cells in the heart muscle generate electrical impulses that are transmitted (conducted) through the heart to stimulate contractions. This electrical activity can be seen on an electrocardiogram or ECG.

36. a. Bones, cartilage, ligaments, and tendons are all forms of connective tissue. Bones are different from other connective tissues in that they are hardened by calcium.

37. b. Cartilage allows smooth movement at the joints.

38. c. The radial pulse is palpated distally on the lateral (thumb) side of the forearm.

39. b. The patient can tell you whether he feels dyspneic (short of breath), or you may be able to see when a patient is experiencing dyspnea. *Apnea* is absence of breathing, *tachypnea* is rapid breathing, and *tachycardia* is rapid heart rate.

40. b. The elasticity of the skin (turgor) indicates the patient's state of hydration. When the skin is pinched, it should return to its original shape quickly. If the skin remains pinched or the natural contour returns slowly, this is called *tenting* (decreased skin turgor) and indicates dehydration.

41. b. All ribs attach to the spine in the back. In the front, pairs 1 through 10 attach to the sternum with cartilage, but the last two pairs do not articulate with anything. This makes it difficult to fracture these ribs; however, they can cause serious injury to the underlying organs of the upper abdominal quadrants (e.g., lungs, liver, and spleen).

42. d. *Masticate* means to chew; a *machete* is a large knife; *crunch* could be the noise of a bone fracturing (though it is not a medical term). *Crepitation* is the term for broken bone ends rubbing against each other.

43. d. Smooth muscle is found in the lower airways, blood vessels, and intestines. Smooth muscle can relax or contract to alter the inner lumen diameter of the vessels.

44. d. The ileum, pubis, and ischium are parts of the pelvis and the acetabulum is the socket on the external surface of the pelvis that receives the head of the femur.

45. b. The three divisions of the sternum from top to bottom are the manubrium, sternum, and xiphoid process.

46. b. The humerus is the bone of the upper arm. The lower arm contains the radius and ulna, and the lower leg contains the tibia and fibula.

47. d. The CNS includes the brain, brain stem, and spinal cord. The peripheral nervous system (PNS) includes everything outside of the CNS.

48. c. HEENT is a mnemonic for head, eyes, ears, nose, and throat.

49. d. The nervous system is subdivided into voluntary and involuntary. The autonomic nervous system manages the involuntary nervous system and glands and is further subdivided into the sympathetic and parasympathetic nervous systems.

50. b. Sensory nerves carry impulses from the brain to the body and from the body back to the brain. Specifically, afferent neurons carry impulses from the body to the brain and efferent neurons carry impulses from the brain to the body.

51. a. The autonomic nervous system manages the involuntary nervous system and glands and is further subdivided into the sympathetic and parasympathetic nervous systems. When the sympathetic nervous system is stimulated, the heart rate increases.

52. a. Skin is an organ that covers the entire body. It is the largest organ of the human body and accounts for about 15 percent of body weight.

53. a. The second layer of skin, the dermis, contains blood vessels, sensory nerves, sweat glands, oil glands, and hair follicles.

54. a. The thyroid produces hormones that tell the body how fast or slow to work and use energy.

55. c. The epidermis contains four layers, except for the palms of the hands and the soles of the feet where the epidermis is thicker.

56. c. The endocrine system produces secretions (hormones) that are released and distributed by way of the bloodstream.

57. b. The pancreas produces insulin; the adrenal glands produce epinephrine and norepinephrine; the thyroid releases hormones that regulate metabolism, growth, and development; gonads produce hormones for reproduction and sex attributes.

58. a. The ovaries and testes (or gonads) collectively produce sex attributes and reproductive hormones.

59. b. Diabetes mellitus is a chronic disease of the endocrine system. The number of people affected by this disease is growing in alarming numbers each year and so are the EMS calls related to diabetic emergencies.

60. a. Kidneys do not produce or release hormones. The pituitary is the master gland, the thymus produces hormones that help in the development of the immune system, and the adrenal glands produce epinephrine and norepinephrine.

61. d. The diaphragm is the major muscle of breathing. It is dome-shaped and separates the chest and abdominal cavities.

62. b. The trachea extends from the larynx to the bronchi.

63. c. Smooth muscle or involuntary muscle is located in the respiratory tract, blood vessels, and most of the intestines and urinary system.

64. a. Gas exchange occurs in the alveoli and pulmonary capillaries that surround them.

65. d. The epiglottis is a flap of cartilage that closes over the trachea during swallowing to prevent aspiration into the lungs.

66. a. The primary respiratory center controlling the stimulus to breathe is located in the medulla oblongata in the brain stem.

67. b. The body eliminates carbon dioxide during exhalation.

68. d. *Hypoxia* is the absence or shortage of oxygen in the tissues (cells) of the body.

69. b. The major functions of the skin include temperature, water, and electrolyte regulation; protection from the environment; and sensing touch.

70. a. One of the major functions of the skin is to protect the body from the environment, by keeping bacteria and other sources of infection out.

71. a. The intercostal muscles (muscles between the ribs) are skeletal muscles.

72. d. The contraction of a muscle results in movement of a body part.

73. a. The majority of blood cells are formed in the bone marrow located within bones (e.g., ends of long bones, flat bones of the head and pelvis, ribs, and vertebral bodies).

74. b. The skull, thorax, and spinal column protect the vital organs of the body (e.g., brain, heart, and lungs).

75. b. A *pathological fracture* is a fracture of a bone weakened by disease such as osteoporosis.

Chapter 5: Principles of Pathophysiology

1. c. An uncomplicated fracture of the tibia, fibula, or humerus can result in a blood loss of 500 mL over the first two hours, whereas a femur fracture can cause a 1,000-mL loss.

2. b. A sprain is a sudden and sometimes severe twisting of a joint with stretching or tearing of ligaments.

3. c. A heart attack occurs when heart muscle dies from lack of oxygenation. Stroke, seizure, and spinal cord injury (SCI) occur as a result of an event affecting the brain, spinal cord, or both.

4. a. A knee dislocation can completely disrupt the blood supply to the lower leg when the tibia is displaced to the posterior, compressing the posterior tibial artery. The elbow, when dislocated, can threaten the brachial artery and blood supply to the arm.

5. a. A recent infection and the distinctive seal-like barking cough are classic signs of croup.

6. c. Bronchiolitis affects the lower airways. Croup and epiglottitis affect the upper airway, and emphysema does not appear in children less than 2 years old.

7. d. Wheezing is caused by constriction of the lower airways and may be heard on both inspiration and exhalation.

8. c. Pneumothorax means air in the chest. This is an abnormal condition that can progress to a life-threatening condition called tension pneumothorax, with a collapse of one or both lungs.

9. c. A pulmonary embolism is the blockage of a pulmonary artery by foreign matter such as a piece of blood clot that has broken away from a pelvic or deep leg vein.

10. a. When cardiac pumping is insufficient to meet the circulatory demand of the body, it is called cardiac or heart failure. Two major problems that occur with failure are that cardiac output decreases and blood backs up in the venous system.

11. c. Hypertension is a devastating disease that affects the cardiovascular system in two ways. It increases the workload on the heart and enlarges the left ventricle, and it accelerates coronary artery disease.

12. d. A TIA or mini-stroke is a temporary occlusion of an artery to the brain caused by a blood clot. The major difference between a TIA and a stroke is that the TIA has no lasting effect.

13. b. A seizure is a sudden temporary change in behavior, sensory, or motor activity due to an excessive or chaotic electrical discharge of one or more groups of neurons in the brain.

14. c. Compensated shock is characterized by signs and symptoms of shock with normal or high blood pressure. Decompensated shock is characterized by signs and symptoms of shock with hypotension. Irreversible shock is characterized by severe hypotension and shutdown of major organs. Neurogenic shock produces hypotension.

15. a. Cardiogenic shock is associated with tachycardia or bradycardia. The slow heart rate is typically associated with a heart attack.

16. a. The formula for blood pressure is: BP = CO × SVR

17. c. People with diabetes either do not produce enough insulin (hormone) to regulate the blood sugar level (type I) or are relatively resistant to whatever insulin is produced (type II). Because of a hormonal imbalance, the blood sugar level may become too high (hyperglycemia) or too low (hypoglycemia).

18. a. In addition, insulin prevents the breakdown of fat tissue in the body. Glucagon and epinephrine have the opposite effects, raising the blood sugar. Norepinephrine produces effects that increase the heart rate and blood pressure.

19. d. A concussion is a mild closed-head injury that results in a transient loss of brain function (stunned) with or without a loss of consciousness. Anyone who has a concussion should be seen by a physician for an evaluation of the extent of the injury.

20. d. Diabetic neuropathy causes sensory deficits from chronic nerve damage. The loss of pain sensation in the feet is why they often develop ulcers that are far advanced before they seek treatment. Similarly, a diabetic patient may suffer atypical symptoms from myocardial ischemia.

21. d. A dark, black, or tarry stool may indicate upper gastrointestinal bleeding or the ingestion of iron or bismuth preparations, such as antacids.

22. a. Abdominal trauma often goes unrecognized because the MOI is often not fully appreciated or goes unrecognized. The solid organs when injured create large blood loss. Therefore, when a patient has shock with an unexplained source, assume there is an abdominal injury.

23. b. The major cause of COPD is cigarette smoking. Industrial inhalants, air pollution, and tuberculosis also contribute to the condition.

24. c. People with asthma have extra-sensitive bronchial airways that are easily irritated. When irritated, bronchospasm, increased mucus production, swelling, and edema create partially or complete reversible acute airflow obstructions in the lower airway.

25. c. Rales is fluid in the lungs, peripheral edema is fluid in the extremities, and rabies is a viral disease that causes inflammation of the brain.

Chapter 6: Life Span Development

1. d. Adolescents have the same respiratory rate range as adults.

2. b. The basics of language are usually mastered by the age of 36 months.

3. a. The normal heart rate at birth is 100 to 160 beats per minutes. It gradually slows to an average of 120 beats per minute during the first year of life.

4. a. Adolescents have the same respiratory rate range as adults.

5. c. Primary teeth are lost, and replacement with permanent teeth begins, in the school-age group.

6. a. Infants have higher metabolic and oxygen consumption rates. Thus, they have higher respiratory rates that may lead to rapid heat and fluid loss through exhaling condensation and warm air.

7. a. During the first month of life, the infant grows by approximately 30 grams per day. As a result, the infant's weight should double by 4 to 6 months, and triple by 9 to 12 months.

8. a. Normal vital signs depend on the patient's physical and health status. The normal temperature remains 98.6 degrees Fahrenheit.

9. b. Though some adolescents continue growing into their 20s, girls are mostly done growing by age 16, boys by age 18.

10. a. Separation anxiety is a normal milestone during the toddler period at about 18 months.

11. c. School-age children lose the primary (baby) teeth and replace with permanent teeth.

12. d. The secondary sexual characteristics are the external physical characteristics of sexual maturity resulting from the action of sex hormones.

13. b. As a general rule, all body systems are at optimal performance in early adulthood between 19 and 26 years of age.

14. c. Statistically, accidents are the leading cause of death in this age group.

15. c. Vision predictably changes in middle adulthood and hearing decreases, but to a variable degree among people.

16. d. In late adulthood, changes result in decreased excretion of fluid, salts, and waste products. Often it becomes necessary to decrease dosages in medications to avoid toxicity.

17. a. Decreased iron levels from poor nutrition or malabsorption further decrease the levels of red blood cells making low-grade anemia relatively common (though not normal) in late adulthood.

18. a. The myocardium (heart muscle) is less able to respond to exercise because the muscle is less elastic. This leads to an increased workload on the aging heart.

19. a. Blood vessel walls thicken, often due to arteriosclerosis. The result is increased peripheral vascular resistance with variable reduction in organ blood flow.

20. c. Some medical considerations common during middle adulthood include cardiovascular disease, cancer, difficulty in controlling weight, and beginning of menopause in women (usually in the late 40s and early 50s).

21. c. Virtually all sensory systems exhibit decreased responsiveness during late adulthood. Nondescript abdominal pain in an older patient may be due to a serious disease, and they may be unable to sense the pain appropriately.

22. b. Normal aging results in a loss of neurons and neurotransmitters. The clinical effects are variable and generally the sleep–wake cycle is disturbed.

23. a. Diminished visual acuity combined with decreased kinesthetic (body position) sensation results in falling. In addition, decreased vision and hearing make driving potentially dangerous.

24. a. Older persons often have an ineffective cough reflex due not only to the weakened chest wall and diaphragm, but also due to weakened bone structure in the ribs, vertebrae, and sternum.

25. a. Death of friends and companions is another major concern.

Chapter 7: Lifting and Moving Patients

1. b. Back injury from improper lifting is the number one physical cause for leaving the EMS profession.

2. b. *Supination* means to turn or move to a face-up position; *proprioception* is the body's awareness of itself in respect to its surroundings; *hydraulics* refers to practical applications of liquid in motion.

3. a. Keeping the back straight and locked with lifting is an example of good body mechanics.

4. b. Keeping the weight close to the body is another example of good body mechanics.

5. a. The higher the center of gravity, the easier it becomes to tip the load.

6. b. The four-person lift is not always possible or necessary, and therefore is not commonly used. The lift-in stretcher with one EMT on each side is still utilized with older model stretchers, but is not common anymore. Today, numerous roll-in-type stretchers are available and used to help reduce the risk of back injury.

7. d. The age and weight of a patient are important factors in considering which type of carrying device to use, but a suspected spinal injury is the most critical factor. A carrying device with spinal immobilization is needed to protect a patient from further spinal injury.

8. c. Patients who are apneic, pulseless, or have a suspected spinal injury should be moved with a long backboard. A patient contaminated with hazardous materials can ambulate if possible, or will be carried on a long backboard through a decontamination area.

9. b. Another example of good body mechanics is to avoid leaning to the opposite side when carrying an object with one hand.

10. c. The actions in each of the other answers require two hands to perform.

11. c. Securing a patient to a carrying device before moving her up or down stairs significantly helps to reduce the risk of injury to both rescuers and patient.

12. c. Most basements have a stairway access. Using a stair chair for a conscious patient is ideal for this type of move. Moving a patient on stairs using a Reeves stretcher or long backboard may cause the patient to slide on the device, creating stress for the patient and possible injury to the rescuers who must compensate for the slippage.

13. d. Twisting while lifting, reaching, or moving is dangerous and is never recommended.

14. a. Keeping the load close to the body when reaching and lifting is an example of good body mechanics.

15. d. When reaching is necessary, keep the back straight and locked, the distance to reach short, and the time spent reaching very short.

16. c. When reaching is necessary, keep the back straight and locked, the distance to reach short, and the time spent reaching very short.

17. c. Good body mechanics for lifting include keeping the weight of the load close to the body.

18. a. Pulling or pushing anything while reaching overhead is dangerous and is not an example of good body mechanics.

19. b. *Urgent* and *nonurgent* are the two terms typically used to describe moves carried out by the EMT. A patient with a rapidly deteriorating condition would warrant an urgent move.

20. d. In the absence of a suspected spinal injury, most EMTs will allow the patient to assume a position of comfort.

21. a. *Urgent* and *nonurgent* are the two terms typically used to describe moves carried out by the EMT.

A patient who is at risk or has a rapidly deteriorating condition would warrant an urgent move.

22. c. Rapidly moving this patient out of the hot environment is appropriate management. A seizing patient lying on the floor, an entrapped patient in a stable vehicle with a non-life-threatening injury, and an infant crying in a car seat are all relatively safe and do not require urgent moves.

23. d. The question describes a device called a *flexible* or *Reeves* stretcher.

24. b. The question describes a scoop stretcher.

25. b. The logroll, basket stretcher, and short spine board can be employed without causing further injury to a patient with a suspected spinal injury.

Chapter 8: Airway

1. c. The carina, bronchi, and bronchioles are part of the lower airways.

2. d. The epiglottis is a cartilage flap, the diaphragm is a large muscle that separates the chest and abdomen, and alveoli sacs are located inside the lungs.

3. c. The carina and bronchi are well down into the lower airway. The diaphragm is a muscle of breathing located between the abdomen and chest cavities, and is not part of the airway.

4. b. The mediastinum contains the great vessels and is located in the center of the chest between the lungs.

5. b. Absence of a gag reflex is a reliable indication that the patient cannot protect her own airway.

6. a. An oral pharyngeal airway or OPA would be inserted at this point to keep the tongue from becoming an obstruction in the airway.

7. b. Standard precautions, including gloves, eye protection, and a facemask, must be utilized with either simple or advanced airway techniques, because the risk for exposure is very high.

8. d. The NPA is an excellent airway adjunct for seizing patients or any patient with clenched teeth and an altered mental status.

9. a. Position the head and open the airway with a chin lift. It is fast, easy, and noninvasive.

10. b. If an unresponsive patient is not supine initially, place him in this position as soon as possible to prevent him from falling. The patient can be moved to a long backboard afterward. If the patient is maintaining his airway, then the recovery position is appropriate. A prone or face down position is not appropriate. The patient may suffocate and you will not be able to fully assess him.

11. d. The head-tilt chin-lift maneuver is not appropriate for a patient with a suspected cervical injury. Use the jaw-thrust maneuver instead.

12. c. Open the airway using the head-tilt chin-lift maneuver to assess the airway and listen for breathing.

13. a. For the patient with a suspected head injury, cervical injury must be suspected as well. Maintain manual stabilization of the spine and use the jaw-thrust maneuver to open the airway.

14. d. Cervical stabilization must be maintained until the patient is immobilized on a long backboard. The jaw-thrust maneuver should be used to open and maintain the airway. If the patient loses his gag reflex, an oropharyngeal airway (OPA) should be inserted.

15. d. The jaw-thrust maneuver is a technique used to jut the jaw forward without moving the cervical spine. This is accomplished by the EMT placing his fingers on the angle of the patient's jaw just below the ears and pushing the lower jawbone forward.

16. c. The jaw-thrust maneuver is a technique used to jut the jaw forward without moving the cervical spine.

17. d. By placing both elbows on the same surface as the patient's head, the EMT can stabilize the cervical spine while opening the airway.

18. c. Rigid-tip catheters are not designed to remove large objects such as chunks of food, teeth, or foreign bodies.

19. a. Aspiration is detrimental for any patient. Aspiration causes an immediate problem by creating an airway obstruction and later by causing respiratory infection, permanent lung tissue damage, and in some cases death.

20. a. A rigid-tip catheter is easy to manipulate within the upper airway. The soft-tip or French catheters are better for endotracheal suctioning.

21. c. To avoid depleting a patient of the residual tidal volume, suctioning should be performed after inserting the catheter and while the catheter is being drawn out. Suction for no more than 15 seconds at a time.

22. d. Suctioning is a messy procedure that carries a high risk of exposure for the EMT. At a minimum, anyone who is near the airway while suctioning is

being performed should be wearing gloves, eye protection, and a mask.

23. a. Oxygen delivery is stopped during suctioning. The patient should be suctioned for no more than 15 seconds at a time.

24. c. The rescuer needs to be able to see the patient's airway to observe for vomitus, blood, or other secretions to prevent possible aspiration.

25. d. The length of the distance from the center of the patient's lips to the angle of the jaw is approximately the same distance as from the lips to the back of the throat.

26. a. Properly sized OPAs are designed to keep the tongue from blocking the airway. If the OPA is too small, it will not keep the tongue from obstructing the airway; if it is too large, it will become an obstruction itself.

27. b. Absence of a gag reflex is the indication for use of an OPA. Seizing patients often have clenched teeth, so a nasopharyngeal airway (NPA) is better for them.

28. c. A lubricant is needed to insert an NPA, and a water-soluble jelly is preferred. Petroleum jelly is harmful to lung tissue.

29. b. Stridor is an abnormal breath sound associated with obstruction. The patient is getting air in, but the cyanosis indicates that not enough oxygen is reaching the tissues.

30. a. For a partial obstruction with poor air exchange, the patient needs help clearing the obstruction. Perform the Heimlich maneuver.

Chapter 9: Respiration and Artificial Respiration

1. a. Oxygenated blood from the lungs returns to the heart by way of the left atrium; from there it is pumped into the left ventricle and out into the body.

2. c. Prolonged exhalations are associated with air trapping (as seen in patients with chronic lung disease) and grunting is an abnormal sound that occurs primarily in infants and small toddlers when the child breathes out against a partially closed epiglottis. Grunting is usually a sign of respiratory distress.

3. d. The EMT will assess by looking for signs of distress such as the use of accessory muscles to breathe, irregular breathing patterns, and poor skin color. Then he will listen for audible abnormal breath sounds, auscultate the lungs, and feel for skin temperature and abnormal chest wall movement.

4. d. The pulse oximeter tool is not reliable for every patient in every situation. Take a good look at the patient, too. Slow, deep, and snoring respirations are normal during sleep.

5. b. Follow the ABCs: make sure the airway is open and will remain open, then assess breathing and circulation. With a conscious patient, this usually means just watching to see that the patient is able to maintain his own airway.

6. b. COPD is chronic lung disease, epistaxis is a nosebleed, and diaphoresis is sweating.

7. a. A good mask seal covers both the nose and the mouth of the patient.

8. b. An adult bag mask device can deliver approximately 1,200 mL of air when fully squeezed with two hands. Blowing through a facemask, an adult could deliver a larger volume if needed.

9. a. The recommendation for ventilating a child is to deliver each ventilation over 1 to 1.5 seconds without an oxygen source.

10. b. To avoid any movement of the cervical spine while ventilating a patient with a bag mask device, one rescuer should ventilate and one rescuer should maintain stabilization of the head and neck.

11. b. The AHA recommends at least 800 cc volume during ventilation without supplemental oxygen and a minimum of 600 cc volume with supplemental oxygen.

12. b. Positive pressure ventilation with a bag mask device is indicated when a patient's ventilations are inadequate.

13. a. The jaw-thrust maneuver is used on patients with suspected or actual cervical injury.

14. c. Using a bag mask device requires two hands and often two rescuers. Bag mask devices are disposable and do not require cleaning. Larger volumes of air can be provided through a pocket facemask.

15. c. Bag mask devices are available in adult, child, infant, and premature neonate sizes.

16. a. Nasal prongs are part of the nasal cannula.

17. c. Obtaining a proper mask seal often takes two hands.

18. a. Hyperventilation is no longer recommended. The patient should be hyperoxygenated with ventilations provided once every five seconds and the bag mask device connected to a high-flow oxygen source.

19. d. Before providing ventilations, the airway should be suctioned and an airway adjunct inserted as needed.

20. a. Improved skin color is a sign of improved oxygenation. Rapid breathing, patient resistance, or air movement out of the mouth and nose do not indicate anything about the adequacy of the ventilations.

21. a. Chest rise with equal expansion is a good indication that the ventilations being provided are adequate.

22. c. Auscultating lung sounds during ventilations is the most reliable method of assuring that ventilations are adequate. Pulse oximetry readings can be unreliable and the filling of the reservoir bag only means that the bag is full. Good compliance during squeezing is one indication that ventilations are adequate, but listening directly to the lungs is more reliable.

23. a. Check to see if an airway adjunct has been inserted properly. The tongue is the most common cause of airway obstruction in any patient.

24. a. An inadequate mask seal will cause leaking. It is common for one rescuer ventilating with a bag mask device to have a problem making a good mask seal.

25. c. Decreased or absent lung sounds, no chest rise, and difficulty squeezing the bag are clear indications that ventilations are inadequate and some adjustments should be made quickly.

26. c. Making an adequate mask seal requires the rescuer to use both hands. This technique should be attempted first.

27. a. The use of a FROPVD can cause a pneumothorax and gastric distention. However, an audible alarm will sound when the relief valve is activated.

28. d. The device does have to be cleaned, the parts are not inexpensive, and the device does use a lot of oxygen.

29. d. Gastric distention and barotrauma (pneumothorax) are major disadvantages to the use of the FROPVD.

30. b. The rate is 1.5 to 2 seconds for adults and 1 to 1.5 seconds for infants and children. With an oxygen source attached, deliver the ventilation over 1 second for all patients.

31. b. A partial stoma means that the patient's airway is still partially open through the oropharynx and during ventilations the openings must be sealed to prevent a leak.

32. d. Mucus plugs and thick secretions can cause an obstruction, which is often the reason EMS is called.

33. a. All oxygen cylinders must be hydrostatically tested on a regular basis.

34. c. The oxygen cylinder only stores oxygen; the bag mask device, pocket facemask, and pressure regulator are oxygen delivery devices.

35. d. Suction and airway adjuncts are not considered components of an oxygen delivery system.

36. a. The patient receives oxygen from both the reservoir bag and the supply line (oxygen tubing).

37. d. Patients with apnea, respiratory arrest, and cardiac arrest require assisted ventilations.

38. c. The non-rebreather mask (NRB) delivers approximately a 90 percent concentration of oxygen.

39. c. There is a mask made to fit over stomas; however, a NRB can be placed over the stoma and is the preferred oxygen delivery device for a stoma patient with respiratory distress.

40. c. There is no need to distress a patient further by trying to force a facemask on. When a patient adamantly refuses a mask, administer oxygen with a nasal cannula.

41. d. A sick, crying child gets blow-by oxygen; a newly born with poor respiratory effort one minute after birth gets assisted ventilations; a woman in active labor with nausea gets a cannula. Until the reason for the fainting is discovered, the COPD patient gets high-flow oxygen by NRB if tolerated.

42. c. Unless the patient is injured or has a serious condition that requires extra oxygenation, the patient can be left on the same liter flow as found.

43. d. Severe hypoxia, mouth breathing, and poor respiratory effort are relative contraindications for use of a nasal cannula.

44. b. The nasal cannula is easy to use, is more comfortable than a facemask, and does not cause nausea or require weaning.

45. b. For the unresponsive patient with a gag reflex, an NPA is the appropriate airway adjunct. The patient requires assisted ventilations once every five seconds. Hyperventilation is no longer recommended; hyperoxygenate instead.

46. c. Cricoid pressure or Sellick's maneuver is commonly used during an intubation attempt to better visualize the patient's vocal cords.

47. a. Shallow respirations, tenderness on the chest, and the mechanism of injury (MOI) suggest that the patient may have rib fractures in addition to the chest bruising. Shallow respirations are a form of guarding that occurs because of the pain that is present with each breath.

48. b. With the possibility of injured ribs, the chest should be splinted. Administer high-flow oxygen and coach the patient to improve ventilations by taking a deep breath regularly.

49. c. You can expect the SpO_2 reading to be high, but most likely it would be inaccurate. CO binds to hemoglobin 200 times better than oxygen, which means that some portion of the blood will be better oxygenated than the rest. The pulse oximeter does not give a reading on this distinction. It only measures the portion of blood with the highest readings.

50. a. The most obvious answer is the best answer. The longer the exposure, the more severe you would expect the symptoms to be.

Chapter 10: Scene Size-Up and Primary Assessment

1. d. It is the EMT's responsibility to complete a scene size-up and ascertain what type of standard precautions are needed; recognize actual or potential safety issues; and attempt to identify the MOI, NOI, or both.

2. b. The EMT should first maintain a high suspicion of danger for this scenario. You would expect a resident who has called EMS late at night to have a light on, unless the resident is blind, unable to reach a light, or the call was made by a third party.

3. d. The symptoms of headache and nausea reported by each household resident suggest the possibility of the flu, food poisoning, or carbon monoxide (CO) poisoning. CO poisoning must be ruled out quickly and corrected if necessary. Call the fire department to obtain CO readings.

4. b. When there are downed powerlines at the scene of an MVC, the EMT must assume that they are live and very dangerous. Automobiles are grounded, so the occupants are safe as long as they stay inside the vehicle.

5. a. Based on the dispatch information, a minimum level of protection will include the use of gloves. Once at the scene, the EMT can decide what additional PPE is needed.

6. a. Pets can be a significant hazard for responders. The EMT may be attacked by a pet that is trying to protect its owner, or the EMT may be distracted from completing an assessment or obtaining information at the scene, or the pet could be injured if it is underfoot during the patient move.

7. c. The term "secure scene" is used by the police once they have attempted to make an actual or potentially violent scene as safe as possible so EMS providers can enter.

8. b. First make sure that the vehicle is turned off, that it is shifted into park, and that the parking brake is applied. This will prevent the vehicle from moving accidentally while you are gaining access to the patient. Letting the air out of the tires is another fast and easy way to stabilize a vehicle and should be considered after ensuring that the engine is off. The use of seat belts or unlocked doors does not affect stabilization of the vehicle.

9. c. Stabilizing an overturned vehicle with cribbing (e.g., blocks of wood) is the appropriate step to take before the fire department arrives. Attempting to move the vehicle could further injure the vehicle occupants or even the responders.

10. b. A burn is a traumatic injury or MOI rather than an illness or NOI.

11. a. The primary injuries you would expect to find from this type of MOI involve the head, face, and neck. Injuries to the chest, abdomen, or extremities would be secondary injuries.

12. b. When an automobile strikes a child pedestrian, the classic injury pattern seen is a blow to the torso, followed by a blow to the legs, and then a head injury when the head is slammed on the hood or the ground.

13. a. Initially, for the safety of the crew and patients, the couple must be kept separated to prevent another escalation. They both need medical attention, but should not be transported in the same ambulance.

14. c. With only one unconscious patient visible and a broken-out windshield, there is no way of knowing if there were any passengers. It is necessary to search the area for other victims.

15. b. The incident commander (IC) will need an accurate count of patients to determine what additional resources will be needed. The triage officer should be triaging patients at this point and will continue to do so. You can get the current patient count and get the information back to the IC, allowing the triage officer to finish his task.

16. b. Scene size-up begins with assessing the scene for safety, including standard precautions, personal safety, crew member safety, and patient and bystander safety. You then determine the MOI/NOI; count or estimate the number of patients; and finally determine what additional resources (if any) are needed.

17. a. There are a number of ways to manage this situation, none of which should include leaving the spouse alone for any amount of time. When it is not possible to wait for someone to come and stay with the spouse, take the spouse along to the hospital.

18. c. With a two-person crew, one ambulance is needed for each critical patient and one ambulance for the two stable patients, for a total of three ambulances.

19. b. Each responder is responsible for personal safety. You should enter the residence and conduct a scene size-up the same as with any other call. Four eyes are better than two, so when your partner approaches and enters the residence he should also conduct a scene size-up.

20. d. The elements of the scene size-up are dynamic and can change quickly. For example, while you are caring for a patient, the spouse may become so distressed that he develops chest pain—and now there are two patients. Reconsideration of the elements of the scene size-up is ongoing during the time spent on the scene.

21. c. In most cases, the decision to call for additional help or to restrain the patient is made after the primary assessment. The fact that police are on the scene does not guarantee your or your partner's personal safety. During the primary assessment of a patient in this type of scenario, it is practical to assure an unobstructed exit.

22. d. Each state has a mandatory reporting procedure for suspected child abuse or neglect. The specific way to report may vary slightly from state to state, but the initial prehospital approach is the same: get the child to the hospital for care and never confront the parent or caregiver with your suspicions.

23. a. This information must be passed on to the ED so that the patient is not returned home before a home assessment is made and the residence is determined to be safe or improved. Some communities have additional resources available to help residents in this type of situation, and EMS can activate those resources.

24. c. A picture is worth a thousand words. Taking a photograph to the ED is an excellent way to help the physician understand the MOI.

25. a. Working in traffic is one of the most dangerous aspects of the EMS field. Rubbernecking is contagious, and the result has often been fatal for rescuers, because the rubbernecking driver becomes distracted by the collision and does not see the rescuers.

26. d. Forming a general impression of a patient means getting a sense of the patient's level of distress and appraising it as mild, moderate, or severe. Threats to life are typically discovered during the initial assessment, whereas MOI, NOI, and scene safety are assessed during the scene size-up.

27. a. Unless the patient is experiencing an allergic reaction, allergy information is not pertinent to forming a general impression of the patient. It is, however, very helpful in making treatment decisions involving the administration of medications.

28. d. AVPU is used to assess mental status. When you see that a patient is aware of you by her watching you, that patient is considered *alert* (A); if the patient is unaware of your presence and you have to speak to get a response, this is considered *verbal* (V); when the patient requires a physical stimulus, this is considered *painful* (P); *unresponsive* (U) is when the patient does not respond to any stimulus.

29. c. When a physical stimulus is required to draw a response from the patient, the rating is P for painful.

30. d. Unless you know the patient, it is difficult to determine the patient's normal or baseline status. It will be necessary to speak with someone who does know the patient to establish if something is different today.

31. d. Unless the child's state is unresponsive, the most reliable information about the child's baseline behavior will come from a parent or caregiver.

32. b. Drooling and epistaxis (nosebleed) can create potentially serious airway problems in unconscious patients; the concern with active TB is disease transmission. Facial fractures raise an immediate and potentially serious concern about airway problems. The injuries may obstruct the airway with swelling, bleeding, or protruding bones, and injured nerves can paralyze facial muscles.

33. c. Look, listen, and feel are the methods used to assess a patient. You are looking to see if the airway is open. The indication of an open airway is the ability of air to enter and exit. If it is not open, you will look to see if there is an obstruction. When a patient is able to talk, you can assess mental status and respiratory effort. When a patient is unconscious or has an altered mental status, you will need to assess the airway by looking, listening, and feeling.

34. a. Absence of pain in the cervical area following a significant MOI does not mean there is no cervical injury. The patient may be distracted by pain in another location, or just stunned by the event and not aware of a minor pain. It is possible to injure the spine without feeling pain immediately.

35. b. Unless the patient has an altered mental status or loss of consciousness, the patient is usually the most reliable source of information regarding the MOI. Often there are no witnesses and not enough information available from the surroundings (environment).

36. a. *Retractions* are increased use of the accessory muscles for breathing. When retractions are present, the patient is working hard to breathe. Labored speech rather than slow speech is associated with inadequate breathing. Stand-alone delayed capillary refill or a low pulse oximeter reading are not reliable findings for inadequate breathing.

37. a. Oxygenation and perfusion status are assessed by looking at the skin and checking for a pulse. Look in the mouth and nose for airway patency.

38. c. Breathing is adequate with a clear airway, a rate in the normal range, and good skin color, temperature, and condition. However, seizures often produce a brief period of apnea, so oxygen administration is appropriate during a seizure and for a short time following a seizure.

39. d. The recumbent position is appropriate for an unresponsive patient who has a clear airway with adequate breathing and circulation. In this position, any secretions that develop will drain out of the mouth.

40. b. The child is wheezing and using accessory muscles (nasal flaring) to breathe, and the skin is pale,

indicating respiratory distress. The child needs oxygen, but it is key to keep the child calm. Upsetting the child may worsen the condition quickly. Begin by administering blow-by oxygen and allow the parent or caregiver to assist.

41. d. The patient most likely has bruised and/or fractured some ribs. This injury produces pain with each respiration, which causes the patient to take shallow respirations and possibly hypoventilate. Administer oxygen by NRB and coach the patient to take deeper inspirations intermittently.

42. d. Yellow is associated with jaundice; moist skin is associated with warm temperatures, overexertion, a stress reaction, or shock; pale skin could be a result of cold, hypoxia, or shock. Cyanosis is clearly a sign of deoxygenation.

43. b. From birth through the first four weeks of life, an infant is an obligate nose breather. Secretions or nasal congestion can be a significant airway obstruction at this age.

44. c. Grunting on expiration, particularly in children, is abnormal and indicates distress.

45. d. Provision of adequate ventilations begins with making a good mask seal and assuring that the chest rises with each squeeze of the bag. The presence of equal breath sounds and improved color also indicate that ventilations are adequate.

46. a. Infants have softer and more flexible airways, and the lung tissue is fragile. With age, the cartilage in the trachea becomes more rigid. The airway tissues in the elderly shrink and lose normal mucous membrane linings. Years of exposure to pollutants inevitably lead to decreased diffusion of gases through the alveoli and a generalized decrease in lung capacity.

47. a. The brachial artery is palpated by pressing the artery against the bone in the medial aspect of the upper arm.

48. b. The steps in the AHA "quick check" for the professional rescuer include: check for responsiveness; if unresponsive, open the airway and check for breathing; if there is no breathing, give two breaths and check for a carotid pulse.

49. d. Arterial bleeding can be life-threatening and must be managed quickly after ensuring that there is an airway and the patient is breathing.

50. a. When a life-threatening problem is identified, it must be managed quickly after ensuring that there is an airway and the patient is breathing.

51. b. Jaundice manifests as yellow eyes, skin, or certain body fluids; it is caused by excess bilirubin (a yellow pigment produced by the normal breakdown of red blood cells) in the blood.

52. b. Sometimes, assessing skin color can be difficult because people come in so many different tones and shades. The sclera of the eyes, the lips, and the nail beds will reveal abnormal skin color (e.g., cyanosis or jaundice) in a person of any color.

53. a. Flushed, hot, and moist skin in an ill patient who has been in warm ambient temperature suggests that he is febrile.

54. d. Cold exposure, infection, pain, or fever can produce these findings.

55. b. In the absence of exposure to cold, a capillary refill time of more than two seconds is delayed and is considered an abnormal finding in a child.

56. a. Because children usually have excellent circulation, delayed capillary refill indicates a circulation problem (e.g., hypoperfusion).

57. a. The goal of the primary assessment is to find and correct life-threatening conditions, prioritize patient care, and make a transport decision.

58. b. Some patients need the definitive care of an ED or OR quickly. Prioritizing the care for a patient and making a transport decision is where the EMT-B can make life-saving decisions for the patient.

59. a. The loss of distal pulses and the finding of a weak central pulse is a clear indication that the blood pressure is very low.

60. b. The airway is open already. Immediate spinal precautions are warranted for this patient because of the MOI and chief complaints.

61. a. When a patient states that he is having difficulty breathing, even though he does not appear to have labored respirations, you must believe him and begin treatment by providing high-flow oxygen. Not treating a patient or incorrectly treating a patient (such as by breathing into a paper bag) may produce serious hypoxia.

62. b. The symptoms are what the patient tells you is concerning him today, and are referred to as the *chief complaint*. Your general impression of the patient, coupled with your objective findings, may support the chief complaint and bring about a field diagnosis.

63. a. It appears that this patient was asleep. When you awoke her, she answered questions appropriately. Not knowing the date without looking at a calendar is normal for any of us. The patient is alert.

64. b. Begin prioritizing the patient based on the more serious problem. Establish a baseline, reassess, and trend your information. From there, you can reprioritize the patient's status.

65. c. The GCS is used to assess the best motor, verbal, and eye-opening responses.

Chapter 11: Vital Signs and Monitoring Devices

1. c. Vital signs are clinical measurements of the respiratory rate, pulse rate, temperature and blood pressure. Other diagnostic measures used in the prehospital setting include pulse oximetry, blood glucose, and capnography.

2. b. Temperature is often referred to as the fourth vital sign. It is an especially important vital sign in children and the elderly. ECG and pulse oximetry readings are diagnostics rather than vital signs.

3. c. Infants use their abdominal muscles for breathing because their chest wall muscles are immature. Watching the belly rise and fall is an easy way to obtain the breathing rate of an infant without touching or disturbing the child.

4. b. Counting the respiratory rate while palpating a pulse is a common method for obtaining an unguarded breathing rate.

5. c. Pulse oximetry is a noninvasive technique that involves an electrode placed on the patient's fingertip and an infrared light beam to measure the oxygen saturation of the blood.

6. d. Pulse oximetry may give false high or low readings under certain conditions. Readings may be falsely high in the presence of carbon monoxide. Chronic smokers have elevated carbon monoxide levels secondary to smoking.

7. c. The normal reading is 95 percent or greater. Look at the patient, not the number. If the patient looks sick and the pulse oximetry reading looks good, then the patient is still sick.

8. d. Severe respiratory distress is defined as increased work of breathing with signs of inadequate oxygenation. Any of the conditions described in the other answers, combined with labored breathing, indicates severe respiratory distress.

9. d. A sustained rapid heart rate with signs of shock (e.g., moist and pale skin) is a serious finding. A slow heart rate in a nondistressed, healthy person is a normal finding. A rate of 160 for a crying newborn is normal, as is a slightly elevated heart rate in a toddler with a fever.

10. c. Palpating the umbilical stump is the quickest and easiest method for obtaining a pulse in a newly born. The pulse should be obtained at 1 and 5 minutes after birth as part of the APGAR score used for assessing a newly born.

11. b. Whenever possible, avoid taking a blood pressure reading on an extremity that is painful, injured, has a shunt or fistula, or on the post-mastectomy side as it can cause pain and as well as inaccurate readings.

12. c. The loss of distal pulses in a pediatric patient is a finding associated with poor perfusion or cold temperatures. When the ambient temperature is warm, consider poor perfusion and look for other findings associated with poor perfusion, such as decreased mental status, bradycardia, and respiratory failure.

13. d. The apical (apex or point of the heart) pulse is typically auscultated on the chest over the heart. In some patients, especially newborns and infants, the apical pulse may be palpated.

14. b. An irregular pulse should be assessed for one full minute to obtain an accurate rate. An irregular pulse does not necessarily indicate shock, and an irregular pulse will be the same on both sides. The term *pulse deficit* is associated with an ECG showing an electrical rate that is faster than the pulse rate.

15. a. Flushed skin is caused by vasodilation; jaundice, or yellow skin, is associated with liver dysfunction; and blood vessel constriction causes skin to become pale and cool rather than hot.

16. d. D-CAP-BTLS stands for deformity, contusion, abrasion, puncture/penetration, burn, tenderness, laceration, and swelling. These are all possible findings associated with the skin. The SAMPLE and OPQRST mnemonics are used for obtaining a focused history and information about pain, respectively. HAZMAT is an abbreviation of *hazardous materials*.

17. c. Evaluation of skin CTC is a direct measure of a patient's circulatory status.

18. a. Pressing on the skin or nail bed will initially cause it to blanch; it should return to normal color within 2 seconds after release of pressure. A capillary refill time of more than 2 seconds is considered abnormal.

19. b. Deoxygenated blood and tissues will appear cyanotic (bluish). *Flushed*, *hot*, and *clammy* are terms associated with vasodilation, and jaundice (yellowing) is associated with liver dysfunction.

20. b. Jaundice is typically seen first in the eyes, where normally they are white. Later, yellowing can be seen in the skin and nail beds.

21. a. An extremity that is red and hot to the touch suggests a local infection. Diabetics are prone to poor distal circulation and vascular disease, which puts them at increased risk for wounds, ulcers, and infections in the lower extremities.

22. d. Persons who are experiencing a new onset of fever are most likely to feel hot, and they could feel dry or moist if they have been sweating. Cool and clammy or cold and moist indicate poor perfusion, whereas warm and pink is normal.

23. b. The longer an extremity has had impaired circulation, the cooler you can expect it to feel.

24. d. Newly developed deep frostbite will cause severely impaired blood flow to the affected area. You can expect the skin to look white or waxy and feel cold and hard to the touch. Discolorations, including black, come later on.

25. a. Severe anaphylactic reaction is shock. The skin color, temperature, and condition (CTC) will be pale, cool, and moist.

26. b. Any patient who has had a loss of consciousness, is still unconscious, or has a new onset of altered mental status should have their blood sugar reading obtained. Finding and correcting low blood sugar is a priority and lifesaving care.

27. a. Infants have great circulation; this is why skin signs, including capillary refill, are very reliable assessment findings.

28. c. Shading both eyes from the ambient light will allow the pupils to dilate in response to the darkness. This is an appropriate method for stimulating a pupillary reaction.

29. a. The size of the pupil is measured in millimeters. Many pocket guides and references include a scale to help measure the exact pupil size in millimeters.

30. a. One of the normal responses of the pupils is to dilate or constrict simultaneously, even if a stimulus is given to only one. This is called the *sympathetic response*.

31. For most people, blood sugar ranges are 80 to 120 mg/dl upon wakening and before meals. Blood sugar charts will show slightly varying ranges based on fasting, after meals, and bedtime. Many protocols use the 80 to 120 mg/dl range.

32. a. A small percentage of the population has unequal pupils as a normal status. Before making any treatment decisions based on abnormal physical findings, remember to first ask the patient if this is normal for her.

33. b. It is very common for elderly patients to fall when they are suffering the effects of a stroke. The fall combined with a new onset of unequal pupils makes the possibility of stroke one of the first things to consider with this patient. Head injury, infection, and medication problems are other possibilities.

34. d. A concussion, fright, and pink eye do not cause a nonreactive response to light. A blinded eye or an artificial eye would have a nonreactive response to light. Remember to first ask the patient if this is normal for him.

35. d. Obtaining an accurate blood pressure with both systolic and diastolic readings is always preferred, in order to establish trends and make good treatment decisions. When this cannot be accomplished because of loud ambient noise, it is reasonable to take a blood pressure by palpation.

36. a. The systolic reading is the first sound and the diastolic reading is the last sound heard. Cardiac output is determined by heart rate x stroke volume, and stroke volume cannot be measured in the prehospital setting.

37. a. The systolic blood pressure is the pressure created within the walls of the arteries when the ventricles (predominately the left) of the heart contract and eject blood out through the aorta.

38. b. The systolic blood pressure is the pressure created within the walls of the arteries when the ventricles (predominately the left) of the heart contract and eject blood out through the aorta.

39. c. The diastolic blood pressure is the pressure created within the walls of the arteries when the ventricles (predominately the left) of the heart are refilling with blood.

40. d. Mercury/glass sphygmomanometers are antiquated now, but the unit of measure mm Hg (millimeters of mercury) is still used today with electronic and tympanic BP devices.

41. c. End-tidal CO_2 (EtCO$_2$) is the concentration of carbon dioxide (CO_2) in the exhaled gas at the end of exhalation. The normal range is 36 to 44 mm Hg.

42. a. A blood pressure obtained by auscultation is more accurate and no more difficult than obtaining the BP by palpation.

43. d. The "E" in SAMPLE is a reminder to inquire about the events leading up to the current call for 9-1-1.

44. d. When it is not possible to get a reliable SAMPLE history from the patient, the EMT-B should attempt to obtain one from family, a caretaker, the patient's personal physician, or anyone else who may have knowledge of the patient's medical history.

45. b. A *symptom* is something the patient tells you about and a *sign* is a finding you detect.

46. b. A *symptom* is something the patient tells you about and a *sign* is a finding you detect.

47. b. *Trending* is the process of obtaining a baseline assessment, repeating the assessment multiple times, and using the information to determine whether the patient is getting better, worse, or not changing. Trending is an important tool in patient care.

48. c. Time and manpower permitting, vital signs should be obtained every 5 minutes on an unstable patient and every 15 minutes on a stable patient.

49. b. In many cases, patients are told to place the Vial of Life in the refrigerator for EMS and other health care professionals (home health aides or nurses) to use as needed.

50. d. The EMT often has a unique perspective in that he can see the way a patient lives at home. When there is evidence that a person is not able to adequately manage activities of daily living, whether due to a condition of new onset or a deterioration of a chronic problem, the EMT has an ethical obligation to report this information to the ED. Some communities have services that the EMT can refer the patient to in an effort to help improve home living conditions.

Chapter 12: Assessment of the Trauma Patient

1. c. Many MOIs are associated with predictable injury patterns. The EMT is trained to visualize the forces that were applied to the body and to look for specific injury patterns, even when injury is not immediately visible or apparent or the patient does not complain of any pain.

2. c. Appreciating the severity of an MOI does not mean that the EMT will be able to recognize all potential injuries or what the patient's final outcome will be. The EMT recognizes shock from findings in the physical exam, not the MOI.

3. a. Critical patients need definitive care at the emergency department rather than on staying on scene. Noncritical patients can be fully assessed on scene prior to transport.

4. a. It is important to talk to the patient and determine his mental status, chief complaint, and level of distress as soon as possible.

5. c. The mechanism of injury (MOI) was significant. He is alert with no loss of consciousness and stable ABCs. The bump on the head is concerning and must be observed closely and the spine immobilized. At this point, he is not a critical patient.

6. b. The secondary assessment is a more detailed exam, which covers the entire body.

7. c. For the patient involved in an MVC who has no apparent injuries or complaints, but has sustained tachycardia, the EMT must consider the possibility of internal bleeding and treat the patient as a high priority.

8. b. Paradoxical motion is associated with multiple rib fractures that have free motion from the rib cage or flail chest. This type of injury is very painful and can be life-threatening.

9. c. The rapid trauma assessment is a tool designed to help the EMT quickly identify and manage life-threatening injuries, and then make a transport decision. For the critical trauma patient, a short scene time with a rapid transport to the trauma center for definitive care is the goal.

10. b. *Crepitus* is the grinding of fractured bones. To find crepitus in the abdomen, flank, or scalp would be very unusual because there are no bones in these areas.

11. d. The mnemonic D-CAP-BTLS represents deformity, contusion, abrasion, puncture/penetration, burn, tenderness, laceration, and swelling. The SAMPLE and OPQRST mnemonics are used for obtaining a focused history and information about pain, respectively. MOI is an abbreviation for *mechanism of injury*.

12. c. Paradoxical movement is associated with flail chest, a fracture consisting of three or more ribs broken in two or more places. The section of ribs will move independently and opposite of the rib cage during inspiration and expiration.

13. b. The medic alert device was a good find and hypoglycemia should be ruled out as soon as possible. However, it is more important to complete the secondary assessment and be thorough in identifying any possible life-threatening conditions, before locating a glucometer or administering oral glucose.

14. c. Prevent the patient from further injury during a seizure by laying him supine; then administer high-flow oxygen. Suctioning a seizing patient is often difficult because of clenched teeth, and the airway should never be pried open. Consider an NPA for seizure patients.

15. d. It is appropriate to stop the secondary assessment and manage a life-threatening injury as soon as it is discovered. For example, if you discover that the patient has stopped breathing while you are assessing the chest for expansion, you would go back to the airway and assist with ventilations.

16. b. The patient's mental status is confusion, and this is very concerning. Altered mental status could be due to traumatic head injury, intoxication, low blood sugar, dementia, or a combination of any of this or other reasons.

17. a. After assessing the mental status the airway, breathing, and circulation must be assessed. The patient is speaking, therefore the airway is open; lung sounds must be assessed next to assure there is no problem with breathing, and then circulation (i.e., distal pulse and blood loss) must be assessed.

18. d. The patient has confusion with blood loss from the ear and high blood pressure, suggesting a skull fracture, with a significant MOI. The scene time should be no longer than 10 minutes with transport to a trauma center and ALS intercept en route.

19. a. The EMT should consider causes other than a normally uncooperative disposition for the behavior of a victim of a serious MOI. Consider hypoxia, head injury, hypoglycemia, or shock as the possible cause of the patient's behavior.

20. d. *Crepitus* is the grinding of fractured bones; finding crepitus in the abdomen would be very unusual because there are no bones in the abdomen.

21. a. A baseline set of vital signs is needed next to help establish any trends and to make treatment decisions. The decision to transport immediately is a good one and the DPE can be done en route. Repeating the primary assessment at any time is also good.

22. d. If the shot was at close range, there should be evidence of powder residue. The caliber, gender of the shooter, and shell type, even if found, are not as helpful for determining if a wound is an entry or exit hole.

23. c. Paradoxical movement and crepitus are associated with flail chest, which may give an asymmetrical appearance.

24. a. Approximately two liters of blood can be lost in the first two hours from a pelvic injury. To prevent any further damage to internal organs, such as the bladder or rectum, the pelvis should be stabilized quickly. Treat actual and potential life-threatening injuries as they are discovered.

25. d. A severe head injury would have a GCS less than 8, a moderate head injury would be 8 to 12, and a mild head injury would be 13 to 15.

26. b. It is typical for a patient to experience soreness in the days following a MVC. The patient may have an underlying condition of arthritis, osteoporosis, or meningitis that has been aggravated by the new injury, but most likely the pain is from muscle strain.

27. a. The EMT should examine the helmet as part of the MOI determination, and take the helmet to the ED. When a helmet shows evidence of damage, the helmet has done its job by keeping the head from absorbing a great deal of mechanical force.

28. c. Recognizing that many MOIs have predictable injury patterns is what gives the EMT a high or low "index of suspicion" for potential or actual injuries.

29. d. For the patient with signs of shock, but no external bleeding, following a traumatic MOI, the EMT must consider internal bleeding as the problem.

30. a. Life-threatening injuries are managed as soon as they are discovered.

Chapter 13: Assessment of the Medical Patient

1. b. Even though the pain is gone now, the patient's description of pain that was sudden in onset and unlike any pain he had experienced before means that the EMT must presume the pain is cardiac until proven otherwise. Make every effort to convince the patient to get evaluated right away.

2. b. Onset, provocation, quality, relief, severity, and time (OPQRST) are the questions related to the history of the present illness or chief complaint.

3. b. Medications provide significant clues to the patient's medical history. The EMT should use any source available when the patient cannot or will not provide necessary information.

4. b. Feeling tired all the time, increased thirst, and frequent urination are signs and symptoms of a new onset of diabetes.

5. a. A scar in the middle of the chest is consistent with cardiac surgery in most cases. Medication bottles in the refrigerator are usually antibiotics or insulin, and inhalers contain medications to assist breathing.

6. a. A patient with an altered mental status or unprotected airway may aspirate while vomiting.

7. c. When a patient is unresponsive and there is no witness to the event, the EMT must take spinal precautions until a cervical injury can be ruled out.

8. b. The assessment steps for an unresponsive medical patient are to do an initial assessment followed by a rapid physical exam, and then obtain baseline vital signs.

9. a. Airway comes first and gets primary consideration throughout care.

10. b. Fever and/or a new rash are considered infectious and contagious until proven otherwise.

11. d. For conscious patients, the focused history and physical exam are routinely performed concurrently.

12. a. Age is demographic information and not part of the SAMPLE history.

13. c. Complete the physical exam and consider intoxication, but rule out the primary causes of altered mental status such as hypoxia, hypoglycemia, stroke, and trauma.

14. a. Airway comes first and gets primary consideration throughout care.

15. b. The assessment steps for an unresponsive medical patient are to do an initial assessment followed by a rapid physical exam, and then obtain baseline vital signs.

16. b. Limit your questions and ask the most important ones first. Phrase your questions so the patient can answer with a "yes" or "no."

17. b. Each of the remaining questions is very important to the patient's present condition.

18. c. Always follow local protocol. The medicine in the patch may or may not be the cause of unresponsiveness. Manage the ABCs first, finish the assessment including obtaining vital signs. Look for multiple patches on the body, and then contact medical control for further directions.

19. a. First, attempt to ask the patient questions. If the patient seems unreliable, then ask someone close to the patient to confirm or refute.

20. c. *Focused history* and *history of present illness or injury* are two expressions used to describe the information about the current event and what led up to it.

21. b. Baseline vital signs are the first complete set of vital signs obtained on a patient. They are used to establish a trend in the patient's condition. The information is then used to make treatment decisions.

22. a. The symptom that is causing the patient the most distress is considered the chief complaint.

23. b. Chest pain is the chief complaint; pale and sweaty skin are signs that you see. The nausea and dyspnea

(difficulty breathing) are the associated symptoms of the chief complaint of chest pain.

24. a. 9-1-1 was called for a reason. An acute coronary syndrome (ACS) must be ruled out at the ED for patients complaining of chest pain—the sooner the better. Time costs heart muscle, and waiting to see if the pain returns could be a fatal mistake.

25. d. Safety first for the patient. Take any measure necessary to assure that the patient does not get injured during the seizure. Manage the ABCs and call for ALS.

26. c. Pacemakers are surgically inserted under the skin, usually in the upper right or left chest. Automated implantable cardioverter defibrillators (AICDs) are implanted in the abdomen.

27. b. Chest pain and shortness of breath (dyspnea) are often associated symptoms. When a patient has either chest pain or dyspnea, the EMT should routinely ask the patient if he is experiencing the other

symptom. This information is very helpful in making a differential diagnosis.

28. d. The Vial of Life is a brief health history form that includes patient demographics, past medical history, allergies, medications, contacts, and health insurance information. The form is rolled up and placed in a plastic container and is typically kept in the refrigerator for health care providers to use as needed.

29. b. Jaundice is associated with hepatitis; the mode of transmission for hepatitis is through contact with body fluids. Gloves, eyewear, and hand washing are the recommended protective measures.

30. d. When caring for coughing patients, place a mask on the patient and yourself. The patient's mask can be an oxygen mask if oxygen is needed. You could ask the patient if she is contagious, but you cannot be sure that her information is reliable.

Chapter 14: Reassessment, Critical Thinking, and Decision Making

1. a. Abdominal pain with hypotension indicates shock.

2. a. Reassessment is necessary to determine any changes in the patient's condition. The purpose is to assess the effectiveness of your care and to determine the need for changes in treatment priorities. This is done by repeating the primary assessment, vital signs, and the focused physical exam.

3. b. Reassessing the patient is necessary to determine if there has been any changes in the patient's condition. The purpose is to assess the effectiveness of your care and to determine the need for changes in treatment priorities.

4. c. The past medical history is important information that should be documented, but it is not part of reassessment.

5. d. Asking the patient if the pain or cause of distress (e.g., difficulty breathing) is improved, worse, or unchanged is typically what is repeated first and most often in reassessment.

6. a. Reassessment is necessary to determine any changes in the patient's condition. The purpose is to assess the effectiveness of care and to determine the need for changes in treatment priorities.

7. a. Repeated diagnostic findings, such as pulse oximetry, blood sugar readings, and ECGs, are used to establish trends. Medication compliance and events leading up to the current episode are part of the focused history.

8. a. *Trending* is the process of obtaining a baseline assessment, repeating the assessment multiple times,

and using the information to determine whether the patient is getting better, worse, or not changing.

9. c. Decreasing blood pressure associated with internal bleeding is a sign of decompensated shock (hypoperfusion). Additional findings include rapid heart rate, cool and clammy skin, and altered mental status.

10. c. Guarded and shallow respirations are a classic finding associated with fractured ribs, because it hurts to take a breath. Prolonged hypoventilation can cause hypoxia, so the patient must be coached to take deeper breaths despite the pain. Initially the patient will resist and high-flow oxygen is needed to compensate for the guarded breathing.

11. d. Treatment for an isolated extremity injury is splinting. Reassessment includes assessing the adequacy of the splint and reassessing distal pulse, motor, and sensory function.

12. c. Reassessing a COPD patient who is on high-flow oxygen includes observing for a decreased respiratory drive. In COPD patients, the stimulus to breathe is abnormal and is driven by low oxygen levels. Prolonged administration of high-flow oxygen may cause the patient's respiratory drive to slow down, so the patient must be coached to increase the breathing rate.

13. c. One of the effects of nitroglycerin is to dilate the coronary arteries. This often causes a drop in blood pressure. Sometimes the blood pressure drops too much, and this condition could worsen the initial cause of chest pain.

14. b. A new complaint of back pain that develops en route to the hospital, while the patient is immobilized to a long backboard, is common. The pain could be caused by the MVC or from lying on the hard board. Loosen the leg straps and allow the patient to flex her knees. This often helps to relieve the pressure on the low back without compromising the cervical spine.

15. a. Assessing in a head-to-toe manner, each body area is reassessed in more detail, including any areas previously assessed or managed earlier.

16. d. The purpose of reassessment is to examine the effectiveness of care and to determine the need for changes in treatment priorities.

17. d. Any competent EMS provider may reassess the patient. The *most* correct answer is that, with time and manpower permitting, the ongoing assessment should be repeated every 5 minutes for an unstable patient.

18. c. Moving the patient out of a supine position has caused the blood pressure to drop, as evidenced by the pale and moist skin. The fastest way to correct this condition is to lay the patient flat and elevate his legs.

19. c. The more observations you can obtain, the better information you have to establish a trend. The minimum number of observations needed to begin trending is three.

20. d. The more observations (e.g., serial assessments) you can obtain, the better information you have to establish a trend.

21. b. Treating a life-threatening condition affecting any of the ABCs is the priority, and doing so may not leave time to complete a thorough reassessment. An example would be treating a patient who is in respiratory or cardiac arrest. The rescuers may be fully involved in CPR and not have time to reassess.

22. b. The patient is stable with an isolated extremity injury. Reassessing vital signs every 15 minutes is appropriate for this patient.

23. c. Treatment for an isolated injury is splinting. Reassessment includes assessing the adequacy of the splint and reassessing distal PMS.

24. a. Allergies are pertinent *medical* information, rather than diagnostic information.

25. b. The presence of JVD in the supine position is a normal finding. When the patient is sitting up or is in high Fowler's position, the presence of JVD would be an abnormal finding.

26. d. Reassessment is warranted whenever there is a change in the patient's condition; otherwise, it is recommended that the conscious patient who is stable with no serious illness or injury be reassessed every 15 minutes. An unstable or potentially unstable patient should be reassessed every 5 minutes.

27. c. The order of assessment for the trauma patient with a significant MOI, following the primary assessment, is: obtain baseline vital signs and SAMPLE history, begin transport, and perform a secondary assessment en route.

28. d. The secondary assessment is usually performed from head to toe in adults and toe to head in young children. However, repeating the exam in the same manner each time, rather than jumping around to various body areas, does help you to avoid missing any areas of the body.

29. b. The secondary assessment is a more thorough examination of the body and may reveal additional findings that were not noted in the primary assessment.

30. c. There are many causes of chest pain and the EMT must gather information from the patient to determine if the pain is cardiac in nature or possibly from another source. An example of a differential diagnosis of chest pain might include cardiac, muscular, pleurisy, pneumonia, and trauma. The answers to questions gathered from the patient or caregiver together with information learned from the assessment will help the EMT exclude possible causes and perhaps narrow the choices. With this information the EMT can better give the proper care.

31. d. For any given chief complaint (i.e., chest pain, difficulty breathing, abdominal pain), there will be associated signs and symptoms that may be present. The EMT should ask about the presence or absence of these associated signs and symptoms. When the associated sign or symptom is present, it is known as a pertinent positive and when it is absent it is called a pertinent negative. The information learned can help to make a proper differential diagnosis.

32. c. Unequal pupils are an abnormal finding; however, in a small percentage of the population this condition is normal for them. When any abnormal finding is noted, first ask the patient if this is normal for her.

33. c. With a little knowledge about medications, the EMT can look at a patient's prescriptions and figure out if the patient is being treated for common conditions such as hypertension, pain, heart problems, and more.

34. d. After the primary assessment, the EMT should obtain vital signs that focus on the chief complaint and do a secondary assessment of the neck and back, followed by a focused assessment and history for a cause of the fainting.

35. c. The EMT should talk to any witness to the event. Of the choices provided, the customer at the checkout would most likely have the most reliable information regarding the loss of consciousness.

Chapter 15: Communications and Documentation

1. b. Getting any treatment order recorded is the best way to protect the EMT from any possible charges of inaccuracies and to maintain quality assurance.

2. c. State the identifier being followed by your identifier; for example, "Dispatch, this is Medic 1."

3. c. To avoid stepping on (breaking into) another transmission, listen and wait for clear air space, then proceed to key the microphone.

4. a. All the information listed in the question is obtained during the scene size-up so that it can be quickly relayed back to dispatch.

5. c. EMS providers are trained to present patient information in a standard format. EDs are familiar with that format and expect to hear reports in that format. Deviating from the standard format can cause confusion and missed information.

6. b. The typical medical radio report is presented in the following order: patient's age, sex, chief complaint, severity, emergency treatment provided, and ETA.

7. a. Ineffective communications, whatever the cause, can create a delay in receiving the patient at the hospital, which in turn can cause delay in further emergency care.

8. a. Standard radio operating procedures are designed to improve communications and reduce errors.

9. a. Background noise can significantly affect communications, making a message unclear or completely misunderstood.

10. b. Hospital registration needs patient demographics, chief complaint, and insurance information. More specific medical information is not required for patient registration.

11. b. Verbal report is given both over the radio, while en route, and in person to the next health care provider taking over care of the patient. These reports are followed up with a written report (patient care report or PCR).

12. c. This may vary from system to system, but the EMT who is managing the patient is the person best prepared to give report.

13. d. Any of these techniques will improve communication with a patient who has these impairments. Although information from the patient may not be reliable, you can use these techniques to make the patient feel better about the transport.

14. a. The use of clear and brief communication over the radio is professional, proper, and expected.

15. d. Children respond to facial expressions. Always keep a smile on when managing children. Getting down to their height is less threatening for them.

16. a. In most cases, all or part of one transmission will get through when two units transmit at the same time.

17. d. The Federal Communications Commission (FCC) is the agency that controls and regulates all radio communications in the United States.

18. c. Slang terms, vulgarity, or any offensive communications should be avoided in all radio transmissions.

19. d. Using a patient's proper name, with the title Mr., Mrs., or Ms., shows respect. If the patient gives permission to use another name, such as a first name or nickname, then it is acceptable to use that name. However, it is disrespectful to use endearing terms such as "dear" or "honey."

20. c. Help the patient put in the hearing aids and use them. Shouting can distort, and not every person who is hearing impaired can read lips or sign.

21. a. Facial expressions, including eye contact, are a universal form of communication.

22. b. You are there to take the patient to the hospital. This is obvious and can be stated without breaching confidentiality or affecting the patient's privacy.

23. c. It is important to relay accurate information to the patient and the patient's family at the scene, without giving false hope or potential outcomes.

24. d. Unless the patient's family members are health care providers who understand medical jargon, the EMT should explain things in lay terms.

25. a. The appropriate method for obtaining a medication order is to give the patient's chief complaint, pertinent information about the physical exam, and focused history; request the order; and confirm the order back to the physician. If you do not understand any part of the order, you must ask the physician to clarify before administering any medication.

26. a. Dispatch is the official timekeeper for the stages of a call and will acknowledge with a time check after each communication from the ambulance.

27. b. The times typically noted on a PCR include: time of dispatch, time en route, time on scene, time off scene, time arriving at the hospital, and time in service.

28. a. Dispatch is the timekeeper and provides all run times.

29. c. In 1970, the NHTSA was established with the Department of Transportation to provide leadership to the EMS community and states.

30. c. The items listed are examples of patient demographics.

31. a. The body of the report includes assessment findings, emergency care provided, and reassessment information, which is needed by the next health care provider to continue care of the patient.

32. d. PCR styles vary from agency to agency and may include boxes to check off and/or a place for narrative. Billing forms require some information about the emergency care provided so that the agency can properly bill for services rendered.

33. b. Military time is used to standardize timekeeping and to minimize time recording errors.

34. b. The GCS score is a cumulative number obtained from the scoring of three factors.

35. c. The patient's ID is demographic information.

36. d. If further assessment of the child reveals no pertinent findings, allow the mother to refuse transport, but recommend follow-up with the child's pediatrician. A person who has been drinking is questionable for competency; a minor needs a parent's consent to refuse treatment; and a victim of violence requires care and mandatory reporting in some states.

37. c. Assessment findings, MOI, treatment recommendations, and implications for refusal should be both discussed with the patient and carefully documented.

38. d. It is a patient's right to refuse all or any part of care. When this occurs, document and ask the patient to sign off; then continue care as permitted and transport.

39. c. Corrections must be made on all copies, and initials and the date must be placed next to the change. When you cannot obtain all copies, an amended form can be completed with the additional information and then distributed the same as the original.

40. c. A PCR that is incomplete, inaccurate, or illegible gives the impression that proper assessment and care was not provided or was provided incorrectly, and the author is attempting to hide something. This is especially so in a court of law.

41. c. Patient confidentiality is of primary concern for any health care provider, whether information is being transmitted in writing or verbally.

42. b. Reporting requirements as to suspected abuse vary from state to state.

43. a. The reporting of suspected child abuse is mandatory in every state. The specific method of reporting varies from state to state.

44. a. Several types of triage tags, each with different features, are used as the first form of documentation at an MCI.

45. b. The use of medical terminology in charting is appropriate as long as it is used and spelled correctly.

46. d. Another example of a pertinent negative is a patient with shortness of breath, but no chest pain, because the two symptoms are typically present together.

47. b. Time of administration and assessment findings before and after the administration of any treatment should be carefully documented.

48. a. Radio failure may complicate the call (e.g., by delaying response or care) and should be documented on the PCR. An exposure is documented on a special incident report; SOPs and route of transport are typically not documented on PCRs.

49. b. A PCR that is incomplete, inaccurate, or illegible gives the impression that proper assessment and care were not provided or were provided incorrectly, and that the author is attempting to hide something.

50. a. The information documented regarding the use of oxygen includes the type of oxygen delivery device (i.e., cannula, non-rebreather mask), the liter flow, and the patient's response to treatment.

Chapter 16: General Pharmacology

1. a. The liver metabolizes most drugs. Drug effects are temporary because the body works to detoxify and eliminate foreign chemicals such as drugs.

2. c. Benadryl is an over-the-counter medication.

3. b. EMTs may assist a patient to take his own nitroglycerin, under orders from medical control.

4. c. A drug usually affects more than one organ or tissue and varies in degree of desired or undesired effects.

5. c. The official name is the same as the generic name and is followed by the initials USP (United States Pharmacopeia) or NF (National Formulary), denoting its listing in one of these official publications.

6. a. The EMS provider is primarily responsible for knowing the generic and brand names of a drug.

7. a. Seizures can cause hypoxia due to brief periods of apnea. The patient needs oxygen first. Further assessment must be completed before determining the need for any additional pharmacological treatment (e.g., glucose for low blood sugar).

8. a. With a history of asthma, a chief complaint of difficulty breathing, and assessment findings of wheezing, anxiety, and confusion, it is appropriate to assist the patient with her own albuterol. Chest tightness is a symptom frequently associated with dyspnea from asthma or an exacerbation of a respiratory condition and is different from cardiac chest pain.

9. d. The signs and symptoms described indicate anaphylactic shock. The airway swelling is of primary concern, making epinephrine the treatment of choice.

10. a. Glutose is a brand or trade name for oral glucose.

11. a. The brand or trade name is a name assigned by the manufacturer, which usually registers the name as a trademark to protect it. One drug may have several trade names. A registered trade name begins with a capital letter and may be followed by the symbol ®.

12. b. Albuterol is the generic name. Ventolin, Proventil, and Combivent are trade names.

13. a. Solutions are liquids that contain dissolved drugs (e.g., eye drops).

14. a. A tablet is a single dose that is shaped like a disc and can be chewed or swallowed whole (e.g., baby aspirin).

15. d. Suspensions are liquids with solid particles mixed in but not dissolved (e.g., activated charcoal).

16. a. Any patient with respiratory distress should receive oxygen first. For the patient with an asthma history and signs and symptoms consistent with an asthma attack, assisting the patient with her own inhaler is appropriate if medical control allows it.

17. d. In anaphylaxis, epinephrine is the primary treatment. It works as a bronchodilator and it decreases vascular permeability.

18. c. Activated charcoal is used to absorb ingested poisons to prevent absorption into the body.

19. a. Epinephrine decreases vascular permeability by constricting blood vessels; this helps to increase the blood pressure. Epinephrine is also a bronchodilator.

20. d. The six "rights" of medication administration are: right patient, right drug, right dose, right route, right time, and right documentation.

21. c. The *classification* of a drug is a categorization based on how the drug works or what it is made of.

22. d. A *contraindication* is something that makes a particular treatment or procedure inadvisable (e.g., giving nitroglycerin to someone who is hypotensive).

23. d. Drugs and drug products are derived from several sources. Epinephrine and insulin are derived from both animals and humans.

24. c. Immunization is the creation of immunity against a particular disease.

25. c. Sublingual drugs are dissolved under the tongue and absorbed across the mucous membrane of the mouth.

26. b. A side effect may be considered desirable or undesirable, depending on the effect it produces. Some of the most common undesirable side effects include headache, nausea, and dizziness.

27. b. Epinephrine increases the heart rate and increases the workload on the heart. In a patient with a pre-existing heart condition or an acute condition such a heart attack, this side effect is significant.

28. b. Nitroglycerin dilates coronary vessels. This increases the blood supply to the heart, thus improving oxygenation to the heart and reducing pain.

29. a. Bronchodilators (e.g., albuterol and epinephrine) increase the heart rate.

30. a. Activated charcoal is used to absorb ingested poisons to prevent absorption into the body.

31. b. A known allergy to bee stings, signs and symptoms of allergic reaction, and hypotension indicate anaphylactic shock.

32. b. Anaphylactic shock is progressing in this patient. Perhaps the auto-injector was not administered correctly or the reaction is severe. Airway management and additional epinephrine are the treatment needed that the EMT can provide.

33. d. Tremors are a side effect of the medication. It is not uncommon for the MDI to be abused and used too much when someone is in distress. When obtaining a focused history, remember to ask how many times the inhaler was used before EMS arrived.

34. b. When a patient experiences an adverse reaction or an undesired side effect, the first thing to do is stop the medication and then provide supportive care for the symptoms. In this case, assist ventilations with high-flow oxygen. Calling for ALS is also appropriate.

35. b. Reassessing a COPD patient who is on high-flow oxygen includes observing for a decreased respiratory drive. In COPD patients, the stimulus to breathe is abnormal and is driven by low oxygen levels. Prolonged administration of high-flow oxygen may cause the patient's respiratory drive to slow down, so the patient must be coached to increase the breathing rate.

Chapter 17: Respiratory Emergencies

1. b. Listening for lung sounds with a stethoscope is essential for the EMT to assess the patient's respiratory status. Begin by listening to the apices (tops) of the lungs in the upper chest. Compare one side of the chest to the other at the same level. Continue listening side to side from top to bottom (bases). Listening on the back in most patients allows for clearer sounds as compared to the chest.

2. a. For most patients, the back provides better listening with a stethoscope due to less muscle mass and adipose (fat) tissue.

3. b. Stridor is an uncommon finding, but should alert you to the possibility of an upper airway obstruction (i.e., croup, epiglottitis, or foreign body obstruction).

4. a. With a history of asthma, a chief complaint of difficulty breathing and dizziness, and assessment findings of wheezing, it is appropriate to assist the patient with her own albuterol. Chest tightness is a symptom frequently associated with dyspnea from asthma or an exacerbation of a respiratory condition, and is different from cardiac chest pain. The tingling in the hands is likely due to hyperventilating and

will subside when the patient can get her breathing rate back to normal.

5. d. A *symptom* is something the patient describes and a *sign* is something you can observe. You cannot always observe when it is difficult for a patient to take a deep breath.

6. b. Give the patient the benefit of the doubt and treat her symptom. Provide high-flow oxygen and reassess. To do otherwise could be disastrous.

7. b. The patient may have fallen asleep. Check for responsiveness first and then assess the ABCs.

8. d. The NRB is the oxygen delivery device of choice for any patient with respiratory distress who can tolerate a mask and has a good respiratory effort.

9. a. A *contraindication* is something that makes a particular treatment or procedure inadvisable. A nasal cannula on a mouth breather would not deliver the oxygen the patient needs.

10. a. The 14-year-old asthma patient needs a dose of her inhaler; medical direction must approve your assisting her with this medication.

11. b. It is appropriate to place the patient on high-flow oxygen by your NRB, not her home oxygen delivery (which is most likely a cannula), and then consider assisting her with her MDI.

12. d. The patient has signs and symptoms of allergic reaction, with respiratory symptoms indicating a progression to anaphylaxis. The administration of epinephrine is indicated.

13. a. The initial management of this patient includes providing a higher concentration of oxygen with a non-rebreather mask, and supportive care such as position of comfort and warmth. Upon further assessment, additional treatment may be found appropriate. Aggressive airway management (e.g., bag mask ventilations) at this point may worsen his condition, and a liter flow of 8 lpm through a cannula is not appropriate.

14. c. The NPA is a great airway adjunct for anyone with a gag reflex, and ventilating at a rate of once every 5 to 6 seconds is the recommended standard for an adult in need of ventilation assistance.

15. a. The goal is to get the medication into the lungs, but coordinating this skill can be easier said than done. Very often the patient's breathing is fast and labored. Coach the patient to exhale, then suck in the medication while inhaling and hold the breath.

16. a. Chest rise and fall, especially in children, is one indication that the ventilations being delivered are effective. Oximetry readings are not completely reliable. Compliance of the bag while you are squeezing is helpful but not completely reliable. Fighting can mean either that the patient is getting better, or that he is hypoxic or has a head injury, so that is not reliable either.

17. d. Each of the answers provided suggests a decline in the patient's condition, thereby indicating the need for ventilatory assistance.

18. c. Seizure patients are great candidates for NPA use, because they often become apneic for a brief time, have clenched teeth, and usually have a gag reflex. The NPA is a safe and easy method of opening the airway with little effort.

19. a. When you are approaching a patient and forming a general impression, the patient's skin color is one of the first indications of how well the patient is perfusing.

20. a. Making sure the mask is tight on the face and making a good seal is the first step in assuring adequate ventilations using a bag mask device.

21. b. Inability to speak, unilateral breath sounds, and unequal chest rise are more often signs of inadequate rather than adequate air exchange.

22. b. The six rights of medication administration are right patient, right drug, right dose, right route, right time, and right documentation.

23. c. Before assisting with the administration of any medication, vital signs and part or all of the focused history must be obtained. The EMT needs a baseline assessment to determine if the patient is getting better, worse, or not changing.

24. b. Albuterol is a bronchodilator, which means it reduces airway constriction.

25. a. Ventilating at a rate of once every 3 to 5 seconds is the recommended standard for a child who is in need of ventilation assistance.

26. a. Keeping the child calm is key. Providing high-flow oxygen by mask (or blow-by oxygen if the child does not tolerate the mask) is the crucial treatment for a sick child in respiratory distress.

27. c. This is the correct sequence for an FBAO in an infant.

28. b. Difficulty swallowing and drooling, together with difficulty breathing, are the classic signs of epiglottitis.

29. a. Croup is caused by viral or other infections including ear infections, which may cause the tissue of the upper airway to swell. The patient may have a mild or severe seal-like barking cough. There will be no noticeable drooling. When home remedies fail, the family then calls EMS.

30. b. After airway and breathing, circulation should be assessed using skin signs, capillary refill, and blood pressure when appropriate.

31. d. Hyperventilation is a respiratory rate greater than that required for normal body function. It is the result of an increased frequency of breathing, an increased volume of air moved, or both. Many disease states cause hyperventilation.

32. a. Dyspneic persons often sit leaning forward on their hands, with the feet dangling. This is known as the

tripod position and suggests moderate to severe respiratory distress.

33. d. Distended neck veins, peripheral edema, and ascites are the most common manifestations of right-sided heart failure (CHF), whatever the underlying cause.

34. a. The patient's inability to speak freely, his tripod position, his poor skin color, and poor lung sounds clearly represent severe respiratory distress. High-flow oxygen is indicated as soon as possible.

35. a. Without further information the patient should not be moved just yet. Begin with assessing and managing the ABCs. Open the airway, use an airway adjunct if the airway does not stay open, assess breathing and administer oxygen as needed, and assess and manage the circulation.

36. c. The patient is unresponsive, with a very slow respiratory rate and heart rate. All actions are appropriate for this patient; however, assisting his ventilations is the higher priority and should be accomplished first.

37. c. The tripod position is sitting up, leaning forward with both arms extended, with hands on the thighs or sitting surface. This position allows expansion of the rib cage and lungs.

38. b. Grunting is typically associated with respiratory distress in infants and children.

39. c. Kussmaul's respirations are deep and rapid respirations associated with conditions that create acidosis in the body, such as diabetic ketoacidosis.

40. b. Colorful sputum tells a lot. Green or yellow signals infection, and pink, red, or black sputum contains blood.

41. b. Smoking or proximity to second-hand smoke kills 1,200 people per day in the United States; it can worsen any respiratory problem.

42. a. Sounds heard through the posterior (back) of a patient are clearer than the front in most cases. This is because there is little or no fat on the back to diminish sounds.

43. d. The oxygen tubing connects to the regulator at one end and to the reservoir bag at the other end.

44. d. The pulse oximeter is a device that measures the saturation of hemoglobin with oxygen; it provides a percentage reading.

45. b. Patients with COPD function at a certain baseline level until an event occurs that causes decompensation. This is known as an acute COPD episode (exacerbation) and is usually when EMS is called for help.

46. a. It takes years to develop chronic obstructive pulmonary disease (COPD); hence, it is a condition of the elderly.

47. b. An asthma attack is bronchospasm and/or bronchoconstriction combined with increased production of mucus, airway swelling, and inflammation.

48. b. Prolonged hyperventilation causes too much carbon dioxide to be blown off. When this happens, the patient begins to experience symptoms of anxiety, dizziness, rapid heart rate, and numbness or tingling in the mouth, hands, and feet.

49. a. Any traumatic injury to the chest can cause difficulty breathing and respiratory distress.

50. c. *Retractions* is a term for the excessive use of respiratory muscles of the neck and chest.

Chapter 18: Cardiac Emergencies

1. a. The aorta is the largest artery in the body.

2. b. The right ventricle pumps blood from the heart to the lungs and the left ventricle pumps blood from the heart out to the body.

3. d. The atrioventricular (tricuspid and mitral) and semilunar (pulmonic and aortic) valves of the heart open and close alternately to promote forward flow of the blood through the heart; this valve action creates the classic heart sounds (lub-dub).

4. a. Unless the patient is hypotensive, let the patient assume a position of comfort.

5. d. Until a cardiac problem can be ruled out, consider chest pain to be a life-threatening event and give the patient high priority.

6. d. The goal when treating a patient who has cardiac chest pain is to reduce the pain and provide rapid transport to the appropriate hospital. The EMT's role is to provide high-flow oxygen; keep the patient calm, thereby preventing any further stress to the heart; assist with nitroglycerin when appropriate; and get the patient ALS.

7. a. The current guidelines are to attach the AED electrodes to patients who are unresponsive, apneic, and pulseless.

8. a. Use of an AED is indicated for a patient who is unresponsive and has no signs of circulation (e.g., apneic and pulseless).

9. a. Use of an AED is indicated for a patient who is unresponsive and has no signs of circulation (e.g., apneic and pulseless).

10. b. The patient is in need of ALS care immediately. Administering oxygen is the priority, and if there are no contraindications, treatment follows with aspirin and assisting with nitroglycerin.

11. a. The patient has all the indications for attaching and turning on an AED: unresponsive, apneic, and pulseless.

12. c. The role of the EMT in the chain of survival is to provide basic life support in the first few minutes of a life-threatening emergency.

13. d. Currently, the standard is to use the same energy settings for defibrillation on all adults.

14. d. Angina pectoris is a severe pain caused by a lack of oxygen to the heart muscle due to a narrowing of one or more coronary arteries. It may be an indication of an impending myocardial infarction. It can occur anytime, even during rest, and should be treated as a medical emergency.

15. a. Fowler's position is the patient lying down, with the upper body elevated at a 45° to 60° angle; in high Fowler's, the upper body is upright, near 90°; in semi-Fowler's position, the patient's upper body is at an angle less than 45°. As this patient has no dyspnea, but does have weakness and dizziness when he mildly exerts himself, his BP may be low, so semi-Fowler's is likely to be the most comfortable position.

16. b. Crackles indicate that fluid is present in the lungs. Fluid responds to gravity, so when you lay a patient down the fluid in the lungs covers more surface area, making oxygen exchange very poor. Sitting upright will be the most comfortable position for the patient and is appropriate unless the BP is very low.

17. d. A decrease in mental status is a sign that the patient is not perfusing adequately. Provide high-flow oxygen and reassess the patient while she is lying down.

18. d. The primary goal in airway management is to make sure that the airway is open, that it stays open, and that the patient is adequately ventilated.

19. b. BLS in a cardiac-arrest scenario begins with assessing for airway, breathing, and pulse; if no breathing or pulse is detected, begin CPR.

20. b. A postarrest patient is unstable even after a successful conversion and requires ALS. Such patients must be closely monitored for the possibility of deteriorating into cardiac arrest again.

21. b. When a cardiac arrest is not witnessed, CPR must be started immediately and continued with little or no interruption. Initially, AED analyses may be performed after two minutes of CPR, with CPR being resumed immediately after delivering a shock or after getting a "No shock" message. Analyses may continue at two-minute intervals with compressors change position.

22. c. V-fib is disorganized electrical conduction that does not allow the heart to produce effective contractions. AEDs are programmed to recognize this rhythm and to indicate "Shock advised."

23. d. The chest pain the patient is describing (pain with breathing in the lower left chest) is not typical cardiac pain. Chest pain with movement such as coughing or deep breathing tends to be muscular pain. Provide oxygen and supportive care.

24. d. The patient should be transported for evaluation even though his chest pain was resolved with nitroglycerin. He may attempt further exertional activity, reproducing the pain or inducing an MI. Oxygen and supportive care en route are appropriate.

25. d. Advanced airway skills and pharmacologic therapy may improve patient outcome in the patient with a cardiac emergency, but they are not a substitute for early defibrillation in a V-fib cardiac arrest.

26. d. The best chance of survival for the patient with cardiac arrest is when advanced airway skills and pharmacologic therapy are available rapidly following cardiac arrest.

27. c. A patient with severe chest pain and hypotension is a critical patient who requires rapid transport and ALS. This patient will not get nitroglycerin even from advanced providers until her BP is higher, but there are other treatments ALS can provide, so begin rapid transport and request ALS en route.

28. a. This patient is unstable and needs rapid transport and ALS. The closest ALS is at the hospital, so begin transport immediately.

29. c. The monophasic defibrillator with escalating doses will provide approximately 200 joules for the first dose. The biphasic defibrillator provides nonescalating defibrillation energy doses of 150 joules. Implanted defibrillators deliver very low energy doses.

30. c. The biphasic defibrillator provides nonescalating defibrillation energy doses of 150 joules.

31. d. A fully automated defibrillator delivers the shock and a semi-automated defibrillator indicates to the user when to provide a shock.

32. d. Fully automated defibrillators have been prescribed for post-discharge cardiac patients for many years. The idea is for a family member to be able to attach the device and turn it on in the event of a cardiac arrest at home.

33. d. Even when the victim of a cardiac arrest has an implanted defibrillator that is firing, the AED defibrillation sequence should not be stopped or delayed. The energy from the implanted defibrillator is not dangerous to caregivers.

34. d. Do not delay early defibrillation. The safest and quickest way to do this is to quickly dry off the patient's chest, attach the electrodes, and begin analyzing.

35. d. Always assess and treat the ABCs in order. Airway—open the airway and insert an adjunct. Breathing—begin ventilations. Circulation—begin CPR if pulseless.

36. d. Every answer provided is a good reason not to attach an AED to a patient who is breathing and/or has a pulse.

37. b. To prevent accidental or inappropriate defibrillation, do not attach an AED to a patient with a pulse or who is breathing.

38. b. The technology used in AEDs today is very good, so it is rare for an AED to give the prompt to shock when the patient does not exhibit a shockable rhythm.

39. c. After a return of spontaneous circulation (ROSC), breathing should be assessed. If spontaneous breathing is not present or is ineffective, assist with bag mask ventilations. Then obtain a blood pressure.

40. a. Do not delay defibrillation. The current recommendation is to complete a two-minute cycle of chest compressions and ventilations prior to analyzing and possibly shocking.

41. b. The recording technology is an advantage of the AED. With this information, the medical director or her designee can review each call for quality assurance.

42. a. There are very few disadvantages to AEDs; the need for ongoing training is the greatest.

43. b. Learning to use an AED is easy for laypersons and health care professionals alike.

44. d. The ventilation to compression ratio in cardiac arrest is 2 ventilations to 30 compressions.

45. b. This technology is referred to as "hands-off" defibrillation because the rescuer presses the "Shock" button without touching the patient.

46. c. Remote or hands-off defibrillation is exceptionally safe for the rescuer.

47. d. Unless there is an acceptable reason to terminate resuscitation, the AED should remain attached and turned on.

48. d. AEDs can be set to recognize ventricular tachycardia (V-tach) as a shockable rhythm. The problem is that this rhythm can produce a pulse for a short time before the patient deteriorates. Technically, this rhythm is shockable when the patient is unstable; however, only advanced EMTs are trained to treat pulsed V-tach this way. This is another reason for not attaching an AED to a patient who has a pulse.

49. d. Finding that the batteries are dead when you need them the most, because you failed to check the AED at the beginning of your shift, is unprofessional and unnecessary.

50. b. Begin CPR as the patient is pulseless. Agonal respirations are ineffective respirations that sometimes present upon dying and when present should not keep you from starting CPR. Many public places such as gyms have an AED as well as staff who have been trained in CPR and are able to help.

51. c. In this scenario, the patient should be shocked when the AED advises.

52. d. Transport should begin as soon as possible, so continue CPR and prepare the patient for transport by placing him on a long backboard. Reanalyze every few minutes.

53. a. In this scenario, the patient should be shocked when the AED advises.

54. c. Refractory V-fib is not uncommon in a cardiac arrest and requires rapid reanalysis and defibrillation as needed.

55. a. For an unwitnessed cardiac arrest, perform two minutes of CPR prior to giving defibrillation.

56. d. This sequence allows the fastest possible delivery of a shock for a victim of cardiac arrest.

57. d. The next pulse check should occur after a set of three shocks, or if the AED reads "No shock advised" before the set of three shocks is delivered.

58. a. Aspirin is a blood thinner that can increase blood flow through the coronary arteries.

59. c. Nitroglycerin is an antianginal drug that relaxes vascular smooth muscle, resulting in peripheral vasodilation. This, in turn, decreases myocardial workload and myocardial oxygen demand and decreases the pain.

60. d. Each chain is only as strong as its weakest link, so each link must have functional and practiced coordination with the next link.

61. c. After a return of pulses, the airway and breathing should be reassessed and assisted if necessary. Following an electrocution, it is common for the patient to remain apneic, because the electrical shock often temporarily paralyzes the breathing muscles.

62. a. Refractory V-fib is not uncommon in a cardiac arrest and requires rapid reanalysis and defibrillation as needed. Until the patient is placed on an ECG monitor and ALS begun, the patient should remained attached to the AED with the unit turned on.

63. c. Always revert to the ABCs. Assure an open and patent airway and assist ventilations if needed.

64. d. Hypoxia, hypothermia, and vomiting are associated with near-drowning.

65. a. Giving a patient's family false hope is never appropriate.

66. c. Every victim of cardiac arrest will need some form of ALS support and follow-up.

67. d. Hands-on practice with a coach yields the best results when training to use an AED.

68. a. Frequent hands-on practice with a coach yields the best results for staying proficient in the use of AEDs.

69. d. Any EMS provider who carries an AED should check it regularly, preferably at the beginning of each shift.

70. a. Dead batteries are the primary reason for AED failure when it is needed to treat a cardiac arrest.

71. b. EMS systems with ACLS-trained personnel. Ideally, for citizens in a community to have the best chance of surviving a cardiac event, as many citizens as possible

should be trained in CPR and AED use, and AEDs should be located in all public areas.

72. b. The links in the AHA "Chain of Survival" are early access, early CPR, early defibrillation, and early ACLS.

73. d. An agency's medical director is the only one who can authorize agency use of the device. Any member of the agency who will use the device must meet the training requirements of the medical director.

74. d. This is the role of the medical director; if she wishes to be more directly involved, that is her option.

75. c. Reviewing each AED case for quality assurance is a great tool for improving future training and patient care.

76. d. Talking with the supervisor is a good and often quick way of getting reassurance about your performance on a call, based on the patient care report. However, discussing the call with the medical director following a full case review can give you more specific feedback and thus help you improve your performance on the next call.

77. d. This is a point of discussion for an advanced provider with knowledge of ECGs and how they correlate to specific pathophysiologic findings.

78. c. ACLS integration with BLS providers is the most likely answer. However, any of these examples, and more, could be discussed with your medical director during review of a cardiac arrest call.

79. a. This is an example of what can be assessed and/or improved as a result of a quality improvement review.

80. c. The goal of the quality improvement team is to identify aspects of the system that can be improved and to develop and implement plans to resolve any weaknesses.

81. b. When an irregular pulse is detected, the EMT should count the pulse for a full minute to obtain an accurate rate.

82. a. Not every patient who gets an implanted defibrillator has had a heart attack in the past, and in many the heart's natural pacemaker still works. The problem is that the sick heart has a tendency to fire irregularly and can change the rhythm to a lethal one.

83. d. Laying the patient down is the right treatment for a drop in blood pressure. The patient needs ALS, so rapid transport is also appropriate. If ALS cannot meet you en route, call medical control to discuss the patient's condition.

84. a. Always follow your local protocols.

85. d. The EMT follows local protocols and medical control, not the orders of the patient's physician.

86. a. These are classic signs of cardiac chest pain.

87. a. The patient's blood pressure is too low; this is a contraindication for the use of nitroglycerin in this patient.

88. d. A drop in blood pressure can cause the patient to feel dizzy or light-headed. Placing him on the stretcher before administering nitroglycerin is an excellent idea.

89. d. Although there are many different brands, the operation of each AED is very similar.

90. d. Always follow the manufacturer's recommendations for use, care, and maintenance.

Chapter 19: Diabetic Emergencies and Altered Mental Status

1. b. Type 2 patients are non-insulin-dependent. Though they may require insulin injections for optimal regulation of blood sugar levels and the prevention of complications, insulin injection is not routinely necessary.

2. b. Insulin requires refrigeration, so check the refrigerator quickly to confirm. Searching for needles or syringes could take a lot longer.

3. b. After forming a general impression, the next step is to complete a primary assessment.

4. b. Until a cervical injury can be ruled out, the EMT should take C-spine precautions, while assessing and managing the ABCs. This should be followed up with a rapid trauma exam and then a baseline set of vital signs. If a glucometer is available, get a blood sugar reading.

5. b. For the patient with AMS and a diabetic history, the safest approach is to assume that the blood sugar is too low and begin treatment. Hypoglycemia is the

more serious condition and can quickly become life-threatening. Of course, calling for ALS, if it is available, is also appropriate.

6. d. Any of the answers are appropriate for this scenario.

7. a. With no further information about the patient's medical history, it is practical for the EMT to expect that the patient might vomit during transport, and to be alert for a potential airway problem.

8. b. Seizing patients tend to clench their teeth, drool, experience brief periods of apnea, and sometimes bite their tongues. The NPA is an excellent adjunct for maintaining the airway until the patient becomes alert enough to remove it on his own.

9. c. Hot, dry skin, together with the sudden change in mental status and weakness, suggest an infection such as a urinary tract infection. With more information, you can rule out other sources of infection (i.e., respiratory or sepsis).

10. c. Patients with acute onset of altered mental status must be assessed first for hypoxia and low blood sugar. Then assess for stroke and cardiac problems.

11. d. Each of these products contains a high concentration of glucose and is commonly used to raise the blood sugar in diabetics.

12. d. The *buccal area* is the space between the cheek and gum. This area and the area under the tongue (sublingual) are highly vascular, which allows for rapid absorption.

13. a. If the patient is not fully alert at this point, transportation should be started. However, many diabetics will refuse transport and the EMT will need to stay on the scene and provide additional care until the patient is fully alert and able to sign a refusal form.

14. b. Always follow local protocols!

15. b. The unresponsive diabetic needs glucose fast. If available, request ALS to meet you en route, provide high-flow oxygen, and begin transport. If ALS is not available, call medical control while en route. Do not administer oral glucose to an unresponsive patient, as this may cause airway obstruction or aspiration.

16. c. The combination of too much insulin and not enough food causes the blood sugar level to drop.

17. a. Appropriate care for the hypoglycemic patient by the EMT includes the use of oral glucose under specific criteria and local protocols.

18. d. Left untreated, hypoglycemia can progress to unresponsiveness, seizures (damage to brain cells), coma, and death.

19. a. Insulin moves sugar molecules from the blood into the cells.

20. d. Febrile seizures are very common in the toddler age group. At this age, the thermoregulatory system is still immature and unable to prevent a fever from rising too quickly. It is the rapid change or spike in temperature that causes the seizures.

21. a. The EMT should be alert for another seizure with a patient who has just experienced a seizure. This is true whether or not the patient has a history of seizures.

22. c. Seizures are a disruption in one or more neurons in the brain. Prolonged seizures can cause brain damage and must be stopped quickly.

23. b. Infection, dehydration, and new-onset diabetes can also cause AMS, but the history makes this patient a high risk for TIAs and stroke.

24. c. The patient has symptoms of stroke and a history that puts him at high risk for stroke. He needs high-flow oxygen, supportive care, and rapid transport to a stroke center.

25. a. The family has described the patient as having stroke symptoms. The fact that the symptoms are resolving quickly are an indication of a mini-stroke (TIA).

26. a. When the body fights an infection, a lot of energy is expended. The diabetic patient can easily use up her glucose reserves when sick or fighting an infection.

27. b. A sudden sickness with fever and AMS suggests an infection. However, hypoglycemia should be ruled out in any patient with AMS.

28. d. The first two conditions to rule out in any patient with an AMS are hypoxia and hypoglycemia.

29. c. With any seizure there is a possibility of traumatic injury. Until you can determine if there was a traumatic injury or not, you must take cervical spine precautions.

30. c. A seizure occurs when there is an excessive or chaotic electrical discharge of one or more groups of neurons in the brain. High-flow oxygen is the appropriate treatment for seizures.

31. b. The fainting (syncope) and loss of speech are stroke symptoms. Continue the focused physical exam and include a stroke score.

32. a. Serial vital signs and neurological assessments (e.g., stroke score) are especially important in making a diagnosis with any neurological event.

33. c. The history, together with the patient's presentation, suggests that the patient may be hypoglycemic and hypothermic. Oral glucose is indicated; however, it is appropriate to administer oxygen and move the patient off the cold floor, provide warmth, and to obtain vital signs first. By the time these actions are completed, ALS will have arrived.

34. a. The patient is presenting with stroke symptoms even though she appears to be young and healthy. Strokes can occur at any age for a variety of reasons.

35. a. The stroke score assesses for facial symmetry, arm (pronator) drift, and abnormal speech.

Chapter 20: Allergic Reaction, Poisoning, and Overdose

1. a. Stridor is associated with the upper airway; wheezing, bronchospasm, and pulmonary edema are associated with the lower airways.

2. c. Signs and symptoms indicating that an allergic reaction *is* progressing to anaphylaxis include respiratory problems, shock, and AMS.

3. b. Benadryl or diphenhydramine is the most common non-prescription antihistamine that is helpful to reverse the effects of histamine release in an allergic reaction. Antihistamines should not replace the administration of epinephrine when indicated.

4. b. Gloves with powder contain the proteins responsible for latex allergies. Studies indicate that 8 to 12 percent of health care workers who are regularly exposed to latex become sensitized and experience a reaction, such as a rash, to the latex.

5. a. Swelling of the lips can progress to swelling of the airway and should be watched carefully.

6. b. The primary assessment and baseline vital signs indicate that the patient is stable. However, the patient is stating that she is having some type of reaction. Provide supportive care and transport her for further evaluation.

7. a. The patient's airway is open and patent, so begin with the basics. Administer high-flow oxygen by NRB and monitor the airway carefully.

8. d. This patient has serious signs indicating that her allergic reaction is progressing to anaphylaxis. It is important to keep her calm and in a position of comfort while you administer high-flow oxygen. This patient is going to need epinephrine and may deteriorate to a state that requires ventilatory assistance. The EMT must anticipate and be prepared for this.

9. a. An unresponsive patient with inadequate respirations and cyanosis is in need of aggressive airway management. Begin by opening the airway; insert an airway adjunct to make sure it stays open, and assist ventilations with a bag mask device.

10. d. EpiPen Jr. is the trade name of a pediatric-dose epinephrine auto-injector.

11. c. The generic name is often an abbreviated form of the drug's chemical name.

12. c. Epinephrine is the main treatment in the management of anaphylaxis, because it is a bronchodilator.

13. a. The epinephrine auto-injector has a safety cap over a recessed needle, so the cap must be removed first. The device is placed against the patient's thigh muscle (preferable with clothing removed). When the device is pressed against the thigh, a spring-activated plunger pushes the needle into the thigh and injects a dose of the drug. It takes a few seconds to empty the container. Record the time of administration and dispose of the injector in a sharps container.

14. b. The form of epinephrine used for injection is a liquid.

15. c. Signs and symptoms of shock and/or respiratory compromise are indications for calling medical control as soon as possible.

16. a. A history of allergies alone is not an indication for the use of epinephrine as a treatment for allergy. The patient must exhibit signs and symptoms of a severe allergic reaction, such as shock and/or respiratory compromise.

17. a. When the patient is exhibiting any sign or symptom of an allergic reaction that is progressing to anaphylaxis, the EMT should call medical control as soon as possible. Do not hesitate to call right away, as anaphylaxis can develop quickly, within minutes.

18. d. Latex is in nearly every medical product we use (e.g., stethoscopes, gloves, tourniquets, bandages, tape); latex is also associated with allergies to foods such as potatoes, bananas, tomatoes, kiwi fruit, papayas, chestnuts, and apricots. The symptoms of a latex reaction include a skin rash and inflammation, respiratory irritation, asthma, and in rare cases, anaphylaxis.

19. d. Many cases of anaphylaxis progress rapidly—within 20 to 30 minutes—from the time of exposure. However, the reaction time can vary from moments to hours.

20. b. The patient is exhibiting local signs of an allergic reaction; this requires continued observation and follow-up with a physician. Transportation to the ED should be strongly recommended in case the condition worsens.

21. c. Any patient with any type of acute anaphylactic reaction needs to be treated with epinephrine. Epinephrine is the main treatment because it acts as a bronchodilator and decreases vascular permeability.

22. d. Because it is a vasoconstrictor, epinephrine decreases the vascular permeability associated with vascular dilation from anaphylaxis.

23. d. The BLS management of anaphylaxis begins with airway maintenance, position of comfort, oxygen administration, and assistance with the administration of an epinephrine self-injector (if the patient has one). Treat for shock and then transport to the nearest hospital.

24. d. An allergic reaction may quickly progress to acute respiratory obstruction and circulatory collapse or anaphylactic shock. The goal in the treatment of anaphylaxis is to rapidly restore respiratory and cardiac efficiency to prevent death.

25. b. Nausea, vomiting, headache, dizziness, seizure, and tachycardia are signs and symptoms of allergic reaction and anaphylaxis. Epinephrine is a very potent drug and a common side effect associated with it is tachycardia.

26. d. Epinephrine works quickly to relieve bronchoconstriction and improve blood pressure. The patient should breathe easier. However, side effects include tachycardia and palpitations.

27. c. Epinephrine should be used with caution in patients who are more than 50 years old and have preexisting dysrhythmias. However, in a life-threatening situation, there is no real contraindication because the medication could be lifesaving.

28. a. The adult auto-injector contains 0.3 mg and the pediatric auto-injector contains 0.15 mg.

29. c. Epinephrine is a very potent drug that increases the workload on the heart. Tachycardia is common in patients of any age following the administration of

epinephrine; those who are over 50 years of age and who have preexisting heart conditions may experience life-threatening dysrhythmias, including ventricular fibrillation.

30. c. Epinephrine is fast acting, taking effect within seconds, but the effects are short (about 10 to 20 minutes).

31. b. Pediatric ingestions of toxic substances account for a significant percentage of the total number of toxic emergencies in the United States. Unattended children and failure to "childproof" homes are the major reasons that children are at high risk for toxic exposures, especially ingestion.

32. c. Carbon monoxide is a colorless and odorless gas that may be inhaled.

33. b. Pesticides may be ingested by eating unwashed fruits or vegetables or may be inhaled during application. However, by and large pesticides get into the body by absorption through the skin. Lead paint and mushrooms are ingested and CO is inhaled.

34. b. Just about any body system may be affected by a toxic substance. The most dangerous toxic substances affect the nervous system, respiratory system, and the endocrine or metabolic systems. The most significant problems occur when substances cause abnormalities in airway, breathing, circulation, or level of consciousness. The type and amount of toxic substance, as well as length of exposure, will have an effect on the severity of the toxic emergency.

35. d. The most dangerous toxic substances affect the nervous system, the respiratory system, and the endocrine or metabolic systems.

36. d. The most significant problems associated with poisoning are those that affect the airway, breathing, and circulation (ABCs).

37. d. The EMT must consider other causes of altered mental status that can resemble intoxication (e.g., hypoxia, hypoglycemia, or trauma) and attempt to rule them out.

38. c. The ABCs are stable, so a focused history and physical exam are appropriate at this point in the scenario.

39. c. The care of a child often includes supportive care for an adult or caregiver of the child. An upset parent may upset the child! That person is often upset or frightened; may have feelings of misgiving, fault, guilt, or remorse; and may need reassurance and understanding.

40. d. Without contaminating yourself or the crew, the patients should be removed from the possible source of the chemical that potentially caused the symptoms. Administer oxygen while obtaining a focused history. If the patients have any chemicals on their clothing, have them remove the contaminated items. Obtain an MSDS and proceed to treat as recommended there.

41. c. This question would be more appropriate for a patient with an allergy than for a possible poisoning.

42. c. Do not wait for EMS. Pediatric ingestions of toxic substances account for a significant percentage of the total number of toxic emergencies.

43. c. As always, begin with the ABCs. Insert an airway adjunct and assist with ventilations, as this patient's respiratory rate and effort are too low.

44. d. The primary assessment of this patient shows an unresponsive patient with snoring respirations and good circulation. Consider taking C-spine precautions until more information is obtained. Unless the patient is deeply unresponsive with no gag reflex, an NPA is the best adjunct.

45. c. Any chemical exposure in the eyes requires quick treatment, with continuous irrigation right through to arrival at the ED. Remove the patient's shirt and any other clothing that may have chemical product on it.

46. d. The generic name of a drug is often an abbreviated form of the drug's chemical name.

47. a. Activated charcoal is administered in a liquid slurry (syrup) form.

48. c. At this point you are out-resourced, with five patients and one ambulance. Declare an MCI, triage the patients, request the appropriate resources, and then begin treatment and transport.

49. a. Call for medical direction whenever you have a concern about a specific treatment. If you know what the product is, calling poison control is another option.

50. c. Calling medical direction for advice is appropriate, but not before managing the ABCs. Consider the use of an NPA for a seizing patient; administer high-flow oxygen and be prepared to suction and ventilate as needed.

51. c. Activated charcoal is a treatment option for aspirin overdose, with orders from medical direction. The patient must be alert and able to swallow to administer activated charcoal.

52. b. Without a blood test, it is not possible to know how much of the toxin was eliminated from the body. Activated charcoal is indicated in this case, with orders from medical direction.

53. c. Medical control may have more specific treatment options for the patient.

54. c. Activated charcoal binds immediately to a variety of substances, inhibiting GI absorption thereof.

55. b. After the primary assessment, it is appropriate to obtain vital signs while you obtain a focused history and proceed with a focused physical exam.

Chapter 21: Abdominal Emergencies

1. d. The hollow organs contained in the abdomen include the stomach, bladder, duodenum, gallbladder, and small and large intestines.

2. c. The peritoneum is the serous membrane that forms the lining of the abdominal cavity; the visceral layer covers and supports many of the abdominal organs; and the parietal layer lines the abdominal cavity. The space between the layers contains a serous (lubricant) fluid.

3. a. Referred pain is pain originating from one area that is sensed in another area. This occurs when the nerves for both areas originated from the same structure in embryonic development. An example of this is diaphragmatic irritation being felt in the shoulder.

4. d. Black stool or blood (melena) suggests at least 100 cc of rapidly lost blood. The source is usually duodenal or jejunal. It must be retained in the gut for eight hours to turn black.

5. b. Patients who are vomiting blood (hematemesis) should be transported with the head and upper body elevated to prevent aspiration. The patient needs oxygen and a mask could cause aspiration if it is not removed quickly. A cannula is safe and effective for vomiting patients.

6. a. The pain associated with kidney stones is acute and severe, often with nausea and vomiting. The pain continues until the stone passes. Typically, patients have flank pain that radiates into the anterior lower quadrant on the involved side. People with kidney stones tend to writhe about in pain, unable to find any comfortable position.

7. b. Numerous conditions that do not originate in the abdomen may also result in acute abdominal pain. Thoracic conditions include pneumonia, spontaneous pneumothorax, and myocardial infarction (MI).

8. b. People with inflammatory conditions such as appendicitis tend to lie quietly because movement usually aggravates their pain.

9. c. There are two major reasons why people with GI emergencies should get nothing by mouth. The first is to rest the GI tract because ingesting food or drink causes the release of digestive enzymes that often worsen most abdominal conditions and the second is to minimize stomach contents in the event surgery is required.

10. a. The physical exam may reveal signs of hypovolemic shock. It is important to distinguish between immediate life-threatening problems and acute problems that are managed in the emergency department.

11. a. Ectopic pregnancy must be ruled out in females of childbearing age presenting with abdominal pain. Ectopic pregnancy is at risk for rupture, which carries a high mortality. Assume it has already ruptured if she is in shock.

12. d. The approach to all GI emergencies is similar regardless of the cause. Administer oxygen, give nothing by mouth, treat for shock when signs of shock are present, consider pain management (call for ALS), and transport by the most appropriate means to the appropriate health care facility.

13. c. Signs and symptoms of an inguinal hernia are no pain, pain or discomfort, nausea or vomiting, and a mass or bulge in the groin or scrotum that can appear gradually over time or suddenly while lifting, bending, straining, coughing, sneezing, or laughing.

14. d. Inguinal hernias require surgical repair. The initial treatment is to let the patient assume the most comfortable, but safe position he can. Lying flat may reduce the bulge and provide relief of pain. Consider getting pain management (ALS) for the transport to the hospital.

15. d. Eating fat causes the gallbladder to contract, releasing vile. Bile contains special enzymes to digest fat so that it may be properly absorbed in the small bowel. If a person has a gallbladder disease, contraction of the gallbladder may lead to distention and pain or an acute attack (cholesystitis).

16. b. Deciding that epigastric pain and "indigestion" are due to gastritis or "heartburn" when they really indicate acute coronary syndrome (ACS) is one of the most commonly missed diagnosed conditions.

17. c. The primary assessment steps are the same for any patient. Assess general appearance, mental status, airway, breathing, and circulation.

18. b. The patient is hypovolemic from GI bleeding and must be treated for shock. Give oxygen, keep the patient warm, raise his legs, and call for ALS, if available, to meet you.

19. c. After forming a general impression of the patient, complete the primary assessment, obtain vital signs, and process with a secondary assessment while obtaining a medical history.

20. a. When a patient has a change in her condition, the EMT should reassess the patient. With the information gathered in the reassessment, the EMT can either maintain or modify the treatment plan.

21. d. The aneurysm formation weakens the wall of the artery; if the aneurysm leaks or ruptures, severe abdominal and back pain as well as shock results. The patient may easily bleed to death. The other conditions listed can cause back pain, but are not associated with a pulsing mass in the abdomen.

22. b. If the patient has not already pulled the oxygen mask away, remove it immediately to prevent possible aspiration.

23. d. The presence of rebound tenderness indicates peritoneal irritation.

24. c. Metabolic problems that may cause abdominal pain include black widow spider bite, lead poisoning, kidney failure anaphylaxis, and diabetic ketoacidosis.

25. c. The most common infection is due to viruses. Patients present with nausea, vomiting, diarrhea, general malaise, and variable degrees of dehydration.

Chapter 22: Hematologic and Renal Emergencies

1. a. Anemia may occur due to any of a number of processes including blood loss, chronic disease, or iron deficiency.

2. d. People with sickle cell anemia have spontaneous sickling of red blood cells (RBCs) in response to low-grade hypoxia, infection, or sometimes no apparent reason at all. The result is a painful and potentially deadly sickle cell crisis.

3. b. Sickle cell anemia is a lifelong disease inherited from both parents.

4. c, Severe pain is the most common symptom in crisis. Between crises, patients may experience minimal symptoms related to severe anemia.

5. d. The immune system is significantly weakened, causing increased risk of infections from certain forms of bacteria (i.e., flu, pneumonia, and salmonella).

6. a. Normal hematocrit (Hct) levels indicate a normal number of RBCs. A high Hct means too many RBCs (polycythemia), and a low Hct level means too few (anemia).

7. d. Hemoglobin is the part of the red blood cell that contains iron and carries oxygen to the lungs and tissues.

8. c. Hemophilia is a rare bleeding disorder in which a clotting factor (XIII) is missing or deficient.

9. d. Red cells, white cells, and platelets are formed in the bone marrow. In adults, active marrow is confined to specific areas of bones. In children, active marrow is also present in the shafts of the long bones.

10. a. About 1 in 5,000 males with hemophilia are born each year.

11. a. People with hemophilia are missing or deficient in clotting factor.

12. c. Bleeding control is the same for any patient. Apply direct pressure, a dressing and bandage, and elevation. An ice pack may be used to help slow bleeding and reduce swelling.

13. c. Mature RBCs circulate in the blood for 120 days. After that they are absorbed by tissues of the reticuloendothelial system (i.e., spleen, tissue macrophages).

14. a. Men have approximately 70 cc's of blood per kg of body weight, whereas women have slightly less, 65 cc per kg. In an adult man, this amount equals approximately five or six liters of blood.

15. c. White blood cells are an important part of the immune system. Infections and high stress can cause high counts of white blood cells.

16. d. Platelets are formed from stem cells in the bone marrow. They form the initial "hemostatic plug" following vascular injury. Clotting proteins then "toughen" and complete the blood clot.

17. a. Suspended within the pale, straw-colored plasma are several types of blood cells (the "formed elements") and dissolved chemicals, minerals, and nutrients.

18. b. Other complications include anemia, hemorrhage, hypotension, chest pain, severe hyperkalemia, and air embolism.

19. b. In patients with enlarged prostates, a sudden onset of urine retention may be precipitated by prolonged attempts to retain urine, immobilization, exposure to cold, and taking certain medications.

20. a. Hypotension is common during and shortly after hemodialysis and can result from a number of causes (i.e., reduction of intravascular volume, changes in electrolyte concentrations).

21. b. Dialysis is a general term for a method, involving a semipermeable membrane, used to separate smaller particles from larger ones, in a liquid mixture. Medically, this refers to hemodialysis. Another form of dialysis is peritoneal dialysis, used on a less sick patient and involves fluid placement into the peritoneal cavity. In this case, the peritoneum itself serves as the dialysis membrane.

22. b. Sometimes if a patient complains of typical flank pain associated with radiation into the anterior lower quadrant, nausea, and vomiting, the most likely possibility is a kidney stone. Similarly, if there is burning with urination and suprapubic pain, a UTI is likely.

23. b. People with a kidney stone are usually unable to find any comfortable position. Pain management and antiemetic for nausea are most helpful in this case.

24. a. Taking a blood pressure on or around the fistula may damage the device or vein.

25. c. Urinary tract infections (UTI) are one of the most common infections encountered in the emergency department. In institutionalized men and women, the incidence of UTI increases markedly. Clinically, a UTI is suspected on the basis of symptoms, painful urination, frequent urination, immediate need to urinate, pain over the bladder, fever, and among the elderly, loss of appetite, and change in mental status to confusion or increased confusion.

Chapter 23: Behavioral and Psychiatric Emergencies and Suicide

1. b. A suicide gesture is something done by a person to ask for help, rather than to die. A suicide attempt occurs when the patient has a true desire to die. A common clinical myth is that people who engage in suicide gestures never really attempt suicide. This is a naïve and potentially deadly assumption.

2. d. A *behavioral emergency* is a display of abnormal behavior, which typically results from a perceived crisis in a person's life.

3. a. An *emotion* is a psychological and physical reaction that is subjectively experienced as a strong feeling.

4. c. Women tend to have better support systems (i.e., family friends). Support systems are an integral part of a person's coping skills.

5. a. Each state, and sometimes locality, has specific regulations governing the handling of mentally ill individuals, including patients who exhibit self-destructive behavior.

6. a. This statement is a classic example of something a person experiencing a behavioral emergency might say or agree to, if asked. The remaining selections involve the patient's history, and a history alone does not indicate that the patient is currently experiencing a behavioral emergency.

7. d. Any major stress or accumulation of minor stresses can lead to psychological crisis (e.g., behavioral emergency).

8. a. A *crisis* is an emotionally significant event or radical change of status in a person's life.

9. b. Any injury or illness creates some form of psychological stress for the patient. How well the patient manages that stress is based on many factors, including past experiences and level of distress. The remaining statements are inaccurate.

10. a. Paranoia is a personality disorder in which the affected individual tends toward excessive or irrational suspicion and distrustfulness of others.

11. d. Any patients who have indicated that they want to harm themselves or have attempted to harm themselves must be transported for evaluation.

12. c. Depression is a dejected state of mind accompanied by feelings of sadness, discouragement, and hopelessness. Patients often exhibit reduced activity levels, an inability to function, and sleep disturbances. Depending on the patient, severe depression may also be accompanied by lack of self-care. This, by itself, could worsen any underlying medical condition. Studies have also shown that depressed people have a higher incidence of cardiovascular disease.

13. c. Numerous cases in the medicolegal literature report serious patient injury from inappropriate restraint techniques. Face down restraint carries a high risk of patient suffocation, especially if the patient is violent.

14. d. Always follow the directions of medical control, as well as your local protocols.

15. a. Personal safety and the safety of the crew is always the first priority. Protecting the patient and bystanders comes next.

16. a. Rapid intervention is necessary for a behavioral emergency, but intervention does not always mean rapid transport. Unless the patient is also experiencing a medical emergency that requires rapid transport, the EMT should be prepared to spend extra time with the patient to avoid further agitating the patient.

17. d. Organic problems can cause or worsen an emotional illness. Be alert for organic or emotional causes (e.g., drug-induced sedation or psychosis).

18. d. Any injury or illness creates some form of psychological stress for the patient. The stress may cause minor behavioral changes or total crisis following a trauma or illness, so the EMT must assess the patient thoroughly to rule out a physical cause.

19. d. The EMT may provoke a violent action by the way she is dressed (e.g., uniform similar to that of a police officer) or behaves (e.g., rushed or aggressive).

20. b. Behavioral clues indicating that a patient could become violent include yelling, cursing, clenched fists, nervous pacing, or verbal or physical threats.

21. d. Aggressive or violent behavior by a patient is classically an attempt to gain control of the situation.

22. a. Physical and chemical restraints are dangerous for the patient and a high risk for the person restraining the patient. Numerous cases in the medicolegal literature report serious patient injury from inappropriate restraint techniques.

23. c. The EMT should attempt to calm the patient by establishing a rapport with the patient using therapeutic interviewing techniques. Despite the need for physical restraint, attempt to help the patient maintain his dignity, and ask for permission to assess him. Limit the physical assessment to vital signs and any other absolutely necessary evaluations.

24. d. During an anxiety or panic attack, the patient will feel as though she is overwhelmed and has lost control. The EMT must assure the patient that he is here to take care of her now and will help her to begin to regain control.

25. c. Restraint options vary from system to system. Always follow medical control and local protocols!

26. a. During a behavioral emergency, the patient may feel overwhelmed or that he has lost control. The EMT must demonstrate control in a calm, professional, and nonthreatening manner to help the patient begin to cope with the present situation.

27. d. The patient's appearance, hygiene, and dress can all provide clues to a possible behavioral or psychiatric disorder. Some people with behavioral problems (both organic and psychiatric) exhibit an abnormal lack of regard for their own personal hygiene.

28. c. Rapid intervention is necessary for a behavioral emergency, but intervention does not always mean rapid transport. Unless the patient is also experiencing a medical emergency that requires rapid transport, the EMT should be prepared to spend extra time with the patient to avoid further upsetting the patient.

29. a. Therapeutic interview techniques include engaging in active listening while limiting interruptions, being supportive and empathetic, and centering questions on the immediate problem.

30. a. Males tend to use more violent means of suicide, and that makes them more successful than females. For the same reason, females make more attempts at suicide than males.

Chapter 24: Bleeding and Shock

1. b. The primary function of the circulatory system is to provide a continuous source of nutrients and oxygen to the tissues.

2. b. The plasma portion of blood carries cells and nutrients to all body tissues.

3. d. The functions of blood include providing nutrients to tissues, sustaining fluid balance, and regulating temperature.

4. a. Venous bleeding is characterized by dark blood with a steady flow.

5. a. Arterial bleeding is characterized by bright red blood with a fast flow that may pulse with each heartbeat.

6. c. Skin abrasions are associated with capillary bleeding, which is characterized by dark blood with very slow bleeding.

7. c. Using gravity to help control bleeding works well. Raising the bleeding extremity above the level of the heart helps to slow bleeding.

8. d. The steps to controlling external bleeding begin with applying direct pressure. If bleeding continues, apply a pressure dressing and elevation of the extremity. A hemostatic dressing may be used if bleeding continues and the last step if all else fails is to apply a tourniquet.

9. d. The EMT should use a tourniquet to control bleeding only when all other methods have failed and the bleeding is life-threatening. Once a tourniquet is applied in the prehospital setting, it cannot be removed.

10. b. Standard precautions are guidelines recommended by the Centers for Disease Control and Preventions for reducing the risk of transmission of bloodborne pathogens and apply to all body fluids and secretions.

11. b. Hepatitis is easily transmitted from persons who exhibit no signs or symptoms of the disease. Health care providers are at risk of exposure when PPE is not used with every single patient.

12. d. Even a large amount of blood poses no risk when there is no contact with it.

13. d. To avoid an airway problem from draining of a nosebleed, have the patient lean forward and instruct him to spit out the blood. Ingested blood causes nausea.

14. d. When a patient who is immobilized to a long board gives notice that she is going to vomit, release the stretcher straps, keep the patient secured to the long backboard, and turn the patient on the board.

15. b. A poor mask seal is the most obvious reason for an air leak.

16. a. The steps to controlling external bleeding include applying direct pressure and elevating the injured area. If bleeding continues, apply a pressure dressing. Ice packs may help to constrict blood vessels and slow bleeding.

17. d. A head, ankle, or spinal injury does not produce enough blood loss to cause shock.

18. d. The diaphragm, liver, large intestine, and right lung are all within reach of a 3-inch knife blade in the URQ of the abdomen.

19. d. Early signs of shock caused by intraabdominal bleeding are persistent tachycardia with normal or low blood pressure. As shock progresses, the blood pressure will drop, and the patient will feel weak, dizzy, or lightheaded and may pass out.

20. b. In the prehospital setting, bowel sounds are not a reliable assessment finding. To properly assess bowel sounds, the evaluator must listen for at least a couple of minutes before the patient moves or any palpation of the abdomen is done. If there is time to listen, the one finding that is significant is complete absence of bowel sounds for at least 2 minutes.

21. c. When a patient is exhibiting signs and symptoms of shock with no apparent reason, the EMT should consider the patient to have intraabdominal bleeding, until it can be ruled out in the ED. Treat the patient for shock!

22. d. This patient is exhibiting signs of decompensating shock. He needs ALS en route to the hospital and will likely require emergency surgery.

23. c. The MOI indicates that the patient needs full spinal immobilization. Any drainage from the ears should not be occluded. The drainage may contain cerebrospinal fluid within blood. The ear should be covered lightly with a gauze dressing that allows nothing in, yet permits continuous drainage.

24. a. The steps in controlling any external hemorrhage begin with applying direct pressure.

25. b. During hypoperfusion, the body shunts blood away from nonvital organs (e.g., skin and intestines) to vital organs (e.g., brain, heart, and lungs). This causes the skin to appear pale, moist, and cool, especially in the extremities and face.

26. c. With severe blood loss, the oxygen-carrying red blood cells are lost and the tissues suffer a decrease in their oxygen supply (hypoxia).

27. c. In an effort to compensate for a loss of blood volume, the body will increase the heart rate and effort and constrict blood vessels to maintain the blood pressure.

28. d. This patient is exhibiting signs of decompensating shock. He needs ALS en route to the hospital, if available.

29. b. The patient could not have lost enough blood from this injury to develop anything but psychogenic shock.

30. d. The blood loss from a single femur fracture over the first hour can be as much as one to two liters. Two femur fractures from a significant MOI like this can quickly produce a state of decompensating shock.

31. c. Studies have shown that patients have the best chance of survival from a significant traumatic MOI if they can reach an OR in less than one hour. This is the "golden hour" concept. Barring extrication, EMS should take no longer than 10 minutes (the "platinum ten") on the scene with this type of patient.

32. d. A significant MOI alone makes a patient a high priority; however, in the less common case when signs of shock are also present, the decision to provide rapid transport is absolute.

33. a. Definitive care of the patient with internal bleeding is most often accomplished in the OR.

34. d. The potential for abdominal trauma is often overlooked or unrecognized in early assessments. This leads to a high mortality for victims of abdominal trauma. The key to correcting this is for the EMS provider to quickly and properly associate certain injury patterns with specific MOIs and make a proper priority treatment decision for the patient. This is one area in which the EMT can make lifesaving decisions.

35. c. The severity of a hemorrhage can best be determined when you can get an estimate of how much blood has been lost.

Chapter 25: Soft-Tissue Injuries and Musculoskeletal Care

1. d. One of the major functions of the skin is to help regulate water and electrolytes in the body. When a large body surface is affected by trauma, such as when it is burned, the patient loses a large amount of fluids; this condition can rapidly lead to hypovolemic shock if fluids are not adequately restored.

2. c. The order of the layers of the skin, from the surface to the underlying tissue or muscle, is the epidermis, dermis, and subcutaneous tissues.

3. d. The subcutaneous tissues are the layers of skin that lie below the dermis and attach the upper layers of skin to the underlying muscles and/or bones.

4. d. Subcutaneous tissue is comprised of fatty tissue and lies below the dermis.

5. a. The first responders have indicated that there is no external bleeding or open wounds. At a minimum, gloves are needed to further assess the patient.

6. a. Abrasions create capillary bleeding, a slow oozing of blood. At a minimum, gloves should be donned prior to examining and treating this patient.

7. c. Scalp wounds can bleed a lot, and any blood in the airway creates a high risk of exposure for the rescuer. Blood that is spit can spray into the rescuer's face. Gloves, eye protection, and a mask are recommended for managing these injuries.

8. a. A soft-tissue injury that involves bone with no broken skin is a closed injury.

9. b. Edema is an abnormal condition that results when fluid leaks into areas of soft tissue.

10. a. A *contusion* is an injury to the soft tissue with no broken skin.

11. a. Facial fractures must be considered. The EMT should palpate the facial bones for stability and crepitus.

12. d. In this case, blood in the eye (*hyphema*) requires no specific treatment by EMS. However, the eye should be examined by a physician to rule out any complications.

13. a. The treatment for soft-tissue injury with a possible fracture includes splinting and applying cold for pain relief.

14. d. An extremity that is red and hot to the touch is a sign of severe infection that requires immediate evaluation and care at the ED.

15. c. A partial-thickness burn covering the upper thigh (less than 9 percent BSA) is classified as a moderate burn.

16. a. The terms *superficial, partial thickness,* and *full thickness* all describe the depth of a burn.

17. b. With no blistering present, this can be called a superficial burn. The BSA involved is the face, at 4.5 percent, and the front of both arms, at 4.5 percent each, for a total of 13.5 percent BSA.

18. a. With no blistering present, this can be called a superficial burn. Because the eyes are involved, however, this is a serious burn that requires the care of a burn specialty unit.

19. b. A superficial or first-degree burn is a mild burn characterized by pain, redness, and heat on the affected area with no blistering or charring.

20. d. The thighs have superficial burns from the splashing; the dermis of the lower legs has been affected, making the injury in that area a partial-thickness burn.

21. b. A second-degree or partial-thickness burn involves the epidermal and dermal layers of the skin.

22. d. The risk for infection comes with damage to layers of the skin below the epidermis.

23. c. The hands are considered a critical body area when affected by burns. The severity of the burn on the hands is also greater than the other areas affected.

24. a. The dermis contains many nerve endings, and a second-degree or partial-thickness burn will produce severe pain in the affected area.

25. d. This will vary depending on the specific body areas involved, but typically a partial-thickness or second-degree burn will not affect subcutaneous fat or blood vessels.

26. a. A full-thickness or third-degree burn involves all the layers of the skin in the affected area.

27. a. The immediate and potentially life-threatening injuries are the airway injuries that resulted from a blast in a confined area. The patient is exhibiting wheezing and may rapidly progress to severe respiratory distress or arrest.

28. c. A full-thickness or third-degree burn involves all layers of the skin in the affected area. The area may appear charred and feel rough. The area around a full-thickness burn may also be affected to a lesser degree and appear blistered and weeping, or may not be affected at all.

29. d. The injury described includes second- and third-degree burns.

30. d. A full-thickness or third-degree burn is characterized as a severe burn that affects all layers of the skin and may affect underlying muscle.

31. a. The description includes partial and full-thickness burns that involve 12% BSA. The most critical factor with this patient is age. The young, the elderly,

and patients with impaired immune systems do not recover well from burn injuries.

32. c. It is not appropriate to remove debris from a burn area, but it is appropriate to flush the area with cool water.

33. b. Determining the source of the burn is part of the scene size-up and identification of the MOI. This must be done before a full assessment can be made and proper treatment begun.

34. b. Management of a superficial burn may include flushing the area with cool water.

35. a. All clothing, including socks and shoes, should be removed, because they could contain some of the chemical and continue the burning process.

36. c. When such a large BSA is affected, a clean and dry sheet can be used to cover and protect the patient during treatment and transport. Always follow local protocol.

37. d. Quick removal of these items is appropriate because they can retain heat and continue to burn. The jewelry (especially rings) must be removed before tissue swelling from edema impairs circulation.

38. b. A circumferential burn on an extremity can constrict blood flow to the distal portion of the extremity, creating a limb-threatening condition.

39. c. Stop the burning process! Flush with water until the chemical is completely removed.

40. a. A bandage is used to keep a dressing in place.

41. a. Never rupture a blister that has developed from a burn. The risk of infection increases significantly when blisters are disturbed.

42. c. In addition to controlling a bleed, the use of a bandage will help reduce the risk of further contamination and possible infection.

43. a. The management of an abdominal evisceration includes the use of a large trauma dressing to cover the contents. The dressing should be moistened and kept warm to help preserve the bowel.

44. a. A blood pressure cuff inflated to occlude venous flow only (no greater than 70 mm Hg) may be used to help control bleeding from an extremity when other methods have not worked.

45. d. The steps for controlling continuous bleeding are direct pressure, elevation, pressure bandage, the use of a hemostatic dressing, and last a tourniquet.

46. d. Wheezing is a sign of respiratory distress. In this case, the MOI is significant (working on a fire scene). Firefighters tend to initially downplay or ignore injury or illness while on the job, and this can cause both a delay in recognizing early signs and symptoms and a delay in treatment.

47. d. Increased tissue damage is a major complication commonly associated with improperly applied dressings. Loss of limb and death may occur, but are not common.

48. b. The use of a tourniquet is a method of last resort for controlling a severe arterial bleed. The tourniquet

should be placed above the open wound. A strap or wide band of cloth can be used to occlude arterial blood flow. Do not use any smaller object, such as string, rope, or wire, as it can cause additional tissue damage at the site where it is applied. Once a tourniquet is applied, it cannot be removed in the prehospital setting; the ED should be notified immediately.

49. b. Keep the extremity elevated above the level of the heart and apply an ice pack.

50. c. Protect yourself first by applying the appropriate PPE for the situation.

51. d. Removing an impaled object from an extremity can cause further damage to blood vessels, nerves, and muscles.

52. d. Control the bleeding and, whenever possible, bring the amputated body part with the patient to the same hospital for possible reattachment or reimplantation.

53. a. The use of dry ice on an amputated body part can cause irreversible tissue damage and failure of reattachment or reimplantation.

54. d. Wet or dry ice should never be placed directly on an amputated part. Freezing can occur and cause irreversible tissue damage, and the opportunity for reattachment or reimplantation may be lost.

55. b. The lenses must be removed as soon as possible. Leaving them in can hold chemical product or residue in and further injure the eye.

56. b. Pepper spray is an oily substance that can be difficult to remove. Do not allow the victim to rub it. Instruct the victim to spit if it is in the mouth, blow the nose, and reinforce the instruction of "no rubbing." Then blot the oil off and flush the area with water.

57. a. Manage the ABCs first! This type of injury can result in respiratory and/or cardiac arrest.

58. b. Do not put yourself in danger. High-voltage wires are commonly buried underground. Call for additional help.

59. a. Most likely, the patient was standing while working on the electrical box. Electricity looks for ground, so check the feet first. Also assess the patient from head to toe in the rapid trauma exam.

60. d. Arc and flash burns can cause external injuries and steam can reach the upper airways. Chemical burns can reach the lower airways.

61. c. Think of the eye as an eviscerated organ. Keep it covered with a moist, sterile dressing and keep it warm.

62. c. A circumferential burn around the chest is a serious injury that can keep the chest wall from expanding properly during breathing.

63. b. The sources of electrical burns are flash, contact, and arcing.

64. a. Management of an avulsion injury includes placing the avulsed tissue back over the affected area and applying a dry sterile dressing and bandage.

65. b. The steps for controlling a continuous bleed are direct pressure, elevation, and pressure dressing. There is no pressure point to use for this type of bleeding.

66. c. Cartilage, tendons, and ligaments are all types of connective tissue, and their function is to aid muscles in movement of the skeleton.

67. c. Phalanges are finger bones.

68. a. The shoulder girdle is made up of the clavicle, humerus, and scapula.

69. a. Musculoskeletal injuries are classified as open or closed.

70. a. A soft-tissue injury with deformity and no opening in the skin is a closed injury.

71. a. A soft-tissue injury with deformity and no opening in the skin is a closed injury.

72. a. Long bones should be splinted in a straight or neutral position to prevent additional damage to bones, vessels, and muscle tissue.

73. d. Dislocations are typically splinted in the position they are found. The patient will be guarding in the best position of comfort for that patient and injury.

74. d. Long bones should be splinted in a straight or neutral position without causing further injury.

75. c. The goal in splinting a dislocation or fracture is to immobilize the bone ends and the joint both above and below the injury.

76. c. The ongoing assessment of an extremity fracture includes reassessing the splint to assure a proper fit and reassessing distal pulse, motor function, and sensation.

77. b. Distal pulses, motor function, and sensation are assessed before and after splinting and during reassessment.

78. b. When a patient experiences tingling and numbness after splinting, the most likely cause is that the splint was applied too tightly. Loosen the splint and reassess.

79. b. A splint that is applied incorrectly, either too tight or too loose, can cause further damage and increased pain and swelling.

80. d. Increased back pain or new back pain is a common complaint of patients who have been immobilized to a long backboard.

81. a. The patient is stable with an isolated extremity injury. This injury should be splinted on the scene.

82. b. At the very least, the patient is going to increase swelling and pain without the proper attention. If the injury is severe, bearing weight will increase the risk of bleeding and loss of function, either temporarily or permanently.

83. d. The injury is not life-threatening and should be assessed and managed accordingly on the scene. The patient needs some psychological support in addition to the care of the traumatic injury. Reassure the patient that you are taking the appropriate measures in the care of her injury.

84. d. A sling and swathe is very effective and commonly used to splint shoulder, humerus, elbow, and forearm musculoskeletal injuries.
85. d. Injuries to the elbow carry a high probability of blood vessel and nerve damage. The brachial artery is the largest blood vessel in the elbow joint.
86. b. The fact that splints can easily be made from many different materials is not an advantage of splinting.

87. b. Splinting and hemorrhage control can be done simultaneously with this type of injury.
88. a. The application of cold helps to reduce and minimize swelling, which helps to reduce pain.
89. b. The MOI and the patient's signs and symptoms suggest rib fractures. Use a sling and swathe to splint her left arm to the chest.
90. c. The carpals and metacarpals are the bones of the hands.

Chapter 26: Chest and Abdominal Trauma

1. b. Fractures of the lower left ribs are often associated with splenic rupture and lower-right ribs with hepatic injury.
2. a. Patients with rib fractures may have deformity to the chest wall. When examined, there may be a feeling of crepitus or an audible crunching noise, the so-called "snap, crackle, pop" of Rice Krispises®.
3. d. Stabilize the flail segment with wide tape extending from stable portions of the chest wall, over the flail segment, and to other stable portions.
4. a. An occlusive dressing provides an airtight seal over a penetrating injury to the chest, back, or abdomen.
5. b. A pericardial tamponade is a condition in which fluid fills the sac around the heart. This sac does not expand, so the fluid keeps the heart from effectively filling during contractions. If this condition is not quickly recognized and managed, the patient will die.
6. a. A penetrating wound to the chest can create what is referred to as a sucking chest wound. Each time the patient inhales, air is drawn into the chest through the wound. The air does not reach the lungs, but instead fills the chest, creating a pneumothorax. An occlusive dressing should be applied quickly.
7. a. An occlusive dressing should be applied immediately to help prevent the development of a pneumothorax or tension pneumothorax.
8. a. The object should be immobilized in place with bulky dressings to prevent further movement of the object.
9. b. For an open wound that is bleeding, direct pressure and bandaging is appropriate. If you suspect that the chest cavity has been penetrated, then apply an occlusive dressing.
10. c. Exposed bowels should be kept moist with a moist dressing and warmth. Never attempt to replace bowel in the abdomen in the prehospital setting.
11. b. In addition to a penetrating abdominal injury, a gunshot wound can also create any of these associated injuries: chest trauma, rib or spinal fractures, and spinal cord injury. The EMT must be highly suspicious of and alert for these potential injuries.
12. c. The knife is not long enough to reach the cervical spine, trachea, or rectum. Spinal injury in other areas should be considered.

13. d. Manage the ABCs, immobilize the patient, and begin rapid transport. Request ALS, if available, to meet you en route.
14. a. Stabilize impaled objects in place unless they interfere with the patient's airway or CPR.
15. c. Cover eviscerations with moist sterile dressings and keep the area warm. Never attempt to replace eviscerated organs.
16. b With impaled objects, the rule is to stabilize impaled objects in place unless they interfere with the patient's airway or CPR. In this case, CPR is needed and the impaled object must be removed to perform chest compressions.
17. b. Trauma affecting any of the components of the urinary tract can lead to bloody urine.
18. a. When the mechanism of injury is blunt, the potential for injury is often underappreciated or not recognized at all.
19. a. Rebound tenderness is the response that occurs when the sudden release of pressure hurts more than the pressure itself.
20. c. The patient's vital signs may reflect early shock, significant pain, or both. At this point, she should assume any position of comfort, which is also safe to transport.
21. d. To properly auscultate bowel sounds, it is necessary to listen for several minutes in a quiet setting. In the prehospital setting, there is often no time for this and the ambient noise is too great.
22. c. Position of comfort, a padded ice pack, and pain management (ALS) and transport.
23. b. Peritonitis is associated with severe pain and abdominal wall muscle spasm.
24. a. Guarding is reflex muscle tensing over an injury or inflammation of the peritoneum. The legs may be drawn up in an effort to reduce the tension of the abdominal muscles.
25. A patient with abdominal trauma should be getting high-flow oxygen by non-rebreather mask. The EMT should be alert for nausea and vomiting and help the patient remove the mask when vomiting occurs.

Chapter 27: Trauma to the Head, Neck, and Spine

1. d. The brain, brain stem, CSF, and spinal cord make up the central nervous system. The peripheral nervous system includes 31 pairs of spinal nerves.
2. a. The brain, brain stem, CSF, and spinal cord make up the central nervous system.
3. d. The autonomic nervous system is the part of the nervous system that controls involuntary muscles and glands.
4. d. One function of cerebrospinal fluid (CSF) is to act as a shock absorber to cushion and protect the brain and spinal cord within the skull and spinal canal.
5. c. The vision control areas are located in the occipital area of the brain.
6. b. The brain stem extends from the brain to the spinal cord.
7. b. The spinal nerves originate in pairs from the spinal cord and extend out to the extremities and trunk of the body.
8. a. The spinal canal is located in the openings of the spinal vertebrae.
9. b. The spinal cord originates at the brain stem and extends down the spinal canal.
10. d. When intracranial pressure (ICP) rises due to a hemorrhage, it can cause the brain to shift downward through the skull.
11. c. It is possible for a patient to have a significant injury (e.g., fractured cervical spine or spinal injury) without any immediately obvious physical or neurological deficits. Various MOIs are associated with certain injury patterns. The EMT must recognize the potential for these injuries and manage the patient with a high index of suspicion for these injuries based on the MOI.
12. c. Being placed on a long backboard, in most cases, is uncomfortable for the patient and may worsen preexisting injuries. Filling the voids when splinting can help make the patient more comfortable during the time spent immobilized.
13. d. The inline neutral position allows the most space in the spinal canal for the spinal cord, thus making this position the safest for moving patients with suspected spinal injury.
14. b. Do no harm! The primary goal in caring for patients who have suspected spinal injury is to get them to the ED without compromising them further.
15. a. Pain or tenderness, especially upon palpation, is a clear indication for immobilizing a patient.
16. b. When you detect an abnormal finding in your assessment, remember to ask the patient whether this is normal for her or is new.
17. c. You may not detect tenderness unless you palpate for it. When an appropriate MOI is present, routinely examine the spine by palpating each vertebra for deformity, crepitus, pain, or tenderness.
18. b. The MOI is significant in this case, so the patient should be immobilized.
19. d. The MOI and the age of the patient are significant factors for deciding to immobilize. Remember, it is possible for a patient to have a significant injury (e.g., fractured cervical spine or spinal injury) without any immediate physical or neurological deficits.
20. c. This scenario can be challenging, especially when the patient is unconscious. A patient who requires suctioning and needs to be immobilized is going to need very close attention. Tilt the board and suction as often as needed. When the patient is alert and can follow instructions, allow the patient to suction as needed.
21. b. After one unsuccessful attempt to place the patient's neck in a neutral position, it is then appropriate to splint it in the position found. Never force the cervical spine into a splint!
22. c. Manual stabilization of the head and neck is maintained until the patient is properly secured to an immobilization device.
23. d. Instruct the patient not to move her head while manual stabilization is undertaken and a cervical collar is applied.
24. b. An isolated extremity injury alone does not indicate a need for cervical immobilization.
25. a. Because the patient is sitting in her vehicle when you reach her, it now becomes appropriate to have her remain still while manual stabilization of her cervical spine is held, a cervical collar is applied, and a short-board device is applied.
26. d. The decision to immobilize the cervical spine can be determined from the MOI and/or a patient's signs and symptoms.
27. c. Swelling or edema is associated with soft-tissue injuries.
28. c. Head injuries can cause a patient to become nauseated and vomit. When a patient has an altered mental status and vomiting, there is a high risk of aspiration. The EMT must be alert for this and be prepared to manage the airway.
29. a. Reassess the ABCs frequently for the unconscious patient, and pay a lot of attention to the airway and breathing. Head injuries can cause a patient to become nauseated and vomit. When a patient has an altered mental status and vomiting, there is a high risk of aspiration. The EMT must be alert for this and be prepared to manage the airway.
30. b. Cervical collars can be difficult to apply on babies and infants due to their short necks. A rolled towel is soft to the touch, easy to apply around the neck, and works effectively in place of a rigid cervical collar.

31. b. The more experience you have with immobilizing patients, the better you can estimate the size of a patient for fitting into various splinting devices. Until then, you should place the device next to the patient and size it for proper fit based on the patient's weight and height.

32. c. Pediatric equipment is typically selected based on the weight and height of the patient.

33. b. When immobilizing a patient with a suspected cervical or spinal injury, the rescuer holding stabilization of the head and neck makes the call to move the patient; she first checks with each rescuer to see that they are all ready, then all rescuers count and move the patient as a team.

34. d. Distal PMS is assessed before and after immobilizing the spine or an extremity.

35. b. When immobilizing the spine, remember the phrase "bone to board." Use the body's bones (shoulders, thorax, hips, legs, and head last) to move and secure the body to the device.

36. a. When immobilizing the spine, use the body's bones (shoulders, thorax, hips, and legs) to move and secure the body to the device.

37. b. The body is secured before the head.

38. a. When immobilizing the spine, remember the phrase "bone to board." Use the body's bones (shoulders, thorax, hips, legs, and head last) to move and secure the body to the device.

39. d. Smoke or fire is an example of a hazard that would prompt a decision to rapidly extricate a patient.

40. c. A short spine board device would allow the least amount of movement for the patient and therefore create the least amount of pain. A rapid extrication onto a long backboard would not be inappropriate, but might cause more pain and injury for the patient.

41. c. The patient is stable following a MVC. The MOI is not described as being significant, so a short spine board is an appropriate device for this patient.

42. b. The short spine board device is used to move a patient from a location where a long backboard will not fit. The patient must be secured to a long backboard device prior to being transported.

43. d. Before placing the short spine board device behind the patient, the rescuers will move the patient forward to allow enough room for the device to fit.

44. b. Manual stabilization of the head and neck is maintained until both the torso and the head are secured to the immobilization device.

45. a. The patient is unstable and had a significant MOI, so rapid extrication is appropriate for this patient.

46. c. The indications for performing a rapid extrication include: unstable patient condition, a patient who is blocking access to an unstable patient, and unsafe scene.

47. d. A cervical collar is applied before the patient is moved.

48. b. Minimal cervical movement is the key to preventing any further injury to the patient with a suspected cervical spinal injury.

49. b. The EMT must have special training and practice to remain proficient in rapid extrication.

50. a. After one unsuccessful attempt to place the patient's neck in a neutral position, it is then appropriate to splint it in the position found. Never force the cervical spine into a splint!

51. a. The patient is conscious, alert, and stable and can be immobilized with the helmet on. Football players wear shoulder padding that elevates the back from the long backboard. If you need to remove the helmet and the shoulder pads are still in place, you will have to place a towel under the head to keep the spine in a neutral position.

52. d. Many types of helmets have face guards that can be removed to give access to the airway while the helmet is left on.

53. b. Bicycle, motorcycle, and auto racing helmets have the classic chinstrap.

54. a. Helmets used in skiing, snowboarding, and motorcycling are examples of the full-faced style. This type of helmet has a rigid chin guard that is continuous with the rest of the helmet.

55. d. Football players wear shoulder padding that elevates the back from the long backboard. If you need to remove the helmet and the shoulder pads are still in place, you will have to place a towel under the head to keep the spine in a neutral position.

56. b. When a helmet is fitted properly and has a snug fit around the head, the EMT can leave the helmet in place and immobilize the patient with it on.

57. d. When removing a full-face-style helmet, sometimes it is necessary to tilt the helmet slightly to avoid mashing the nose, but you must do so without moving the head or neck.

58. a. The airway, breathing, and circulation must be assessed and managed in order. As blood is draining from the mouth the patient will need suctioning, an airway adjunct, and possibly assistance with ventilations.

59. c. Manual stabilization of the head and neck is maintained until the patient is properly secured to an immobilization device.

60. c. The rescuer should ensure that the airway remains open by using a jaw-thrust maneuver.

61. b. The usual response to brain injury is elevated BP due to loss of cerebral autoregulation. This is the only way that the body can continue perfusion to the injured brain tissue. The "Cushing's reflex" of hypotension and bradycardia occurs at a late stage, and only lasts four to six minutes. Death follows shortly thereafter.

62. b. The patient who is immobilized with a helmet left on will not get a cervical collar.

63. c. Only the stretcher straps holding the patient on the long backboard should be unfastened. Keep the patient secured to the long backboard and turn the patient on the board.

64. d. The neutral position allows for the most space for the spinal cord within the spinal canal. This is the most stable position for the spinal column, reducing instability.

65. d. The short spine board device is used to keep the spine from moving when a long backboard cannot be used as the first immobilization device. Once the patient is moved out to an area where she can be moved onto a long backboard, the patient is secured with both devices.

66. c. The short spine board device is used to keep the spine from moving when a long backboard cannot be used as the first immobilization device (e.g., when the patient is seated in an automobile).

67. a. The indications for performing a rapid extrication include: unstable patient condition, a patient who is blocking access to an unstable patient, and unsafe scene.

68. b. The use of rapid extrication increases the risk of further spinal injury for any patient. That is why this technique is used only in urgent circumstances.

69. b. This is an example of when to use a standing takedown.

70. d. Indications for immobilizing a patient with a helmet on include: the patient is stable, the helmet fits well, and proper immobilization can be accomplished with the helmet on.

Chapter 28: Multisystem Trauma

1. c. The unconscious trauma patient most likely has a head injury; however, with no external bleeding he could not lose enough blood to produce signs of shock (e.g., tachycardia and hypotension), so the blood loss should be presumed to be internal bleeding.

2. c. Every community has different needs and resources available. The patient described has multisystem trauma from a significant mechanism of injury and needs definitive care at a trauma center. Follow local protocols for transport decisions and the criteria and procedure for air-medical transport.

3. b. A significant electrical shock can cause a victim to be thrown or knocked down. The MOI has the potential to cause a head, cervical, or spinal injury in addition to the injury from the shock.

4. a. The potential for a spinal injury is the primary reason for immobilizing this patient to a long backboard.

5. d. Taking cervical precautions, begin with opening the airway.

6. c. A sudden loss of consciousness is an indication to quickly reassess the ABCs. If it becomes necessary to remove the helmet (e.g., to manage the airway), then take the necessary steps to do so safely.

7. a. The indications for performing a rapid extrication include: unstable patient condition, a patient who is blocking access to an unstable patient, and unsafe scene. Both patients in this vehicle meet the criteria for a rapid extrication.

8. d. The rescuer holding stabilization will remove the helmet. The second rescuer supports the head by reaching under the patient's neck and into the helmet to support the back (occiput) of the patient's head.

9. b. When you need to access the airway or assist the patient's breathing, it is appropriate to remove the helmet immediately.

10. b. Bleeding in the brain can put pressure on the brain stem causing posturing such as flexion or extension.

11. b. One characteristic of decerebrate posturing is muscles rigidity with the jaw clenched and the neck and head extended. Getting and maintaining an airway is the priority and can be challenging. Consider using a nasopharyngeal airway adjunct and assist ventilations with a bag mask device until ALS arrives and can continue care.

12. c. If the helmet is going to be taken off, use the best-trained hands. In the field, it is not uncommon to have the assistance of athletic trainers who are very knowledgeable about the technique for removal and the specific brand of sports helmet they use for their team.

13. d. The energy that can be absorbed by the body during an impact produces damage to the patient's body. The extent of the damage caused by this energy depends on the specific organs that have been affected.

14. a. These patients have very little to no chance of survival. This is why they are transported to the nearest hospital by ambulance.

15. a. The transfer of energy from the bullet to the tissues pushes them apart, creating a cavity. If the bullet is small, the cavity may be temporary. This is why bullet holes are often missed during assessment.

16. c. Getting a complete and accurate account of the incident is the best way to suspect injury patterns and look for injuries that may not be apparent at first.

17. a. The transfer of energy from the bullet to the tissues pushes them apart, creating a cavity. As the bullet continues to move through the body it may exit, leaving a larger hole.

18. a. The "golden hour" is the first hour after the injury occurs. In serious trauma situations, the best chances of survival for the patient are a result of reaching the hospital operation suite and having the bleeding controlled within that hour. EMTs can do their part to achieve this goal by limiting scene time to a "platinum ten" minutes. That means ten minutes for assessment and management at the scene for a critical trauma patient.

19. a. Early recognition of the mechanism of injury and the possible injuries associated with those forces can help save the patient's life.

20. b. a, c, and d are either contraindications or relative contraindications for air-medical transport.

21. d. Rapid acceleration occurred with the rear-end collision and rapid deceleration occurred when her vehicle struck the vehicle in front.

22. b. The "golden hour" is the first hour after the injury occurs. In serious trauma situations, the best chances of survival for the patient are a result of reaching the hospital operation suite and having the bleeding controlled within that hour. EMTs can do their part to achieve this goal by limiting scene time to a "platinum ten" minutes. That means 10 minutes for assessment and management at the scene for a critical trauma patient.

23. a. The injuries to the upper airway are relatively minor and not a risk unless the patient becomes unconscious. The possible associated injuries (injury to organs behind the sternum) with a sternal injury can quickly become life threatening.

24. a. Assess airway, breathing, and circulation in that order. Correct any life-threatening conditions as they are discovered. This patient has difficulty breathing and a chest injury. This must be assessed rapidly to determine what type of injury is present.

25. c. The EMT should carefully consider the mechanism of injury suspect and assess for associated injuries to the chest and abdomen.

Chapter 29: Environmental Emergencies

1. d. *Evaporation* is loss of heat at the surface from vaporization of liquid (e.g., sweating).

2. c. *Convection* is the transfer of heat by the circulation of heated particles (e.g., cooling soup by blowing on it).

3. b. *Conduction* is the transmission of heat from a warmer object to cooler objects in direct contact (e.g., lying on a cold surface).

4. a. Deeply frostbitten skin has a white, waxy appearance. It feels hard, as if frozen. Generally there is a complete loss of sensation that does not recover within a short time.

5. a. Diminished coordination and psychomotor function set in quickly and progress rapidly after a sudden and extreme exposure, such as falling into freezing water.

6. c. Decreasing mental status is the most significant indication that a patient's condition is becoming critical, in either a hot or a cold exposure.

7. b. Manage the ABCs first as needed. Then quickly splint the extremity to prevent further damage, gently move the patient out of the cold, remove any wet clothing to prevent further heat loss, and begin to warm the patient.

8. a. The priority is to prevent any further heat loss. Move the patient into a warm environment, remove any wet clothing, and begin to warm the patient.

9. b. The patient should not bear any weight on the extremity, and the EMT should carefully splint it. Presuming that transportation will not take too long, it is appropriate to just keep the extremity from rewarming and let the ED provide additional care for the injury. Follow local protocol!

10. d. The loss of fluid and electrolytes is a significant factor in the development of heat illness. Signs and symptoms of dehydration associated with prolonged heat exposure may include any of those seen with heat illness and a rapid weight loss (typically more than 7 percent of body weight).

11. d. Weak pulse, shock, and altered mental status (AMS) are later signs of more severe heat illness.

12. b. The most significant signs or symptoms are those that affect the ABCs.

13. a. The scenario describes a febrile seizure. The proper steps to take are to remove warm clothing and allow the child to cool off. Provide oxygen to the patient and supportive care to the parents and transport the patient in his car seat for evaluation.

14. d. Each of the steps described is appropriate treatment. The ABCs must be managed first and the patient must be cooled.

15. d. As the body temperature climbs rapidly, to 104°F to 106°F, a life-threatening emergency develops. Treatment must be rapid or the patient will progress from AMS, to convulsions, brain damage or renal failure, and death.

16. d. The MOI, together with the loss of consciousness, indicates the potential for a head or spinal injury. Cervical precautions must be taken immediately and continued until head and spinal injuries can be ruled out.

17. c. A prolonged exposure in any body of water will cause heat loss, leading to hypothermia.

18. b. The patient has symptoms of decompression sickness. The history is key here. Anyone who has breathed compressed air underwater is at risk for

decompression illness. Any patient with a complaint of joint soreness 24 to 48 hours after a dive should be considered for decompression therapy.

19. b. Hypoxia can result from aspiration of any type of fluid, not just during a near-drowning.

20. b. When examining victims of near-drowning, it is important to note that they may initially appear normal, but typically will develop symptoms that affect breathing and respiration (e.g., progressive dyspnea, wheezing, and cyanosis).

21. b. Factors typically associated with drowning include: use of alcohol, male in his 20s, spinal injury, and hypothermia. Frostbite maybe a factor in freezing water.

22. d. Regardless of the patient's age, a human bite that breaks the skin should be evaluated. The patient's tetanus vaccination must be verified or brought up to date, and the wound must be cleaned and dressed to prevent infection.

23. d. When it is not known what type of snake made the bite, the general wound care for this type of injury includes managing the ABCs, splinting the extremity, keeping the patient still, and transporting the patient to the ED.

24. b. After completing your assessment, begin wound care for bites.

25. c. Heat exhaustion often occurs following exertion in a hot, humid environment. Signs and symptoms include: pale skin; profuse sweating; hypotension, especially with positional changes; headache; weakness; fatigue; thirst; and normal or slightly elevated temperature.

26. a. Decompression illness or the bends is a sickness occurring during or after ascent secondary to a rapid release of nitrogen bubbles from the blood.

27 b. There is a higher incidence of heat exhaustion in individuals on water pills. Young children, the debilitated, immobilized, or those having prolonged bouts of diarrhea are also at higher risk.

28. b. Frostbite is the formation of ice crystals within the tissues. These crystals damage the blood vessels and other tissues.

29. c. The young, the elderly, and intoxicated individuals are at a higher risk for developing hypothermia. The young and elderly have immature or failing thermoregulatory systems and intoxicated persons have impaired judgment; these factors predispose these groups to develop hypothermia.

30. a. Small marine animal stings (e.g., Portuguese man-of-war, lionfish, jellyfish, sea urchins) are very painful. Heat is typically more effective than ice in destroying the venom of marine organisms. Generally, unless anaphylaxis is present, no medication is warranted.

31. a. Because the patient did have seizure activity but has no history of seizures, and this episode occurred in the pool, the EMT must consider a possible traumatic injury as the MOI for the seizure. Attempt to get more information about the possible MOI as you begin a rapid trauma assessment.

32. c. A submersion or near-drowning occurs when the process of drowning is interrupted or reversed. The victim of near-drowning may appear normal initially, with symptoms (e.g., difficulty breathing, wheezing, tachycardia, or cyanosis) developing over the next few hours. The patient was also witnessed having seizure activity, though she had no prior history of seizures, and this must be followed up.

33. c. Symptoms of a black widow spider bite include feeling a small sting at the site followed by a dull ache. The patient will develop severe muscle spasms, especially in the abdomen, chest, back, and shoulders. The bite from a tick or brown recluse spider is typically not felt and may go unnoticed for hours. The bite of a fire ant is very painful. The area becomes red, swollen, and the bites produce vesicles that are filled with fluid.

34. a. Abdominal rigidity is another indication of a black widow spider bite. Management of this patient includes wound care, supportive care for shock, and transport.

35. a. Shivering is the body's heat-producing mechanism; it begins when the core body temperature (CBT) is around 95°F and may continue for a few hours until the body's energy reserves are depleted.

Chapter 30: Obstetric and Gynecologic Emergencies

1. c. The umbilical cord, which connects the fetus with the placenta, contains two umbilical arteries and one umbilical vein.

2. b. The placenta is often referred to as the *afterbirth* because it is delivered in the third stage of labor, after delivery of the baby.

3. c. The examiner can best feel contractions of the uterus by placing a hand on the top of the uterus (top of the abdomen). This muscle contraction is quite strong as it pushes the fetus down the birth canal.

4. a. The contents of an obstetric kit are sterile prior to opening the kit.

5. c. The first step to take when a patient suddenly becomes unresponsive is to assess for breathing and a pulse. A pregnant patient in her third trimester may lose consciousness when placed in a supine position. When the large fetus lies directly on the vena

cava, as it does in the supine position, blood return to the heart can be severely restricted, causing a loss of consciousness. The remedy is easy: turn the patient on her side.

6. c. The signs and symptoms of abruptio placenta that distinguish this obstetrical emergency from others are the sudden onset of severe abdominal pain and blood loss that is not always apparent, because it may be trapped behind the placenta.

7. a. The sign and symptom of placenta previa that distinguishes this obstetrical emergency from others is blood loss that can be significant; however, the patient usually experiences no pain.

8. a. Crowning indicates that the baby is ready to be delivered. Stop the ambulance and assist with the delivery. Call for additional help if needed.

9. c. The feeling of having to move her bowels comes from the baby being in the birth canal and pressing on the rectum. This is a reliable sign that the baby is being delivered.

10. a. Contractions that are five minutes apart are an indication that there is enough time to begin transport to the hospital.

11. c. Braxton Hicks contractions, or false labor, are irregular and often painless. These contractions are practice contractions that prepare the uterus for the real thing. They can begin as early as the first trimester, but more often occur in the third trimester.

12. a. Eclampsia is the most serious condition of hypertension during pregnancy, and usually occurs between 20 weeks and 1 week postpartum. Eclampsia is marked by convulsive seizures and coma and is a life-threatening condition for both mother and fetus.

13. a. Request ALS to meet you and provide care as for any other seizure patient. Manage the airway, provide high-flow oxygen, and assist ventilations if needed. Begin gentle but rapid transport.

14. a. Pregnant women are predisposed to nausea and vomiting because of the pressure of the fetus on the stomach. Always be alert for vomiting.

15. c. Allowing the spouse and/or friend to be present during the delivery is an accepted and appropriate practice. This may help to keep the patient relaxed and better able to concentrate on your instructions.

16. d. The patient should be lying back with her head elevated and knees flexed, preferably on your stretcher.

17. d. The third stage of labor is the delivery of the placenta. During this time and after the delivery of the placenta, the patient should be monitored for excessive blood loss and signs of shock.

18. c. Nuchal cord (umbilical cord wrapped around the neck) is not uncommon during childbirth. Immediately after the head delivers, the EMT must look to see if this condition is present. If it is, the cord must be carefully lifted off the neck and over the head without tearing the cord.

19. d. As the head begins to emerge from the vaginal opening, the EMT must place a gloved hand gently over the head to prevent an explosive birth, which can rip and tear the mother's perineum.

20. a. After assessing the neck for a wrapped cord, the EMT can begin to suction the baby's mouth and nose while waiting for the next contraction.

21. d. Once the head is delivered, the EMT can begin to suction the baby's mouth and nose while waiting for the next contraction. The mouth is suctioned first, because the baby takes its first breath through the mouth.

22. b. The most common presentation of the baby through the vaginal opening is face down, although face up is very common, too. From there the baby's head will turn to the side.

23. d. Almost any sterile cutting device may be used, although a sterile blade or scissors is preferable.

24. b. The bleeding must be controlled immediately, because even a little blood loss is a lot for a newborn. Keep the first clamp in place and use a second clamp proximal to the first; then reassess.

25. a. The placenta is a large organ, and when it is inspected it becomes obvious to see a piece missing. Any portion of the placenta that is left undelivered can cause moderate to severe bleeding.

26. d. The contractions that expel the placenta may be as painful as the contractions experienced during delivery of the baby.

27. d. The placenta must be inspected for completeness, because any portion of the placenta that is left undelivered can cause serious hemorrhaging.

28. b. The care for this patient is the same as for any patient with hemorrhagic shock.

29. d. The *perineum* is the area between the anus and the vaginal opening. This area can tear during delivery (especially with the first baby), causing a wound that looks like a laceration.

30. d. For uncomplicated childbirth, postpartum care of the mother includes giving supportive care, making her comfortable, and reassessing her for signs of shock.

31. d. When drying, warming, and suctioning do not stimulate the baby to breathe normally immediately after birth, the EMT should administer oxygen. If oxygen does not improve respiratory effort, ventilations by bag mask device must be started.

32. d. Holding a baby upside down or by the feet is unsafe and not an acceptable practice.

33. d. A heart rate of less than 60 beats per minute at one minute after delivery is critically low and requires cardiopulmonary resuscitation.

34. d. The EMT should assist in the delivery of a breech presentation (buttocks first) by supporting the buttocks and legs as they deliver, to prevent pulling and tearing of the neck muscles as the baby's head delivers.

35. d. This condition is prolapsed cord and it is a true emergency. Begin safe but rapid transport.

36. c. A limb presentation is a complication of childbirth that the EMT should not attempt to deliver. This type of delivery may require cesarean section.

37. c. Identical twins develop from the same cell, are the same gender, and share the same placenta. Fraternal twins develop from two separate cells and each has its own placenta.

38. b. Twin babies are smaller than single babies at birth and often are premature.

39. d. Additional help will be needed to care for and transport twins, but assistance with the delivery is the same as for a single baby. The first baby is usually the biggest and delivers head first. The second baby is usually smaller and breech.

40. d. The aspiration of meconium is dangerous because it causes serious complications in the lungs, including respiratory infection and death.

41. a. The mouth and nose should be suctioned as soon as the head is delivered. If meconium is still present after delivery, do not stimulate the baby until additional suctioning to remove the meconium has been completed.

42. d. Meconium is the baby's first bowel movement, which may occur while in the uterus when the baby is under stress or is overdue for delivery.

43. b. Premature infants are at higher risk than full-term babies for developing hypothermia because they have a very small amount of body fat and a larger body surface area in relation to their weight; also the temperature regulating system of a premature infant is too immature to be reliable.

44. a. A premature baby weighs less than 5.5 pounds or is born before 38 weeks' gestation.

45. c. This patient complaining of abdominal pain has signs of internal bleeding (pale skin, persistent tachycardia); management includes high-flow oxygen and treatment for shock. Pale skin and tachycardia may be associated with severe pain alone, but the EMT should consider the more serious condition of shock first and treat for that.

46. d. The combination of all these symptoms suggests a sexually transmitted disease.

47. d. The EMT should consider any female of childbearing age who is complaining of abdominal pain to be experiencing an ectopic pregnancy (a life-threatening condition) until proven otherwise (e.g., a negative pregnancy test at the ED).

48. c. The consumption of vitamin A supplements during pregnancy has been shown to cause irregular fetal development.

49. c. The body's self-preservation mechanism shunts blood from all areas of the body, including the fetus, to the mother's vital organs (brain, heart, and lungs).

50. d. For the baby to survive, the mother must survive until reaching the ED/OR.

51. b. Full-term gestation is 38 to 42 weeks. Less than 38 weeks' gestation is premature and more than 42 weeks is overdue.

52. c. The amniotic sac is actually a thin fetal membrane that forms a closed sac around the fetus and contains serous fluid in which the fetus is immersed.

53. c. Endometritis may also occur within the uterus, resulting in excess growth of otherwise normal endometrial tissue. Symptoms may include excessive menstrual bleeding and severe cramps.

54. a. Chlamydia continues to be the most frequently reported bacterial sexually transmitted disease.

55. b. The EMT must treat the whole patient and respond to both physical and emotional needs of the patient.

56. d. Uncontrolled internal bleeding from any source can lead to hypovolemia, shock, and death.

57. b. Assume a woman with abdominal pain has a leaking or ruptured ectopic pregnancy, especially if she is in shock.

58. d. In the prehospital setting all abdominal complaints are managed alike: supportive treatment with care for shock. Manage the ABCs, position of comfort or supine, positioning for shock, provide high-flow oxygen, keep the patient warm and calm, and consider rapid transport to an appropriate facility.

59. c. Lacerations, bruising, and tearing are primary injuries of an assault.

60. c. Pelvic inflammatory disease (PID) causes various signs and symptoms. Some women experience nothing and don't even know they have it. Possible signs and symptoms include: acute abdominal pains close to last menstrual period, discharge (yellow or green, and may have an odor), pain during or after intercourse, guarding, fever, nausea, vomiting, and irregular periods.

Chapter 31: Pediatric Emergencies

1. c. The score gives a numerical assessment of how well a newborn infant is responding after birth. APGAR is assessed and given a score of 0, 1, or 2 at one and five minutes after birth.

2. b. The next step in resuscitation of the newborn is to assist with ventilations using a bag mask device. If the heart rate still does not increase, begin chest compressions.

3. a. Meconium is the baby's first bowel movement. If it occurs while the fetus is still in utero, it is considered a sign of fetal distress.

4. c. Signs of respiratory distress can occur within minutes or hours of birth. Signs include tachypnea, sternal retractions, grunting, and cyanosis.

5. a. The essential aspects of care after resuscitation are keeping the baby warm and ensuring oxygen delivery.

6. d. The leading causes of trauma death in pediatrics are motor vehicle crashes, abuse, auto-pedestrian accidents, bicycle injuries, falls, burns, drowning, and firearms.

7. c. Sudden infant death syndrome (SIDS) is also called "crib death," though patients range in age from two weeks to one year. SIDS rarely occurs in infants older than six months. In many cases, the infant has died during sleep and is not discovered immediately.

8. c. An infant's respiratory muscles are immature and fatigue faster than those of an adult.

9. a. *Grunting* is an abnormal respiratory sound produced by a partially closed glottis. Grunting is a characteristic of respiratory distress in children.

10. d. A slow respiratory rate in a child who is in respiratory distress indicates that the child is tiring; this is an ominous sign.

11. d. As the child become more hypoxic from inadequate oxygenation, the mental status will decrease. This is the most significant indication that the child is in failure and progressing to respiratory and cardiopulmonary arrest.

12. a. Secretions, positioning, and foreign bodies are all causes of airway obstruction in pediatric patients.

13. d. When the onset of respiratory distress is sudden, the EMT should suspect and assess for a foreign body, especially when stridor or wheezing is noted.

14. b. Respiratory distress from asthma is characterized by difficulty exhaling and a prolonged expiratory phase.

15. d. The method for opening the airway in any unconscious patient with no suspected injuries is the head-tilt chin-lift maneuver.

16. c. To properly assess an unresponsive patient who may have choked, you should place the patient supine on a flat surface. This position will also help to prevent any further injury from a possible fall.

17. a. The obstruction must be relieved before proceeding with breathing and circulation.

18. c. The steps in the management of a FBAO in an unresponsive infant are open the airway, attempt ventilation, deliver five back blows and five chest thrusts, and then perform a jaw-thrust maneuver and look for the FBAO. Never perform a blind finger sweep on an infant.

19. b. The patient is in need of a bronchodilator. The EMT can assist with a MDI under direct or indirect medical control. Always follow local protocols!

20. a. Mucus and nasal secretions are a real problem for small infants, because they breathe primarily through the nose. The obstruction can be easily relieved with a bulb syringe.

21. a. Further upsetting or agitating the child can cause a rapid deterioration in his condition. The EMT's general approach must be calm and reassuring during the management of such a patient.

22. d. Tachypnea (fast respiratory rate) and delayed capillary refill (poor circulation) in a sick child are signs of decompensated shock.

23. a. The patient's labored effort to breathe suggests distress, but the cyanosis indicates respiratory failure.

24. b. The child appears to have had a febrile seizure. Skin signs indicate that circulation is adequate.

25. a. Mental status, capillary refill, and pulses are direct measures of end-organ perfusion.

26. b. Urine output is an indirect but valid measure of end-organ perfusion in a sick child.

27. d. Cool extremities and a loss of distal pulses in warm ambient temperatures are signs of inadequate perfusion in a sick child.

28. b. Unlike adults, respiratory distress and failure are the primary causes of cardiac arrest in children. When the EMT can recognize respiratory distress and failure, she can act quickly to prevent the child from deteriorating to cardiac arrest.

29. d. Unlike adults, respiratory distress and failure are the primary causes of cardiac arrest in children.

30. a. Febrile seizures are caused when a child's body temperature rises too quickly. Management includes attention to the ABCs; gentle cooling of the child, such as removing layers of clothing; and then transporting for evaluation.

31. c. Febrile seizures are caused when a child's body temperature rises too quickly, which can occur when a child is sick with an infection.

32. a. Traumatic brain injury is a common pathology in children of all age groups.

33. b. BLS care for this patient includes managing the ABCs (e.g., oxygen, suctioning, and transport), and calling for ALS to meet you en route, if possible.

34. a. The patient has a history of seizures and may have another while in your care. The BLS care of this patient includes attention to the ABCs and transport for evaluation. If another seizure occurs, request ALS to meet you en route to the ED.

35. c. Brief periods of apnea are not uncommon with seizures. The EMT should administer high-flow oxygen during the postictal period of a seizure and longer, if needed.

36. c. The heads of children are disproportionately large in relation to their bodies. This leads to more injuries to the head, face, and neck because children tend to land head first.

37. a. The heads of children are disproportionately large in relation to their bodies. This leads to more injuries

to the head, face, and neck because children tend to land head first.

38. c. The growing bones in children are not as calcified and strong those in an adult.

39. c. The use of an OPA is appropriate in any unconscious patient without a gag reflex.

40. a. The patient is unconscious with labored breathing following a traumatic MOI. Manage the ABCs. Ensure that the airway is open and assist with ventilations.

41. a. The patient appears to be stable, so it is both appropriate and safest to immobilize and transport the child in the car seat. Children tend to be less frightened and easier to manage when transported in their own car seats, because the seats are familiar to them.

42. a. Difficulty walking or sitting, anxiety, avoidance of eye contact, and uncooperativeness with certain aspects of assessment, together with other suspicious findings at the scene, may indicate that the child is a victim of sexual abuse.

43. c. Mouth and gum lacerations in a baby are a sign often associated with "baby bottle syndrome." The parent or caregiver repeatedly forces the bottle into the infant's mouth in an effort to stop it from crying.

44. b. Document only your specific findings and facts regarding the call. Opinions are not regarded as professional or reliable.

45. a. Suspected child abuse or neglect reporting is mandatory in every state. The specific method of reporting varies from state to state. However, the next health care provider (e.g., ED staff) to take care of the patient should be informed of your suspicions.

46. c. The EMT has the advantage of observing the conditions of the child's home and the interactions within the home., The EMT should document the specific findings appropriately, without rendering opinions or judgments.

47. a. Child abuse is a crime; reporting suspected child abuse or neglect is mandatory in every state. The specific method of reporting varies from state to state.

48. b. EMS calls involving children can be challenging for any EMS provider. Each person manages stress differently, so you should talk to your partner first and assess his reaction. He may need to take the rest of the shift off, or he may want (and be perfectly able) to return to service.

49. a. Each person manages stress differently.

50. a. Talking about the call with your crew is very helpful in working through the stress of a call like this. However, it may not be enough for everyone. Consider utilizing critical incident stress management (CISM) and other techniques for those who need additional support.

51. d. No one is expected to remember all the ranges of vital signs for each age group. What is expected is that the EMT knows where to find a pediatric reference and how to read it.

52. c. The priority of the ABCs never changes, but the method of assessment should be modified according to the age of the patient. For example, with toddlers and preschool-age children, the toe-to-head direction of physical exam may be less threatening and upsetting than the head-to-toe method.

53. c. Children of grade-school age are typically reliable with information regarding their past medical history.

54. b. Studies have shown that families who are included in the initial and emergency care of a child in cardiac arrest do better in the grieving process. Let the parents or caregivers know that the child is your first priority. Designate a crew member to explain the treatment being provided and answer questions.

55. b. Parents of injured and sick children can experience a wide range of emotions. Often they may feel that the child's pain is somehow their fault. Maintain a professional demeanor, honestly explain any procedures, and keep them informed.

56. d. Parents of injured and sick children can experience a wide range of emotions. Often they may feel that the child's pain is somehow their fault. Reassure her that the bleeding is controlled and permit her to observe.

57. c. EMS calls involving children can be challenging for any EMS provider, and it is common for EMTs who are parents to internalize the stress somewhat more than those who are not parents.

58. b. The experienced and professional EMT knows that a calm and reassuring disposition goes a long way toward establishing trust with patients and parents of patients.

59. c. Utilizing a parent in the management of a pediatric patient is a good practice, but is not always necessary nor appropriate for every call.

60. a. Do not risk losing the patient's confidence by getting involved in disputes or taking sides.

61. d. Cardiac arrests due to MI are more prevalent in adults than in children.

62. d. Further upsetting or agitating such a patient can cause a rapid deterioration in his condition. The EMT's general approach must be calm and reassuring during the management of this child. Let the patient stay in a position of comfort with minimal disturbance.

63. a. Croup is caused by viral or other infections (e.g., ear, throat) and is characterized by a two- or three-day onset of sickness progressing to respiratory distress. The patient may have a barking cough.

64. a. The poor skin signs, loss of distal pulses, and delayed capillary refill indicate hypoperfusion and inadequate circulation.

65. c. BLS management includes management of the ABCs, recognition of the need for ALS, and rapid transport.

Chapter 32: Geriatric Emergencies

1. a. The increased stiffness of the heart muscle leads to an increased workload on the aging heart. Because cardiac reserves become limited, stress is not well tolerated.

2. a. By 80 years of age, there is a 50 percent decrease in blood vessel elasticity, often due to arteriosclerosis. The result is an increase in peripheral vascular resistance with variable reductions in organ blood flow.

3. b. The elderly may have decreased pain perception due to factors such as neuropathy, degenerative nerve pathway, and declining mental status.

4. c. Decreased elasticity of the diaphragm combined with decreased muscle mass and chest wall weakness leads to decreased respiratory function.

5. d. Weakened bone structure in the ribs, vertebrae, and sternum combine with decreased elasticity of the diaphragm contribute to older persons having an ineffective cough reflex.

6. a. The history of a recent respiratory infection together with warm skin (fever) and diminished lung sounds are very likely to be a recurrent respiratory infection (e.g., pneumonia).

7. c. His skin is warm, therefore you can presume he has a temperature (e.g., infection somewhere) without knowing the exact number reading. The pulse oximetry reading cannot rule out any condition. We know the patient is a smoker; the amount he smokes is not useful at this point. A colorful productive cough (e.g., yellow or green) indicates an infection. A clear productive cough or absence of a productive cough does not exclude pneumonia.

8. d. Prolonged periods of immobilization can produce pressure ulcers or bedsores which can become ischemic and necrotic casing damage to the skin, subcutaneous tissue, and often muscle. The wounds occur over boney surfaces such as the sacrum, elbows, knees, and ankles.

9. c. Changes in renal function have a major effect on the metabolism of many drugs in the older patient.

10. d. Insulin production decreases, leading to abnormalities in glucose metabolism.

11. c. Alzheimer's can run its course in just a few years or last as long as 20 years; the average is 9 years. It is associated with the development of abnormal tissues and protein deposits in the brain.

12. d. Dementia can occur to anyone at any age as a result of brain injury or oxygen deprivation.

13. a. Abusers can be anyone that an older person comes in contact with. Most commonly, the abusers are family members with the spouse being primary and children secondary abusers.

14. b. Neglect, either passively or intentionally failing to provide for the physical, psychological, and/or social needs of the older person is the most common form of elder abuse.

15. b. With decreased muscle mass and weakened bones, the older patient can be very fragile. Bones can be easily fractured during a move.

16. c. Osteoporosis is a disease distinguished by low bone mass and the deterioration of bone tissue. This condition leads to the bones becoming fragile and at risk for fractures, especially the hips, spine, and wrists.

17. c. Patients with hearing deficits often take out their hearing aids or routinely do not wear them. Look for them and have the patient use them and bring them to the hospital.

18. c. As the brain shrinks, the subdural space enlarges and veins become stretched. When the patient experiences rapid acceleration or deceleration forces, the brain and the vessels tear on the sharp, bony edges inside the skull. Bleeding leads to a subdural hematoma.

19. b. Blood thinners or anticoagulants medication suppress the body's formation of clotting factors. People taking these medications will bleed easily and longer than people who do not. When an injury occurs, especially to the head, these patients should be transported for evaluation of internal bleeding.

20. d. People on blood thinners are at risk for a life-threatening bleed as a result of even a minor head injury and should be transported for further evaluation. The EMT should attempt to convince the patient to go using recourses at their disposal. However, a patient who is alert and orientated can still refuse any or all treatment.

21. a. Because of a decrease in the function of the thermoregulatory system and the body's impaired ability to maintain homeostasis, even a modest elevation or subnormal temperatures are indications for concern, especially when it is associated with confusion, loss of appetite, or there are behavioral changes. Slight temperature changes are consistent with pneumonia, urinary tract infections, and sepsis.

22. c. Hypoxia and hypoglycemia should be ruled out first in ANY patient who has a sudden change in mental status.

23. d. Patients with abnormalities of the head, neck, and spine must be packaged very carefully to avoid making an injury worse or creating a new injury.

24. c. Medications such as beta-blockers keep the heart rate slow even when the body is under stress from injury or illness.

25. a. Nearly all cases of COPD are caused by long-term smoking or exposure to smoke. It is not a young person's disease.

Chapter 33: Emergencies for Patients with Special Challenges

1. b. The victim of abuse may fear things will get worse if they tell.

2. a. Neglect is a form of abuse whereby the caregiver does not provide necessary care.

3. a. Domestic violence is a crime and the EMT may need to work within a crime scene. Preserving evidence is a component of cooperation with law enforcement.

4. a. Dialysis shunts are implanted under the skin. Failure of this type of device includes signs of infection at the site (i.e., redness, swelling), hemorrhage, hemodynamic compromise, angina, or signs of embolus.

5. d. In the case of obvious death, it would not be appropriate to begin CPR. It is important to console the family. In this case, help the family contact hospice staff and the funeral home as they wish. When police arrive, you can turn the body over to them.

6. c. Child abuse is a crime. It is highly recommended that the EMT document all of her assessment findings on the prehospital care report and provide the emergency department with all findings. Assess and treat the child as you would for any other ill or injured child. Avoid judging the family or caretaker, avoid confrontation, and do not make any accusations.

7. b. The other examples are clues to physical abuse rather than neglect.

8. c. An ill infant or a developmentally delayed or a chronically ill child may cause enough stress in the family to induce an abusive situation. The biggest risk is being the sibling of an abused child or having a parent who was abused as a child.

9. d. The EMT should be aware of cultural differences, but not to the point of limiting your thinking about the person as a patient.

10. c. A regular sized BP cuff will falsely elevate the pressure reading if the person's arm is large. This is true whether the patient is obese or simply muscular. Always have a variety of different sized cuffs available to choose from.

11. d. Some EMS systems have contingency plans prepared in advance for obese patients.

12. a. Apnea monitors are used by parents of babies that have infantile apnea and by adults who have sleep apnea.

13. c. Ostomy bags are designed for those who have had a stoma created in their abdomen for excretion of stool away from the normal path to the rectum.

14. a. Problems that arise with ventilators are due to power failures and pressures that are either too high or too low.

15. b. Airway devices found in the patient's home include nasal cannulas, facemasks, tracheostomies, and suction devices to clear airways. Problems arise with airway devices when they are improperly placed or become obstructed, when oxygen tubing becomes blocked or the oxygen runs out.

16. Hospice also provides services for the patient's family.

17. c. The goals of palliative care or "comfort care" are to alleviate pain and other distressing symptoms for patients with potentially life-threatening illnesses and their families and friends.

18. a. The airway adjunct for a tracheostomy contains an outer tube, an inner tube, and a phalange that rests against the neck. Typical problems that arise with this type of air adjunct in which EMS may be called to help with include the following: the outer tube may slip out and the patient or caregiver is unable to put it back in, the inner tube becomes obstructed and needs to be suctioned and cleaned, or the opening in the neck starts bleeding.

19. c. The EMT must put on sterile gloves and withdraw the sterile catheter from the protective sleeve and maintaining sterility, insert the suction catheter with no suction applied until resistance is met, then pull back about 1 to 2 cm before applying continuous suction as the catheter is smoothly withdrawn from the airway.

20. d. With this in, the EMT should include this topic in the past medical history of the patient.

21. c. Developmental disabilities begin anytime during development up to 22 years of age and are chronic and lifelong. People with developmental disabilities have problems with learning, language, mobility, self-help, and independent living.

22. a. The child may or may not be able to communicate with strangers, but should be talked to as though he or she can understand. Look at the child when you speak, and listen to the parent/caregiver and allow extra time for the child to answer questions.

23. a. Some patients with autism do not have normal sensations and may not feel cold, heat, or pain in a typical manner and may fail to recognize pain in spite of significant pathology being present.

24. c. With little or no access to preventive care, homeless people generally wind up suffering from several ailments simultaneously. The problems are often complex and interrelated.

25. b. The homeless population can have serious health problems including conditions that pose a risk of infection for health care providers if standard precautions are not taken. Some of these conditions include tuberculosis, bronchitis, pneumonia, HIV/AIDS, and skin and wound infections just to name a few.

Chapter 34: EMS Operations

1. b. A penlight is of little value in a cache of extrication equipment.
2. a. The exposure control plan also states how personnel should clean up a blood spill in the ambulance.
3. d. A stretcher mount is not considered part of an emergency vehicle's mechanical system.
4. a. Unless there are special circumstances (e.g., prolonged scene time with extra personnel), the scene of a call is not where the EMT would typically be checking the equipment or restocking the ambulance.
5. a. Permission to assess and treat a patient should be obtained before you touch the patient. In most cases, this will occur on the scene of a call.
6. a. The decision on which priority response to use is made at the time of dispatch in most cases.
7. c. State vehicle and traffic regulations do not typically approve the use of emergency lights and audible devices for drills, training, or when returning from calls.
8. c. An ambulance is not exempt from leaving the scene of an accident, even when a patient is on board.
9. b. The driver of an emergency vehicle must drive with extreme care and due regard for other drivers. The proper action in this case is to wait for a safe location to pass the vehicle on the left.
10. d. The driver of an emergency vehicle is held to a higher standard than other drivers and must drive with extreme care and due regard for other drivers. If the driver of the ambulance continues with lights and sirens, the family member will most likely continue his unsafe driving. Ideally, the ambulance operator should stop and warn the family member to readjust how he is proceeding behind the ambulance.
11. a. Having completed an emergency vehicle operator course (EVOC) or ambulance accident prevention seminar (AAPS), driving course is an excellent method of obtaining training and practice in operating emergency vehicles. It does not, however, provide any immunity or confer special driving privileges.
12. b. The driver of an emergency vehicle is held to a higher standard than other drivers and must drive with extreme care and due regard for other drivers.
13. b. The ambulance is a much heavier vehicle than a personal vehicle. The EMT uses the skills learned in an emergency vehicle operator course (EVOC) when driving at any level of response.
14. a. The driver of an emergency vehicle is held to a higher standard than other drivers and must drive with extreme care and due regard for other drivers.
15. b. Use of escorts is dangerous and has caused many collisions. Whenever possible, avoid the vehicle escort scenario.
16. c. In this situation, each vehicle operator should use a different siren, to prevent confusion for other vehicle operators.
17. a. Courtesy to and safety of other drivers is the responsibility of the emergency vehicle operator.
18. a. This is the definition of operating an emergency vehicle with "due regard."
19. a. Safety of other drivers is the primary responsibility of the emergency vehicle operator.
20. a. This information is not typically documented on the prehospital care report (PCR).
21. c. This situation describes a third-party caller.
22. c. Enhanced 9-1-1 also displays the caller's telephone number and location, and can locate the actual room where the call was made within a large building.
23. a. A *repeater* is a device that receives transmissions from low-power sources and retransmits them at a higher power on another frequency.
24. c. If the patient is able to sit up, the stair chair is a valuable piece of equipment for spaces such as that described in the question.
25. b. At this point, the patient can be placed directly on a stretcher.
26. c. The long backboard is the ideal piece of equipment in this situation. It acts as a splint, and once the patient is secured and padded on the board, further patient movement is significantly reduced or eliminated.
27. a. The long backboard is the ideal piece of equipment in this situation. It acts as a splint, and once the patient is secured and padded on the board, further patient movement is significantly reduced or eliminated.
28. a. For the patient who is able to sit up, the stair chair is a valuable piece of equipment for moving through tight spaces. This patient should not walk or lie down, because of her condition.
29. b. Routinely documenting this information is a good practice. Some agencies routinely document the name of the nurse or physician to whom the patient was turned over.
30. c. The EMT who routinely completes patient care reports in a timely fashion, using accurate and complete information with no misspelled words, demonstrates professionalism.
31. a. The PCR contains administrative information, patient demographics, vital signs, patient narrative, and treatment.
32. d. The steps you take to prepare your ambulance for going into service will help to ensure the safety and health of you, your crew, and the patient.
33. b. The crew is responsible for cleaning and restocking as much of the ambulance as possible while at the hospital and before returning to service.

34. b. These are the OSHA-recommended steps for disinfecting an ambulance in such a situation.
35. b. Each of the other steps is necessary on every exposure call.
36. b. Verification of proper immunizations should be done well before you report to work.
37. c. These are the OSHA-recommended steps for disinfecting equipment in such a situation.
38. b. This product is designed for low-level disinfection.
39. b. *Sterilization* kills all forms of microbial life on medical instruments.
40. a. *Cleaning* is the process of removing dirt from the surface of an object with soap and water.
41. d. These are the OSHA-recommended steps for disinfecting an ambulance in such a situation.
42. c. A solution of bleach and water in a dilution of 1:100 is the OSHA-recommended concentration.
43. c. Yellow bags are used to transport reusable items, such as blankets or other equipment, back to the station for cleaning. The yellow indicates that the items are contaminated with possible infectious body fluids other than blood (e.g., urine, vomit, feces).
44. d. A complete verbal report is the standard for transferring patients from one health care provider to the next. A face-to-face report helps to minimize errors and missed information.
45. b. No emergency department appreciates the surprise of an emergency patient arriving without notice. Prearrival notice to the ED is standard practice and helps the staff to be prepared for the patient when that patient arrives.
46. d. This will vary from agency to agency. In many agencies, the EMT is responsible for checking fluid levels on a regular basis, but the agency's vehicle mechanic performs the maintenance.
47. a. Each of the answers is a valid reason for completing a daily ambulance checklist. However, the *primary* purpose is to have the vehicle prepared to respond to calls.
48. c. The patient with a head injury and AMS gets the air medical transport. Cardiac arrest victims are not flown, and the toddler and 10-year-old patient are stable and can go by ground transport.
49. d. 100 $\times$ 100 feet is the minimum required landing zone area for a small rotor aircraft.
50. b. 1,500 $\times$ 1.56 = 2,340 $\div$ 10 = 234 minutes.

Chapter 35: Highway Safety and Vehicle Extrication

1. b. Extrication is a method of extracting someone wherever he/she is entrapped.
2. b. The purpose of an extrication is to free the patient and provide care on scene during the extraction.
3. c. This is the definition of *disentanglement*.
4. d. Advanced life support (ALS) is provided by EMS providers with more training than the EMT such as the paramedic.
5. d. After sizing up the scene and managing hazards, the steps of a rescue include: gain access to the patient, assess and begin treatment, disentanglement, extrication, further assessment, treatment, and transport.
6. b. Each EMT is trained to the awareness level, which means they have the knowledge to recognize a hazardous scene, call for more help, and not enter unless they have a higher level of training and the proper equipment.
7. a. The greatest concern is the traffic. Studies show that drivers who are drugged, intoxicated, or tired actually drive right into the emergency lighting.
8. c. When too many lights are used, it is very confusing and blinding to the oncoming traffic.
9. d. When the first emergency vehicle arrives at the scene, flares or cones should be placed to direct traffic away from the collision and anywhere emergency personnel are working.
10. a. Estimating the severity of injuries and patient transport needs is part of the scene size-up, but the estimates may be modified at any point in the rescue.
11. b. Under each vehicle is a catalytic converter (maintaining a temperature around 1,200°F), which is a source of ignition for grass fires.
12. c. After sizing up the scene and managing hazards, the steps of a rescue include: gain access to the patient, assess and begin treatment, disentanglement, extrication, further assessment, treatment, and transport.
13. c. The bumpers on many vehicles have pistons in them and are designed to withstand a slow-speed collision to limit the damage to the front or rear of the vehicle. Sometimes these bumpers become loaded in the crushed position and do not immediately bounce back out. When emergency workers are on or near the vehicle, the bumper may suddenly release causing injury to the workers.
14. d. Electric powered vehicles run very quiet and may not be heard right away. Working in and around a running vehicle is dangerous for obvious reasons.

Vehicles that use natural gas or a high-pressure tank have an increased risk for fire and/or explosion.

15. d. Any of these items will help to protect the patient from the breaking glass.

16. a. Remember to make sure the engine is turned off and, if possible, to set the parking break. If trained to do so, stabilize the vehicle with ropes, chocks, or a come-a-long until the rescue team arrives to assist.

17. a. Sometimes the fastest and easiest method of gaining access is overlooked. Don't forget to check first for an unlocked door.

18. a. Attempt simple access first by trying to open a door that is unlocked before breaking any glass.

19. d. The window furthest from the patient should be the first one broken to gain access to the patient.

20. b. As the name indicates, this is a simple form of access requiring no tools or special equipment.

21. c. This term applies when tools or special equipment are used to gain access to a victim who is entrapped.

22. a. As the name indicates, this is a simple form of access requiring no tools or special equipment.

23. b. The amount of time it takes to gain access is the dynamic factor in rescue operations and is very different from other types of EMS calls.

24. a. Traffic is the greatest hazard for emergency responders.

25. a. The A post supports the roof at the windshield; the B post is the support on the side of the vehicle behind the driver's door.

Chapter 36: Hazardous Materials, Multiple Casualty incidents, and Incident Management

1. c. Each EMT is trained at least to the awareness level, which means they have the knowledge to recognize a hazardous scene, call for more help, and not enter unless they have a higher level of training and the proper equipment. The level of response and participation is predetermined in many communities.

2. b. The EMT must complete a scene size-up at each call, including potential HAZMAT incident scenes.

3. b. Each EMT is trained at least to the awareness level, which means they have the knowledge to recognize a hazardous scene, call for more help, and not enter unless they have a higher level of training and the proper equipment.

4. c. The incident commander has the primary responsibility of ensuring everyone's safety at the scene of an incident. He may designate a safety officer, especially at large incidents, to assist with this task.

5. b. Before work begins at an incident where a hazardous material is present, zones are established to prevent injury and unnecessary exposure to the substance.

6. a. Before work begins at an incident where a hazardous material is present, zones are established to prevent injury and unnecessary exposure to the substance.

7. a. Flammability hazards include: may cause fire or explosion; may ignite other combustible materials; and may be ignited by heat, sparks, or flames.

8. b. In such a case, the victims of a possible exposure should be removed right away. The longer the victims are exposed, the more serious their conditions may become.

9. c. The EMT is trained to recognize a hazardous scene, call for more help, and not enter unless she has a higher level of training and the proper equipment.

10. d. This is the recommendation for approaching and staging at the scene of a HAZMAT incident.

11. b. The EMT is trained to recognize a hazardous scene, call for more help, and not enter unless he has a higher level of training and the proper equipment.

12. b. Safety first for you and your crew!

13. b. The *cold zone* is the furthest outside the incident. It is the safe area for personnel trained to the awareness level or higher.

14. b. Gross decontamination should be completed by the patient if he or she is able.

15. b. One of the duties in a treatment sector (group) is to monitor the HAZMAT teams before and after entry into the hot zone.

16. d. Decon is the process of removing hazardous materials from exposed persons and equipment at an incident.

17. c. Victims who have been in a confined space where smoke and fire were present are at risk for carbon monoxide inhalation and should be evaluated for it.

18. d. Wind directions can change the dynamics of a HAZMAT incident very rapidly. Wind direction is routinely monitored during outside HAZMAT incidents for this reason.

19. d. This rescue is still an extrication for one patient, but now there is a second patient in need of evaluation.

20. c. At the onset, there is the potential for a number of patients here (more than you and your crew can effectively manage), so declaring an MCI (multiple-casualty-incident) is appropriate.

21. d. At the onset, there are a number of patients here (more than you and your crew can effectively manage), so declaring an MCI is appropriate.

22. d. The size and complexity of the incident, including the number of personnel on scene, are the primary factors that help determine how many sectors (groups) will be established at an incident.

23. a. Each EMT is trained to the HAZMAT awareness level, which means they have the knowledge to recognize a hazardous scene, call for more help, establish a safe perimeter, and not enter unless they have a higher level of training and the proper equipment.

24. a. This is the role of the treatment sector (group) officer.

25. a. To *triage* is to sort patients based on the severity of injury and the resources available.

26. a. The use of triage tags helps to reduce or eliminate the need to repeatedly count and get a baseline assessment of each patient.

27. c. This task can be done quickly and possibly help save a life without delaying the triage of other potential patients.

28. a. The size of the incident will determine when and how much logistics are required.

29. b. During a disaster operation, the EMT provides medical and psychological support to those who need it.

30. a. Preplanning and training are the best way to prepare for disaster operations.

31. a. "Keep it simple and clear with plain English" is the concept used in such emergencies.

32. b. Each community needs to have an IMS that has been practiced and is understood by all of the providers in each of the agencies that may be asked to respond to any major incidents.

33. c. The four major components utilized during the management of a large MCI are operations, planning, logistics, and finance.

34. c. An ED with the resources will direct you to take your patient through a designated area in its facility for additional decon.

35. c. The cold zone is the furthest outside the incident. It is the safe area for personnel trained to the awareness level or higher.

36. a. The patient's clothing is removed early as part of the decon process.

37. d. The local fire departments should have all this information, as well as a preplan for possible incidents at the locations.

38. c. Responsibilities can include managing the EMS response, designating the EMS division or sector officers, and establishing a command post and remaining there.

39. a. Unified command is multiple agencies (e.g., EMS, fire department, and police) working together at an incident to contribute to the command process by determining the overall goals and objectives, and using joint planning for tactical activities.

40. b. The unified command post is where the commanders of each agency work collectively to determine the overall goals and objectives for planning tactical activities and maximizing the use of all assigned resources at the incident.

41. d. This patient has minor injuries and none that affect the ABCs.

42. a. This patient is having a breathing problem, which makes her a high priority in need of immediate care.

43. b. Get the ball rolling and declare an MCI. Assess the amount and type of resources needed and request them.

44. c. This is the definition of a *multiple-casualty incident (MCI)*.

45. c. There is not much you can do for these victims until they are extricated.

46. a. Hazardous terrain rescues are categorized as low angle, high angle, or flat with obstructions. A steep slope or "low-angle" terrain is capable of being walked up without using the hands. This terrain can become more dangerous because of difficult footing, especially when you are carrying a patient in a basket on snow, ice, rocks, or mud.

47. b. While wearing a PFD, you can attempt to throw a rope to the victim during the wait for the rescue team.

48. b. A personal flotation device (PFD) is the required minimum personal safety equipment for any rescuer working in or near water. An exposure suit is used when working in cold or icy water.

49. a. Confined spaces may contain very little oxygen or may contain dangerous gases. Rescues in confined spaces require continuous air monitoring during the rescue effort.

50. c. The EMT with the proper training and equipment may participate in any of the phases of a rescue that she is qualified for.

Chapter 37: EMS Response to Terrorism

1. b. An indicator that you have encountered terrorist activities includes finding suspicious items in a vehicle or on a person, such as weapons of an unusual nature, bomb-making materials, or manuals for the manufacture of these items.

2. a. Biological agents are classified into three general categories: viral agents, bacterial agents, and toxins.

3. c. Indicators that a terrorist incident where CBRNE ages have been used include unusual findings such as responders becoming ill, multiple unconscious patients with or without obvious injury, dead animals or vegetation, HAZMAT at the scene, smoke or vapor clouds, evidence of an explosion, and other atypical settings.

4. c. Nerve agents usually overstimulate the release of chemical neurotransmitters, causing muscles and certain glands of the body to overreact.

5. d. This action will assist with protection of responders, treatment, and decontamination.

6. d. Awareness-level training gives the EMT the information to recognize when it is or is not safe to gain access to patients in dangerous situations or environments.

7. b. The EMT working an incident of terrorism basically becomes part of the crime scene. As soon as possible after a response to terrorism, the EMT should compile field notes, organize them, and provide them to investigators.

8. b. The role of the EMT in this type of incident is similar to that in other incidents. Upon arrival at the scene, report to command and then to any area designated by command.

9. c. Radiation can be used as a weapon by using explosives and radioactive materials (in the form of powder or pellets). These radiological dispersal devices are also called "dirty bombs."

10. Some basic ways to reduce exposure to radiation include: increasing the distance from the source, decreasing the amount of time spent near the source, and using a shield as a barrier between yourself/patients and the source.

11. c. ARS is typically caused when a person receives a high dose of radiation to the body in a matter of minutes. It is more likely to occur in a patient receiving cancer treatment than anyone in the event of a dirty bomb explosion. The primary danger of a dirty bomb is the explosion itself.

12. a. Later effects include: continued nausea, vomiting, diarrhea, loss of appetite, weakness, internal bleeding, fever, destruction of bone marrow, seizures, and possible coma.

13. b. Blister agents and some irritant agents are absorbed through the skin.

14. b. Contaminated patients should be located to a restricted area with symptomatic patients in one section and asymptomatic patients in another. Begin gross decon by having the patients remove clothing, shoes, jewelry, and any other items.

15. b. Tear gas, pepper spray, and mace are examples of irritating agents designed to temporarily incapacitate.

16. d. Victims of exposure to biological agents have delayed onset of symptoms. Some early effects may be seen within four to six hours; other effects may take days or weeks.

17. c. Secondary devices are bombs placed at the scene that are designed to have a delayed explosion after the primary explosion. The EMT must be alert to the potential for a secondary device.

18. d. Explosive devices can be designed to broadcast chemical, biological, and radiological agents.

19. a. The first unit on scene will establish command and survey the scene. Then communicate with dispatch and call for additional resources. The next round of providers will be assigned sector/officer roles.

20. b. Care for nerve agent exposure includes airway management, the use of an antidote kit containing atropine and pralidoxime and packaged as Mark 1 Kit, and Valium (diazepam).

21. c. TRACEM-P harms include: thermal-heat sources, radiologic-nuclear bombs, fuels and by-products, asphyxiation (lack of oxygen due to chemical gases/vapors), chemical (toxic or corrosive), etiologic (biological hazards), mechanical trauma from metal, bullets, etc., and psychological (from any event).

22. a. Ricin is a poison found in castor beans and can be made from the waste materials of processing castor beans. It can be formed into powder, a mist, or a pellet and has no antidote. As a terrorist weapon it has been used in London, Paris, Canada, and Minnesota. Ebola, small pox, and yellow fever are viruses.

23. b. Using unnecessary levels of PPE may cause additional hazards for the responders such as heat stress, dehydration, and limited visibility and mobility.

24. a. These devices will have three basic components: an igniter or fuse, a container or body, and an incendiary material or filler.

25. c. A blast lung injury occurs as a result of a blast wave from a highly explosive detonation. Injuries include pulmonary contusion, bleeding, or swelling with damage to alveoli and blood vessels.

Appendix B:
Basic Life Support Review

1. The care provided in the first few minutes of a life-threatening emergency is called:
   a. CPR.
   b. secondary assessment.
   c. basic life support.
   d. reassessment.

2. One of the major changes in the Guidelines 2005, which was again reinforced in Guidelines 2010, was to improve the effectiveness of the delivery chest compressions by:
   a. emphasizing that all rescuers should push hard and fast.
   b. allowing more time between compressions for better chest recoil.
   c. increasing the compression rate and omitting ventilations for the lay rescuer.
   d. adding voice prompts in AEDs and defibrillators, which remind the rescuer to maintain the correct compression rate.

3. The general term that is used to describe the spectrum of disease from acute angina to myocardial infarction is:
   a. heart attack.
   b. acute coronary syndrome (ACS).
   c. unstable angina.
   d. coronary illness.

4. In an effort to maintain the most effective delivery of chest compressions during a sudden cardiac arrest (SCA), it is recommended that the rescuers performing compressions switch positions every _____ minutes.
   a. two
   b. three
   c. four
   d. five

5. For the adult patient who is not breathing, each rescue breath should be provided:
   a. one second per breath.
   b. over two seconds.
   c. every six to eight seconds.
   d. every thirty seconds.

6. The recommendation for one-rescuer CPR is for a compression ventilation ratio of:
   a. 30:2 for all rescuers.
   b. 30:2 for lay rescuers only.
   c. 15:2 for health care providers only.
   d. 30:2 for health care providers only.

7. The goal of the Guidelines 2010 was to develop widely accepted international resuscitation guidelines that were:
   a. based on a majority vote.
   b. based on the least cost to implement.
   c. based on scientific evidence.
   d. easy to read and explain.

8. Guidelines that are supported by very good evidence of effectiveness and safety in humans are class:
   a. I.
   b. IIa.
   c. IIb.
   d. III.

9. The Guidelines 2010 recommend that when attempting defibrillation:
   a. all rescuers deliver one shock followed by immediate CPR for two minutes.
   b. lay rescuers deliver one shock followed by immediate CPR for five minutes.
   c. using an AED, on children one to eight years old, the dose is the same as an adult.
   d. health care providers deliver three shocks followed by immediate CPR for one minute.

10. All health care providers with a duty to perform CPR should be trained, equipped, and authorized to perform defibrillation is a class _____ guideline.
    a. I
    b. IIa
    c. IIb
    d. III

11. For the infant or child patient who is not breathing, each rescue breath should be provided:
    a. over two seconds.
    b. every one to two seconds.
    c. every three to five seconds.
    d. every six to eight seconds.

12. The recommendation for interruptions in CPR for pulse checks should:
    a. occur once every minute.
    b. take less than five seconds.
    c. take less than ten seconds.
    d. not occur more than once every five minutes.

13. When the rescuer performing the chest compressions allows the chest to recoil after each compression, this action:
    a. allows the heart to fill with blood.
    b. allows each ventilation to fill the lungs.
    c. reduces the amount of compressions delivered each minute.
    d. increases the amount of compressions delivered each minute.

14. When providing ventilations without an advanced airway in the patient experiencing cardiac arrest, the rescuer should avoid over ventilation because it:
    a. impedes blood return to the heart.
    b. increases the venous capacity of the heart.
    c. reduces the threshold for cardioversion.
    d. reduces the ventricular fibrillation threshold.

15. When an individual executes his right of self-determination and declares he does not want to be resuscitated if he becomes unresponsive, this is referred to as a(n):
    a. unrecognized determination.
    b. DNAR order.
    c. termination order.
    d. final rite.

16. The Guidelines 2010 are considered:
    a. the legal standard of care.
    b. national regulations.
    c. consensus standards.
    d. international law.

17. The initial dose for shocking ventricular fibrillation using a monophasic waveform for treatment is:
    a. 120 J.
    b. 200 J.
    c. 300 J.
    d. 360 J.

18. After the initial dose, subsequent shocks using monophasic waveform for treatment of ventricular fibrillation are:
    a. 150 J.
    b. 200 J.
    c. 300 J.
    d. 360 J.

19. In the out-of-hospital setting, the 5-year-old child who collapses from sudden cardiac arrest should first receive _____ .
    a. one minute of CPR
    b. two minutes of CPR
    c. ten cycles of CPR
    d. defibrillation with an AED

20. Of all the interventions available to the cardiac arrest patient, which has the most scientific evidence in its favor?
    a. CPR
    b. defibrillation
    c. compressions
    d. high-dose epinephrine

21. The use of the AED is encouraged for all patients over the age of:
    a. fifty.
    b. fifteen.
    c. eight.
    d. one.

22. Where is the best "bang for the buck" in saving cardiac arrest patients?
    a. adding more ALS units
    b. expanding the use of fibrinolytics
    c. removing barriers to implementing PAD
    d. training EMTs to intubate

23. In the Guidelines 2010, updates in health care provider training for CPR on a "child" applies to:
    a. opening the airway.
    b. patients between one and eight years old.
    c. patients from one year old to the onset of puberty.
    d. two-rescuer, two-thumb-encircling-hands technique.

24. In what situation should you phone first instead of phone fast?
    a. a child with previous MI
    b. a child who may have drowned
    c. a child with a possible airway obstruction
    d. when you are not near a phone

25. In adults, when should the rescuer consider phoning fast instead of phoning first?
    a. cardiac arrest caused by electrical shock
    b. preexisting MI
    c. poisoning or drug overdose
    d. patients over sixty years old

26. When using a bag mask, the rescuer should:
    a. enlist a second rescuer to help squeeze the bag.
    b. use the "C"/"E" clamp hand position.
    c. provide breaths over one second.
    d. all of the above.

27. Where is the best position for the ventilator when using a bag mask on a supine patient?
    a. at the patient's side
    b. about 18 inches above the head of the patient
    c. straddling the patient
    d. lying flat on your stomach

28. Which statement is incorrect?
    a. Proper use of the bag mask requires practice.
    b. The jaw thrust can be used with one-rescuer technique on a trauma patient.
    c. Tidal volumes of 400 to 600 ml can be given over one second.
    d. The bag mask should be attached to 100% oxygen.

29. When smaller tidal volumes are used with the bag mask, the:
    a. patient should be hyperventilated.
    b. breaths need to be given faster.
    c. breaths need to be more forceful.
    d. chest should rise visibly.

30. When a victim suddenly collapses and has no signs of circulation, the rescuer should first provide _____ .
    a. two rescue breaths
    b. defibrillation with an AED
    c. one cycle of thirty compressions
    d. five cycles of thirty compressions followed by two rescue breaths

31. What evidence helped researchers recommend dropping the pulse check step for laypersons?
    a. No one checks it anyway.
    b. The patient often still has a faint pulse.
    c. It takes too much time to teach.
    d. They were frequently wrong in their assessment.

32. When biphasic waveform defibrillation is used on an adult in sudden cardiac arrest, the initial shock dose is:
    a. 150 J.
    b. 200 J.
    c. 300 J.
    d. 360 J.

33. If a foreign body airway obstruction is suspected in an adult patient, the health care provider should:
    a. call for the defibrillator.
    b. reposition the neck and reattempt to ventilate.
    c. simply give chest compressions.
    d. perform a blind finger sweep.

34. The initial shock dose for a child in ventricular fibrillation using a monophasic or biphasic manual defibrillator is:
    a. 1 J/kg.
    b. 2 J/kg.
    c. 3 J/kg.
    d. 4 J/kg.

35. If a person has a foreign body airway obstruction (FBAO) and is an adult:
    a. do not do chest compressions.
    b. chest compression may be helpful.
    c. reach down his throat to remove the object.
    d. ventilate twice as fast.

36. Where are the hands placed to do CPR compressions on an adult?
    a. on the bottom of the breastbone
    b. at the top of the breastbone
    c. on the seventh intercostal space
    d. in the center of the chest, between the nipples

37. At what rate should the chest be compressed for an adult patient in sudden cardiac arrest?
    a. 60 per minute
    b. 80 per minute
    c. 90 per minute
    d. at least 100 per minute

38. The compression-to-ventilation ratio for infants and children older than one year, when performed by two health care providers, is:
    a. 5:1.
    b. 15:2.
    c. 30:1.
    d. 30:2.

39. When providing chest compressions on a child in sudden cardiac arrest, the rescuer should use:
    a. the heel of only one hand to compress the lower half of the sternum.
    b. the heel of one or two hands to compress the lower half of the sternum.
    c. one hand to compress to a depth of one-quarter of the chest diameter.
    d. both hands to compress to a depth of one-quarter of the chest diameter.

40. The first choice technique for chest compression in an infant when there are two rescuers is to do the:
    a. two-thumb-encircling-hands chest technique.
    b. two fingers at the center of the chest.
    c. one-handed technique.
    d. two-handed technique.

41. While performing CPR with an advanced airway in place, the rescuer delivering the ventilations should provide _____ ventilation(s) every _____ seconds.
    a. one; six to eight
    b. one; five to six
    c. two; fifteen
    d. two; thirty

42. The Guidelines require training in the use of a(n) _____ by all health care providers.
    a. bag mask
    b. LMA
    c. Combitube®
    d. ET tube

43. CPR is in progress on an adult when you arrive with a defibrillator. You quickly analyze the rhythm, detect pulseless ventricular tachycardia, and administer one shock. The next step is to:
    a. check the pulse, reanalyze the rhythm, and resume CPR for two minutes.
    b. reanalyze the rhythm, check the pulse, and resume CPR for two minutes.
    c. resume CPR for five cycles, then reanalyze the rhythm and check the pulse.
    d. reanalyze the rhythm, resume CPR for five cycles, and then check the pulse.

44. Acute MI and unstable angina are now recognized as part of a spectrum of disease known as:
    a. acute coronary syndromes (ACS).
    b. advanced coronary syndromes.
    c. ACLS disorders.
    d. acute cardiac disorders.

45. Recommended prehospital medications for all patients with ACS include _____ in the absence of contraindications.
    a. aspirin
    b. nitroglycerin
    c. beta-blockers
    d. antiarythmics

Appendix B: Answer Form

	A	B	C	D		A	B	C	D
1.	❏	❏	❏	❏	24.	❏	❏	❏	❏
2.	❏	❏	❏	❏	25.	❏	❏	❏	❏
3.	❏	❏	❏	❏	26.	❏	❏	❏	❏
4.	❏	❏	❏	❏	27.	❏	❏	❏	❏
5.	❏	❏	❏	❏	28.	❏	❏	❏	❏
6.	❏	❏	❏	❏	29.	❏	❏	❏	❏
7.	❏	❏	❏	❏	30.	❏	❏	❏	❏
8.	❏	❏	❏	❏	31.	❏	❏	❏	❏
9.	❏	❏	❏	❏	32.	❏	❏	❏	❏
10.	❏	❏	❏	❏	33.	❏	❏	❏	❏
11.	❏	❏	❏	❏	34.	❏	❏	❏	❏
12.	❏	❏	❏	❏	35.	❏	❏	❏	❏
13.	❏	❏	❏	❏	36.	❏	❏	❏	❏
14.	❏	❏	❏	❏	37.	❏	❏	❏	❏
15.	❏	❏	❏	❏	38.	❏	❏	❏	❏
16.	❏	❏	❏	❏	39.	❏	❏	❏	❏
17.	❏	❏	❏	❏	40.	❏	❏	❏	❏
18.	❏	❏	❏	❏	41.	❏	❏	❏	❏
19.	❏	❏	❏	❏	42.	❏	❏	❏	❏
20.	❏	❏	❏	❏	43.	❏	❏	❏	❏
21.	❏	❏	❏	❏	44.	❏	❏	❏	❏
22.	❏	❏	❏	❏	45.	❏	❏	❏	❏
23.	❏	❏	❏	❏					

Appendix B: Answers

1. c. basic life support.—Together with advanced cardiac life support (ACLS), it is part of the emergency cardiac care provided to patients experiencing symptoms of a heart attack. BLS is used interchangeably with the old phrase basic cardiac life support (BCLS) when discussing cardiac care. BLS is often used to refer to the technique of cardiopulmonary resuscitation (CPR) when managing a cardiac arrest.

2. a. emphasizing that all rescuers should push hard and fast.—The better and faster the compressions, the more blood flow they will produce.

3. b. acute coronary syndrome.—An acute coronary syndrome (ACS) is a catch-all term devised to emphasize that many times it is impossible to tell the difference between unstable angina and infarction.

4. a. two—Studies have shown that the effectiveness of chest compressions deteriorate rapidly as the rescuer tires. The new recommendation is for the rescuers to switch, without interruption, every two minutes.

5. a. one second per breath.—When the adult patient has a pulse, but is not breathing, rescue breaths should be given over one second every five to six seconds.

6. a. 30:2 for all rescuers.—This change emphasizes the importance of maximizing chest compressions without interruptions for all rescuers.

7. c. based on scientific evidence.—This evidence was reviewed and scientific consensus obtained from the international resuscitation community.

8. b. IIa.—An example of a Class IIa treatment is that each rescue breath be given over one second.

9. a. all rescuers deliver one shock followed by immediate CPR for two minutes.—The new recommendation is for single shocks, followed by immediate CPR and rhythm checks assessed every two minutes.

10. b. IIa—Another example of a Class IIa treatment is chest compressions delivered at a rate of 100 per minute.

11. c. every three to five seconds.—When the infant or child patient has a pulse, but is not breathing, rescue breaths should be given over one second every three to five seconds.

12. c. take less than ten seconds.—Interruptions in chest compression should occur as infrequently as possible and take no more than ten seconds.

13. d. allows the heart to fill with blood.—If the chest does not recoil, the heart will not receive adequate venous return and the subsequent compression will not produce adequate cardiac output.

14. a. it impedes blood return to the heart.—Over inflation of the lungs increases intrathoracic pressure, and this prevents adequate filling of the heart with blood.

15. b. DNAR order.—It is the responsibility of the health care provider to search for and honor a DNAR that is deemed valid.

16. c. consensus standards.—They are based on the ILCOR consensus and the science of resuscitation.

17. d. 360 J.—This is a change from the 2000 Guidelines. The recommended dose for initial and subsequent shocks using monophasic waveform is 360 J.

18. d. 360 J.—The recommended dose for initial and subsequent shocks using monophasic waveform is 360 J.

19. b. two minutes of CPR—In the out-of-hospital setting, all rescuers should provide five cycles or approximately two minutes of CPR prior to using the AED.

20. b. defibrillation—Early defibrillation is the single acute intervention that really makes a difference in saving lives from sudden cardiac arrest.

21. d. one—Since 2003, the use of AEDs is recommended for children one year and older in sudden cardiac arrest.

22. c. removing barriers to implementing PAD—Limited funds are better spent on removing the barriers to training the lay public in CPR and public access defibrillation (PAD). Clearly, all the medications do not help save as many patients as getting the defibrillator operator there faster.

23. c. patients one year old to the onset of puberty.—The change applies to victims of cardiac arrest from about one year old to the onset of puberty or adolescence, as defined by the presence of secondary sex characteristics.

24. a. a child with previous ACS—The major exception to the phone-fast rule is those children under eight years old who are known to be at risk for ventricular fibrillation (VF) or ventricular tachycardia (VT), who have a history of cardiac dysrhythmias, or those with congenital heart disease who experience sudden witnessed collapse.

25. c. poisoning or drug overdose—These patients tend to be hypoxic and have the best chance of survival when CPR is provided in the first few minutes of sudden cardiac arrest.

26. d. all of the above.—The technique of providing ventilations with a bag mask requires routine practice and is a fundamental skill that should be mastered by all health care providers.

27. b. about 18 inches above the head of the patient—The ventilator should be positioned approximately 18 inches above the head of the patient; hyperextend the airway and use the weight of the left arm, which is sealing the mask, to hold the airway in the hyperextended position. The other hand can be used to squeeze the bag against itself.

28. b. The jaw thrust can be used for one-rescuer bag mask technique on a trauma patient.—It is not possible to do a jaw thrust, jutting both sides of the jar anterior, with only one hand.

29. d. chest should rise visibly.—With supplemental oxygen attached to the bag mask, smaller tidal volumes (400–600 ml) are acceptable. The rescuer should still be able to see the chest rise and maintain the patient's oxygen saturation at greater than 90 percent.

30. a. two rescue breaths—After the two rescue breaths are given, the rescuer should immediately begin chest compressions in cycles of 30:2.

31. d. they were frequently wrong in their assessment—This step was taking too long to perform and was too often performed incorrectly. The goal now is to deliver chest compressions rapidly and without delays.

32. a. 150 J.—An initial dose of 150 J to 200 J is recommended when using a biphasic truncated exponential waveform, and 120 J for a rectilinear biphasic waveform.

33. b. reposition the neck and reattempt to ventilate.—Blind finger sweeps should not be used on any patient.

34. a. 2 J/kg.—Subsequent doses should be 4 J/kg.

35. b. chest compressions may be helpful.—Chest compressions generated at least as high or higher intrathoracic pressures than abdominal thrusts. Therefore, the chest compressions used in CPR are helpful in dislodging an FBAO in the unresponsive patient.

36. d. in the center of the chest between the nipples—This position has not changed in the new Guidelines.

37. d. at least 100—This rate changed in the Guidelines 2010.

38. b. 15:2.—For infants less than one year old, the compression to ventilation ratio is 5:1.

39. b. the heel of one or two hands to compress the lower half of the sternum.—The placement of the hand or hands should be at about the nipple line.

40. a. two-thumb-encircling-hands chest technique.—The Guidelines still recommend this as the primary method for compressions for the neonate.

41. a. 1: six to eight—Once an advanced airway has been inserted, the rescuer delivers one ventilation every six to eight seconds, and the compressor continues without interruption.

42. a. bag mask—The bag mask provides effective ventilations when used by properly trained providers who practice the skill.

43. c. resume CPR for five cycles, and then reanalyze the rhythm and check pulse.—Pulse and rhythm are not checked after the shock; rather, they are checked after five cycles of CPR, or about two minutes.

44. a. acute coronary syndromes.—An acute coronary syndrome (ACS) is a catch-all term devised to emphasize that many times it is impossible to tell the difference between unstable angina and infarction.

45. a. aspirin—All patients with signs and symptoms of ACS, including non-Q wave MI, should receive aspirin and beta-blockers in the absence of contraindications.

Appendix C: Tips for Preparing for a Practical Skills Examination

During an EMT course, many educators teach the core curriculum and provide enrichment material as time, resources, and experience permit. Near the end of an EMT course, it is typical for educators to change their style of teaching and begin preparation for the exam; that is, they will provide examples of the material to be tested on state and national exams, and give tips on how to take the written exams. The educator may hold one or more practice skills sessions and a mock practical exam to help students prepare. Limited time and resources often do not allow for as much skills practice time as some students would like. Thus, I have included some tips to help you get ready for the practical skills exam.

If you have not done so already, obtain a copy of the skills testing sheets to be used for your practical skills exam, and carefully read the instructions well before the day of the exam itself. Note that each exam skill sheet has items that are identified as critical pass-or-fail items. These items, which are usually bolded for easy identification, include taking or verbalizing standard precautions or scene safety, as well as other critical tasks. National Registry skills sheets also list "Critical Criteria" at the bottom of each sheet. This is a list of items that were not performed and should have been. When an evaluator checks one of these items, the candidate will fail the station.

Often the course instructor will hand out a set of the skills testing sheets to be used for the state and/or registry exam during or near the end of the course, and you will be given an opportunity to practice the skills in lab using the testing sheets. I strongly recommend that you take every opportunity provided during the course to do this. In addition, find one or more students or experienced EMTs to practice skills with. While you demonstrate the skill, have another person use the testing sheet to evaluate your performance. Be tough on each other in a friendly way! Pay close attention to the critical failure items and then focus on obtaining every point available.

Before the day of the practical skills exam, make certain you are familiar with the location of where the exam is being given. Arrive at least 15 minutes early on the day of the exam. Bring a copy of the skills sheets with you to review while you are waiting. On the testing day, be patient and be prepared to be at the testing site for most of the day. Practical skills testing typically takes a lot of time. In addition to bringing the skills sheets to review, bring a book, a drink, lunch, and plenty of patience.

On the day of the practical exam, if you have the option of choosing the order of the testing stations, I recommend using one of two methods. The first one is this: If you are a little nervous and you want to build your confidence, start with a short skill station like AED. This is a skill you will have successfully completed in a CPR class. From there, continue to build your confidence by selecting the stations that you feel you can complete without difficulty.

The second method I recommend is selecting the most difficult stations and completing those first. For most people, the assessment stations seem the most difficult because they have the most steps and take the longest to complete. Once these stations are complete, you can breathe a little easier while completing the remaining stations.

If you do not have the option of choosing the order of skills to be tested, do not worry at this point; you have prepared and are ready for each skill station. During the exam, the evaluators are instructed not to tell you if you have passed or failed a skill station until you have finished testing at all of the stations, so do not expect or ask them to. (The reasoning behind this is that if you fail a station early in the testing, you may become distracted and fail another.)

Once in the station, you will be read a set of instructions and given the opportunity to ask questions for clarification and to check the equipment provided. I recommend that you do this, especially if you are the first candidate of the day coming into a station. The evaluator has been instructed to make sure that the equipment is functioning properly and that there will be no distractions for the candidates. They are not there to trip you up, but occasionally something goes amiss, such as a blood pressure cuff that is broken and is not detected before the exam starts.

In the patient assessment station, I recommend that you ask if the injuries or significant signs that you are supposed to detect are going to be visible with moulage or by another method. This is a common area where problems can develop. Verbalize the steps and tasks you complete as if you were talking to a new partner. After a long day of testing, evaluators become fatigued just like you. If an evaluator happened to have her head turned while you were performing a critical step, she will hear you verbalizing it.

If you should have to repeat a station, know the retest policy and do not overreact. You have spent a lot of time training and should persevere rather than throwing it in over one bad day! Remember, we humans do make mistakes occasionally. The key is how you learn from your mistakes, correct them, and move forward.

Lastly, get some sleep before the examination. Try to get a good night's rest two nights before in addition to the night before. Many people are very nervous about test taking and do not sleep well the night before no matter what. Getting a good sleep two nights before does help.

Best of luck and be prepared!

—*Kirt*

Appendix D:
National Registry Practical Examination Sheets

National Registry of Emergency Medical Technicians®
Emergency Medical Technician Psychomotor Examination

BLEEDING CONTROL/SHOCK MANAGEMENT

Candidate: _____   Examiner: _____
Date: _____   Signature: _____

Actual Time Started: _____

	Possible Points	Points Awarded
Takes or verbalizes appropriate body substance isolation precautions	1	
Applies direct pressure to the wound	1	
NOTE: The examiner must now inform the candidate that the wound continues to bleed.		
Applies tourniquet	1	
NOTE: The examiner must now inform the candidate that the patient is exhibiting signs and symptoms of hypoperfusion.		
Properly positions the patient	1	
Administers high concentration oxygen	1	
Initiates steps to prevent heat loss from the patient	1	
Indicates the need for immediate transportation	1	

Actual Time Ended: _____   TOTAL   7

Critical Criteria

___ Did not take or verbalize body substance isolation precautions
___ Did not administer high concentration of oxygen
___ Did not control hemorrhage using correct procedures in a timely manner
___ Did not indicate the need for immediate transportation
___ Failure to manage the patient as a competent EMT
___ Exhibits unacceptable affect with patient or other personnel
___ Uses or orders a dangerous or inappropriate intervention

You must factually document your rationale for checking any of the above critical items on this form (below or turn sheet over).

(Reprinted with permission of the National Registry of Emergency Medical Technicians.)

National Registry of Emergency Medical Technicians®
Emergency Medical Technician Psychomotor Examination

BVM VENTILATION OF AN APNEIC ADULT PATIENT

Candidate: _____   Examiner: _____

Date: _____   Signature: _____

Actual Time Started: _____

	Possible Points	Points Awarded
Takes or verbalizes appropriate body substance isolation precautions	1	
Checks responsiveness	*NOTE: After checking responsiveness and breathing for at least 5 but no more than 10 seconds, examiner informs the candidate, "The patient is unresponsive and apneic."*	1	
Checks breathing		1	
Requests additional EMS assistance	1	
Checks pulse for at least 5 but no more than 10 seconds	1	
NOTE: The examiner must now inform the candidate, "You palpate a weak carotid pulse at a rate of 60."		
Opens airway properly	1	
NOTE: The examiner must now inform the candidate, "The mouth is full of secretions and vomitus."		
Prepares rigid suction catheter	1	
Turns on power to suction device or retrieves manual suction device	1	
Inserts rigid suction catheter without applying suction	1	
Suctions the mouth and oropharynx	1	
NOTE: The examiner must now inform the candidate, "The mouth and oropharynx are clear."		
Opens the airway manually	1	
Inserts oropharyngeal airway	1	
NOTE: The examiner must now inform the candidate, "No gag reflex is present and the patient accepts the airway adjunct."		
Ventilates the patient immediately using a BVM device unattached to oxygen [Award this point if candidate elects to ventilate initially with BVM attached to reservoir and oxygen so long as first ventilation is delivered within 30 seconds.]	1	
NOTE: The examiner must now inform the candidate that ventilation is being properly performed without difficulty.		
Re-checks pulse for at least 5 but no more than 10 seconds	1	
Attaches the BVM assembly [mask, bag, reservoir] to oxygen [15 L/minute]	1	
Ventilates the patient adequately -Proper volume to make chest rise (1 point) -Proper rate [10 – 12/minute but not to exceed 12/minute] (1 point)	2	
NOTE: The examiner must now ask the candidate, "How would you know if you are delivering appropriate volumes with each ventilation?"		

Actual Time Ended: _____   **TOTAL**   17

Critical Criteria

____ Failure to initiate ventilations within 30 seconds after taking body substance isolation precautions or interrupts ventilations for greater than 30 seconds at any time

____ Failure to take or verbalize body substance isolation precautions

____ Failure to suction airway before ventilating the patient

____ Suctions the patient for an excessive and prolonged time

____ Failure to check responsiveness and breathing for at least 5 seconds but no more than 10 seconds

____ Failure to check pulse for at least 5 seconds but no more than 10 seconds

____ Failure to voice and ultimately provide high oxygen concentration [at least 85%]

____ Failure to ventilate the patient at a rate of at least 10/minute and no more than 12/minute

____ Failure to provide adequate volumes per breath [maximum 2 errors/minute permissible]

____ Insertion or use of any adjunct in a manner dangerous to the patient

____ Failure to manage the patient as a competent EMT

____ Exhibits unacceptable affect with patient or other personnel

____ Uses or orders a dangerous or inappropriate intervention

You must factually document your rationale for checking any of the above critical items on this form (below or turn sheet over).

(Reprinted with permission of the National Registry of Emergency Medical Technicians.)

CARDIAC ARREST MANAGEMENT / AED

Candidate: _____   Examiner: _____

Date: _____   Signature: _____

Actual Time Started: _____

	Possible Points	Points Awarded
Takes or verbalizes appropriate body substance isolation precautions	1	
Determines the scene/situation is safe	1	
Attempts to question bystanders about arrest events	1	
Checks patient responsiveness	1	
NOTE: The examiner must now inform the candidate, "The patient is unresponsive."		
Assesses patient for signs of breathing [observes the patient and determines the absence of breathing or abnormal breathing (gasping or agonal respirations)]	1	
NOTE: The examiner must now inform the candidate, "The patient is apneic," or, "The patient has gasping, agonal respirations."		
Checks carotid pulse [no more than 10 seconds]	1	
NOTE: The examiner must now inform the candidate, "The patient is pulseless."		
Immediately begins chest compressions [adequate depth and rate; allows the chest to recoil completely]	1	
Requests additional EMS response	1	

Performs 2 minutes of high quality, 1-rescuer adult CPR
    Adequate depth and rate (1 point)
    Correct compression-to-ventilation ratio (1 point)
    Allows the chest to recoil completely (1 point)
    Adequate volumes for each breath (1 point)
    Minimal interruptions of less than 10 seconds throughout (1 point)
	5	

NOTE: After 2 minutes (5 cycles), patient is assessed and second rescuer resumes compressions while candidate operates AED.		
Turns on power to AED	1	
Follows prompts and correctly attaches AED to patient	1	
Stops CPR and ensures all individuals are clear of the patient during rhythm analysis	1	
Ensures that all individuals are clear of the patient and delivers shock from AED	1	
Immediately directs rescuer to resume chest compressions	1	

Actual Time Ended: _____   **TOTAL**   18

Critical Criteria

___ Failure to take or verbalize appropriate body substance isolation precautions
___ Failure to immediately begin chest compressions as soon as pulselessness is confirmed
___ Failure to deliver shock in a timely manner
___ Interrupts CPR for more than 10 seconds at any point
___ Failure to demonstrate acceptable high-quality, 1-rescuer adult CPR
___ Failure to operate the AED properly
___ Failure to correctly attach the AED to the patient
___ Failure to assure that all individuals are clear of patient during rhythm analysis **and** before delivering shock(s) [verbalizes "All clear" and observes]
___ Failure to immediately resume compressions after shock delivered
___ Failure to manage the patient as a competent EMT
___ Exhibits unacceptable affect with patient or other personnel
___ Uses or orders a dangerous or inappropriate intervention

You must factually document your rationale for checking any of the above critical items on this form (below or turn sheet over).

(Reprinted with permission of the National Registry of Emergency Medical Technicians.)

National Registry of Emergency Medical Technicians®
Emergency Medical Technician Psychomotor Examination

JOINT IMMOBILIZATION

Candidate: _____   Examiner: _____

Date: _____   Signature: _____

	Possible Points	Points Awarded
Actual Time Started: _____		
Takes or verbalizes appropriate body substance isolation precautions	1	
Directs application of manual stabilization of the injury	1	
Assesses distal motor, sensory, and circulatory functions in the injured extremity	1	
NOTE: The examiner acknowledges, "Motor, sensory, and circulatory functions are present and normal."		
Selects the proper splinting material	1	
Immobilizes the site of the injury	1	
Immobilizes the bone above the injury site	1	
Immobilizes the bone below the injury site	1	
Secures the entire injured extremity	1	
Reassesses distal motor, sensory, and circulatory functions in the injured extremity	1	
NOTE: The examiner acknowledges, "Motor, sensory, and circulatory functions are present and normal."		
Actual Time Ended: _____ **TOTAL**	9	

Critical Criteria

____ Did not immediately stabilize the extremity manually

____ Grossly moves the injured extremity

____ Did not immobilize the bone above and below the injury site

____ Did not reassess distal motor, sensory, and circulatory functions in the injured extremity before and after splinting

____ Failure to manage the patient as a competent EMT

____ Exhibits unacceptable affect with patient or other personnel

____ Uses or orders a dangerous or inappropriate intervention

You must factually document your rationale for checking any of the above critical items on the reverse side of this form.

© 2011 by the National Registry of Emergency Medical Technicians, Inc.
All materials subject to this copyright may be photocopied for the non-commercial purpose of educational or scientific advancement.

(Reprinted with permission of the National Registry of Emergency Medical Technicians.)

National Registry Practical Examination Sheets   **281**

National Registry of Emergency Medical Technicians®
Emergency Medical Technician Psychomotor Examination

LONG BONE IMMOBILIZATION

Candidate: _____   Examiner: _____

Date: _____   Signature: _____

Actual Time Started: _____

	Possible Points	Points Awarded
Takes or verbalizes appropriate body substance isolation precautions	1	
Directs application of manual stabilization of the injury	1	
Assesses distal motor, sensory, and circulatory functions in the injured extremity	1	
NOTE: The examiner acknowledges, "Motor, sensory, and circulatory functions are present and normal."		
Measures the splint	1	
Applies the splint	1	
Immobilizes the joint above the injury site	1	
Immobilizes the joint below the injury site	1	
Secures the entire injured extremity	1	
Immobilizes the hand/foot in the position of function	1	
Reassesses distal motor, sensory, and circulatory functions in the injured extremity	1	
NOTE: The examiner acknowledges, "Motor, sensory, and circulatory functions are present and normal."		

Actual Time Ended: _____   **TOTAL**   10

Critical Criteria

___ Did not immediately stabilize the extremity manually
___ Grossly moves the injured extremity
___ Did not immobilize the joint above and the joint below the injury site
___ Did not immobilize the hand or foot in a position of function
___ Did not reassess distal motor, sensory, and circulatory functions in the injured extremity before and after splinting
___ Failure to manage the patient as a competent EMT
___ Exhibits unacceptable affect with patient or other personnel
___ Uses or orders a dangerous or inappropriate intervention

You must factually document your rationale for checking any of the above critical items on this form (below or turn sheet over).

(Reprinted with permission of the National Registry of Emergency Medical Technicians.)

OXYGEN ADMINISTRATION BY NON-REBREATHER MASK

Candidate: _____   Examiner: _____
Date: _____   Signature: _____

Actual Time Started: _____

	Possible Points	Points Awarded
Takes or verbalizes appropriate body substance isolation precautions	1	
Gathers appropriate equipment	1	
Cracks valve on the oxygen tank	1	
Assembles the regulator to the oxygen tank	1	
Opens the oxygen tank valve	1	
Checks oxygen tank pressure	1	
Checks for leaks	1	
Attaches non-rebreather mask to correct port of regulator	1	
Turns on oxygen flow to prefill reservoir bag	1	
Adjusts regulator to assure oxygen flow rate of at least 10 L/minute	1	
Attaches mask to patient's face and adjusts to fit snugly	1	

Actual Time Ended: _____   **TOTAL**   11

Critical Criteria

____ Failure to take or verbalize appropriate body substance isolation precautions
____ Failure to assemble the oxygen tank and regulator without leaks
____ Failure to prefill the reservoir bag
____ Failure to adjust the oxygen flow rate to the non-rebreather mask of at least 10 L/minute
____ Failure to assure a tight mask seal to patient's face
____ Failure to manage the patient as a competent EMT
____ Exhibits unacceptable affect with patient or other personnel
____ Uses or orders a dangerous or inappropriate intervention

You must factually document your rationale for checking any of the above critical items on this form (below or turn sheet over).

Comments:

(Reprinted with permission of the National Registry of Emergency Medical Technicians.)

National Registry of Emergency Medical Technicians®
Emergency Medical Technician Psychomotor Examination

PATIENT ASSESSMENT/MANAGEMENT – TRAUMA

Candidate: _____ Examiner: _____

Date: _____ Signature: _____

Scenario #: _____

NOTE: Areas denoted by "**" may be integrated within sequence of Primary Survey/Resuscitation	Possible Points	Points Awarded
Actual Time Started: _____		
Takes or verbalizes appropriate body substance isolation precautions	1	
SCENE SIZE-UP		
Determines the scene/situation is safe	1	
Determines the mechanism of injury/nature of illness	1	
Determines the number of patients	1	
Requests additional EMS assistance if necessary	1	
Considers stabilization of the spine	1	
PRIMARY SURVEY/RESUSCITION		
Verbalizes general impression of the patient	1	
Determines responsiveness/level of consciousness	1	
Determines chief complaint/apparent life-threats	1	
Airway -Opens and assesses airway (1 point) -Inserts adjunct as indicated (1 point)	2	
Breathing -Assesses breathing (1 point) -Assures adequate ventilation (1 point) -Initiates appropriate oxygen therapy (1 point) -Manages any injury which may compromise breathing/ventilation (1 point)	4	
Circulation -Checks pulse (1 point) -Assesses skin [either skin color, temperature or condition] (1 point) -Assesses for and controls major bleeding if present (1 point) -Initiates shock management [positions patient properly, conserves body heat] (1 point)	4	
Identifies patient priority and makes treatment/ transport decision (based on calculated GCS)	1	
HISTORY TAKING		
Attempts to obtain sample history	1	
SECONDARY ASSESSMENT		
Head -Inspects mouth**, nose** and assesses facial area (1 point) -Inspects and palpates scalp and ears (1 point) -Assesses eyes** (1 point)	3	
Neck** -Checks position of trachea (1 point) -Checks jugular veins (1 point) -Palpates cervical spine (1 point)	3	
Chest** -Inspects chest (1 point) -Palpates chest (1 point) -Auscultates chest (1 point)	3	
Abdomen/pelvis** -Inspects and palpates abdomen (1 point) -Assesses pelvis (1 point) -Verbalizes assessment of genitalia/perineum as needed (1 point)	3	
Lower extremities** -Inspects, palpates and assesses motor, sensory and distal circulatory functions (1 point/leg)	2	
Upper extremities -Inspects, palpates and assesses motor, sensory and distal circulatory functions (1 point/arm)	2	
Posterior thorax, lumbar and buttocks** -Inspects and palpates posterior thorax (1 point) -Inspects and palpates lumbar and buttocks areas (1 point)	2	
VITAL SIGNS		
Obtains baseline vital signs [must include BP, P, R] (1 point)	1	
Manages secondary injuries and wounds appropriately	1	
REASSESSMENT		
Demonstrates how and when to reassesses the patient	1	
Actual Time Ended: _____ **TOTAL**	42	

© 2011 by the National Registry of Emergency Medical Technicians, Inc.
All materials subject to this copyright may be photocopied for the non-commercial purpose of educational or scientific advancement.

(Reprinted with permission of the National Registry of Emergency Medical Technicians.)

Critical Criteria

___ Failure to initiate or call for transport of the patient within 10 minute time limit

___ Failure to take or verbalize body substance isolation precautions

___ Failure to determine scene safety

___ Failure to assess for and provide spinal protection when indicated

___ Failure to voice and ultimately provide high concentration of oxygen

___ Failure to assess/provide adequate ventilation

___ Failure to find or appropriately manage problems associated with airway, breathing, hemorrhage or shock

___ Failure to differentiate patient's need for immediate transportation versus continued assessment/treatment at the scene

___ Performs other assessment before assessing/treating threats to airway, breathing and circulation

___ Failure to manage the patient as a competent EMT

___ Exhibits unacceptable affect with patient or other personnel

___ Uses or orders a dangerous or inappropriate intervention

You must factually document your rationale for checking any of the above critical items on this form in the space below

Comments:

(Reprinted with permission of the National Registry of Emergency Medical Technicians.)

SPINAL IMMOBILIZATION (SEATED PATIENT)

Candidate: _____   Examiner: _____

Date: _____   Signature: _____

Actual Time Started: _____

	Possible Points	Points Awarded
Takes or verbalizes appropriate body substance isolation precautions	1	
Directs assistant to place/maintain head in the neutral, in-line position	1	
Directs assistant to maintain manual stabilization of the head	1	
Reassesses motor, sensory, and circulatory functions in each extremity	1	
Applies appropriately sized extrication collar	1	
Positions the immobilization device behind the patient	1	
Secures the device to the patient's torso	1	
Evaluates torso fixation and adjusts as necessary	1	
Evaluates and pads behind the patient's head as necessary	1	
Secures the patient's head to the device	1	
Verbalizes moving the patient to a long backboard	1	
Reassesses motor, sensory, and circulatory function in each extremity	1	

Actual Time Ended: _____   **TOTAL**   12

Critical Criteria

____ Did not immediately direct or take manual stabilization of the head
____ Did not properly apply appropriately sized cervical collar before ordering release of manual stabilization
____ Released or ordered release of manual stabilization before it was maintained mechanically
____ Manipulated or moved the patient excessively causing potential spinal compromise
____ Head immobilized to the device **before** device sufficiently secured to the torso
____ Device moves excessively up, down, left, or right on the patient's torso
____ Head immobilization allows for excessive movement
____ Torso fixation inhibits chest rise, resulting in respiratory compromise
____ Upon completion of immobilization, head is not in a neutral, in-line position
____ Did not reassess motor, sensory, and circulatory functions in each extremity after voicing immobilization to the long backboard
____ Failure to manage the patient as a competent EMT
____ Exhibits unacceptable affect with patient or other personnel
____ Uses or orders a dangerous or inappropriate intervention

You must factually document your rationale for checking any of the above critical items on the reverse side of this form.

(Reprinted with permission of the National Registry of Emergency Medical Technicians.)

National Registry of Emergency Medical Technicians®
Emergency Medical Technician Psychomotor Examination

SPINAL IMMOBILIZATION (SUPINE PATIENT)

Candidate: _____   Examiner: _____

Date: _____   Signature: _____

Actual Time Started: _____

	Possible Points	Points Awarded
Takes or verbalizes body substance isolation precautions	1	
Directs assistant to place/maintain head in the neutral, in-line position	1	
Directs assistant to maintain manual stabilization of the head	1	
Reassesses motor, sensory, and circulatory functions in each extremity	1	
Applies appropriately sized extrication collar	1	
Positions the immobilization device appropriately	1	
Directs movement of the patient onto the device without compromising the integrity of the spine	1	
Applies padding to voids between the torso and the device as necessary	1	
Immobilizes the patient's torso to the device	1	
Evaluates and pads behind the patient's head as necessary	1	
Immobilizes the patient's head to the device	1	
Secures the patient's legs to the device	1	
Secures the patient's arms to the device	1	
Reassesses motor, sensory, and circulatory function in each extremity	1	

Actual Time Ended: _____   **TOTAL**   14

Critical Criteria

___ Did not immediately direct or take manual stabilization of the head

___ Did not properly apply appropriately sized cervical collar before ordering release of manual stabilization

___ Released or ordered release of manual stabilization before it was maintained mechanically

___ Manipulated or moved the patient excessively causing potential for spinal compromise

___ Head immobilized to the device **before** device sufficiently secured to the torso

___ Patient moves excessively up, down, left, or right on the device

___ Head immobilization allows for excessive movement

___ Upon completion of immobilization, head is not in a neutral, in-line position

___ Did not reassess motor, sensory, and circulatory functions in each extremity after immobilizing patient to the device

___ Failure to manage the patient as a competent EMT

___ Exhibits unacceptable affect with patient or other personnel

___ Uses or orders a dangerous or inappropriate intervention

You must factually document your rationale for checking any of the above critical items on the reverse side of this form.

(Reprinted with permission of the National Registry of Emergency Medical Technicians.)

Appendix E:
Glossary

A

abandonment Situation in which a care provider assumes responsibility for an incapacitated person and then leaves the patient unsupervised.

ABCs Techniques involved in assessing airway, breathing, and circulation.

abdominal aortic aneurysm (AAA) A weakened area of the aortic wall resulting in a ballooning of the vessel within the abdomen.

abdominal cavity The space between the chest and the pelvis that contains the organs of digestion and elimination.

abdominal thrusts Forceful application of pressure to the upper abdomen, toward the chest, in an attempt to expel a foreign body from the airway.

abduction Movement away from the body.

abortion Premature termination of a pregnancy.

abrasion Superficial scrape to the skin.

absence seizure Seizure characterized by a blank or vacant (absent) stare lasting a few seconds.

acceleration/deceleration Injuries caused by the brain continuing to move back and forth inside the skull after the head has come to a sudden stop.

accessory muscles of respiration Neck, chest, and abdominal muscles that can be used to assist in respiration in times of distress.

accessory muscle use Muscles of the shoulder girdle and chest wall used in addition to the intercostal muscles and the diaphragm in an attempt to improve the flow of air in and out of the lungs in respiratory distress.

acetabulum The socket in the pelvis where the proximal femur meets the pelvis.

acquired immunodeficiency syndrome (AIDS) A group of symptoms, or syndrome, that results from the HIV infection.

acromioclavicular (AC) dislocation Separation of the shoulder and clavicle.

action The effect of a medication on the person who takes it.

activated charcoal Suspension of charcoal in a liquid that has the ability to bind most ingested toxins and prevent their absorption.

active listening An effort to listen for the meaning of a patient's statements.

active rewarming Actions taken to increase body temperature.

activities of daily living (ADLs) Normal functions of self-care that people must be able to perform to live on their own, such as eating, toileting, and dressing.

acute coronary syndrome (ACS) Continuum of conditions affecting blood flow to the heart, including angina and acute myocardial infarction.

acute mountain sickness (AMS) Adverse reaction to high altitude in unacclimated individuals.

acute myocardial infarction (AMI) The death of heart muscle due to an inadequate supply of oxygen-rich blood (hypoperfusion).

acute stress Single event that creates a stress response.

acute stress reaction Exaggerated response due to sympathetic stimulation.

addiction Physical need the body has developed for a drug.

adduction Movement toward the body.

adenosine triphosphate (ATP) High-energy fuel molecule that cells need to function.

advance directive A method to make a patient's wishes about resuscitation known to family and health care providers before the patient becomes incapacitated.

advanced cardiac life support (ACLS) Complex procedures used to treat sudden cardiac death or acute coronary syndrome; typically performed by an ALS provider (i.e., advanced EMTs and paramedics).

Advanced Emergency Medical Technician (AEMT) Emergency medical technician who can not only provide basic emergency care but can also provide some advanced emergency medical care such as advanced airway management, intravenous therapy, and basic medications.

advanced life support (ALS) A broad term applied to emergency medical care rendered beyond basic life support, the hallmark of which is usually special tools and procedures.

advanced lividity Pooling of blood in the dependent portions of the body with a clear line of demarcation.

AEIOU TIPS Mnemonic used to remember the causes of altered mental status: alcohol, epilepsy, insulin, oxygen/overdose, uremia, trauma, infection, psychiatric, and stroke.

aerobic metabolism Process of metabolizing glucose using oxygen that produces large amounts of energy for the cells to use.

affidavit Written testimony.

afterdrop Drop in core body temperature as a result of peripheral vasodilation and shunting of cool blood to the body center during active rewarming of the severely hypothermic patient.

afterload Amount of force the ventricle must overcome to provide blood flow through the circulatory system.

against medical advice (AMA) Patient's refusal of medical care despite a great risk of loss of limb or life.

age of majority Age at which a person may act without parental permission and is generally treated as an adult.

agitated delirium (AD) or excited delirium Combination of agitation, violent or bizarre behavior, insensitivity to pain, elevated body temperature, or increased strength.

air embolism Air that has gotten into a blood vessel, resulting in a blockage of blood flow.

air hunger The feeling a person may have if his or her oxygen level is low or he or she is unable to effectively breathe; indicated by mouth breathing.

airway The passageway for air movement into and out of the lungs.

alert Term used to describe the mental status of a patient who is awake and interacting with his or her environment.

all clear An order that means that nothing, not even the bag mask device, should touch the patient.

allergen A substance that causes an exaggerated response of the immune system (allergic reaction).

allergic reaction An exaggerated response of the immune system upon exposure to a particular substance.

altered mental state A change in behavior due to illness or disease.

alveolar-capillary gas exchange The movement of gases between alveoli and adjacent capillaries.

alveolar ventilation Amount of inhaled air that reaches the alveoli in the lungs for gas exchange.

alveoli Tiny air sacs in the lungs that allow exchange of carbon dioxide and oxygen.

Alzheimer's disease A progressive, irreversible deterioration of intellectual function.

American Academy of Emergency Physicians (ACEP) Association of physicians, specializing in emergency medicine, that was formed in 1968.

American Ambulance Association (AAA) National group that represents ambulance service owners that provide service to 75 percent of the American population.

American Heart Association (AHA) National group of citizens, physicians, and allied health care professionals dedicated to reducing death and disability from cardiovascular disease.

American Red Cross (ARC) Relief organization founded by Clara Barton in the Civil War era; has played a large role in training civilians and rescuers in first aid and CPR.

amniotic sac The membranous sac that surrounds the fetus and placenta within the uterus.

amputation Cutting off of an extremity.

amyotrophic lateral sclerosis (ALS) Neuromuscular disease caused by the degeneration of motor neurons; also known as *Lou Gehrig's disease*.

anaerobic metabolism Process of metabolizing glucose without oxygen, which produces minimal energy.

anaphylactic shock Allergic reaction to an allergen characterized by a severe inflammatory response.

anaphylaxis Exaggerated allergic reaction that can result in life-threatening airway, breathing, or circulatory compromise.

anatomy Study of the structure of an organism.

angina Pain or discomfort that results from insufficient oxygenated blood flow to the heart muscle.

angle of Louis The bony ridge where the manubrium meets the body of the sternum; also called the *sternal angle*.

anisocoria Unequal pupils.

anorexia Absence of appetite.

anoxia No oxygen.

antecubital fossa Anterior surface of the elbow, in the bend of the arm.

anterior Directional term referring to a location toward the front.

antibodies Specialized defense particles within the blood that help to protect against foreign material.

anticonvulsant Any drug intended to control or prevent seizures.

antidote Substance that counteracts or neutralizes the effects of a poison or toxic substance.

anus The end of the digestive tract, which allows for exit of solid wastes.

anxiety disorder Inappropriate or exaggerated response that is abnormal in relation to the situation, formerly called *neurosis*.

aorta Largest artery in the body, which carries blood from the left ventricle of the heart out to the rest of the body.

aortic valve Final valve in the heart that regulates blood flow from the heart into the aorta and the systemic circulation.

apex The point of a triangle; a directional term used to describe the top of the lungs or the bottom tip of the heart.

Apgar Predictive score for measuring the health of newborns at 1 and 5 minutes immediately following birth.

apnea Lack of breathing; breathlessness.

appendicitis Inflammation/infection of the appendix often characterized by the presence of right-lower quadrant pain.

appendicular skeleton Bony extremities composed of the shoulder girdle, arms, pelvic girdle, and legs.

appendix Small saclike portion of the large intestine that may become inflamed in a condition called appendicitis.

arachnoid Weblike middle protective membrane covering the brain and spinal cord.

arterial bleeding Bleeding from an artery, usually under pressure, which can be life threatening.

arteries Vessels that carry blood away from the heart; with the exception of the pulmonary artery, they carry oxygenated blood.

arterioles Smaller arteries that supply blood to the capillaries.

arteriovenous (AV) shunt Bridge or shunt between the artery and vein, usually in the arm, which permits access several times a week to be connected to the hemodialyzer, the machine used to clean the blood.

arteriosclerosis Group of diseases characterized by a loss of elasticity and thickening of artery wall.

arthritis Decrease in the flexibility of joints along with an inflammation within those joints.

artificial pacemaker Man-made electronic device that creates the electrical impulse signaling the heart to beat.

artificial ventilation Method of providing oxygen to a patient who is not effectively breathing; also known as *rescue breathing*.

aspiration Term meaning "to draw into"; refers to foreign material inadvertently being drawn into the airway during inspiration.

assault In civil law, refers to placing a person in fear of being touched through an attempt at treatment without the person having given consent to do so.

asthma Condition consisting of bronchospasm and inflammation in response to multiple stimuli; also known as *reactive airway disease*.

asystole Flatline ECG of the heart in cardiac standstill.

atherosclerosis Disease of arteriosclerosis characterized by plaque buildup on the walls of arteries, causing narrowing and potential occlusion of blood flow.

atlas The first cervical vertebrae that holds the head.

atrial fibrillation Unorganized impulses in the atrial of the heart.

atrioventricular (AV) node Node of specialized cardiac conduction fibers that slow the electrical impulse as it moves from the atria to the ventricles to allow for the mechanical contraction of the heart to catch up to its electrical activity; primarily influenced by the vagus nerve of the parasympathetic nervous system.

atrium Small receiving chamber, one on each side of the heart, that empties blood into its corresponding ventricles to be pumped out of the heart; plural: atria.

auditory hallucination A false perception of the sensation of the ears; hearing something that is not actually there.

aura Sensation or awareness that a seizure is about to begin.

auscultate Term that means to listen.

autism Part of a group of disorders (Autism Spectrum Disorders) characterized by social interaction deficit; impaired communication (verbal and nonverbal); severely limited range of activities and interests of play; and repetitive, obsessive behaviors.

automated external defibrillator (AED) Defibrillator that can "read" the ECG using a logic algorithm stored in a microprocessor; advise the EMT to "shock," or defibrillate; and then deliver that shock to the patient.

automatic implantable cardioverter/defibrillator (AICD) Defibrillator that can be placed within the body.

automatic transport ventilator (ATV) Positive pressure ventilation device that delivers ventilations automatically.

automaticity Ability of the myocardium to self-pace.

autonomic nervous system Collection of nerves that originates in the brainstem and transmits impulses to many organs to allow for many basic body functions.

AVPU Abbreviation to remember the classifications of mental status: alert, voice, pain, and unresponsive.

avulsion Forceful separation of an extremity.

awareness level Ability of EMTs to recognize a hazard, know how to protect themselves, and know how to activate the emergency preplan for such an event.

axial distraction Separation of the spinal vertebrae.

axial loading Compression of the spine by force from above.

axial skeleton Bony skeleton that forms the axis of the support structure of the body; includes the skull, spinal column, and thoracic cage.

axilla Armpit.

axis Second cervical vertebra around which the atlas sits and may rotate.

B

back injury Any injury of the muscles, tendons, or ligaments in the back.

back slaps Firm blows administered to an infant's upper back in an attempt to expel a foreign body from the airway.

bacteremia Bacteria in the blood.

bag-valve-mask (BVM) Device consisting of a refilling bag, a one-way valve, and a mask that is used to ventilate a patient. Also referred to as *bag mask device*.

bandage Strip of cloth applied to a wound.

bariatric medicine The branch of medicine that deals with the diagnosis and treatment of problems of obesity.

bariatric stretchers Special ambulance stretchers designed to carry patients over 700 pounds.

baroreceptors Stretch receptors located in the carotid arteries and aortic arch that send messages to increase or decrease systemic vascular resistance and cardiac output based on the change in blood pressure.

barotraumas Trauma caused by rapid or extreme changes in air pressure.

base Directional term used to describe the bottom of an object, such as a triangle.

base station Main radio transmitter used in a system, frequently located at the base of operations.

baseline vital signs First set of vital signs obtained, used to compare to vital signs obtained later.

basic life support (BLS) Broad term applied to those skills that can be performed by either a citizen or an EMT with a minimum of specialized equipment.

basilar skull fracture Break at the base of the skull (the area behind the face).

basket stretcher Type of stretcher, such as the Stokes basket, that will allow complete immobilization of the patient and protection during a move over rough terrain.

battery In civil law, refers to touching a person without his or her consent.

battle's sign Bruising behind the ears on the mastoid process; indicates a fracture of the skull.

beats per minute (bpm) Measurement of the rate of the heart.

bedroll Stretcher linens wrapped around the patient during transport.

behavioral disability Condition that affects how a child interacts with people, things, and his or her environment.

behavioral emergency Any situation in which a patient exhibits a behavior that is unacceptable or intolerable to one's self, family, or the community.

biceps muscle The muscle that allows flexion of the arm at the elbow; antagonist to the triceps muscle.

bilateral Directional term used to describe points on both sides of the body.

biohazard Short for "biological hazard"; refers to any material that is considered unsafe because of contamination with body fluids.

biological agents Live organisms or natural substances that can kill or incapacitate.

bipolar disorder Psychiatric disorder characterized by cyclic mood changes, ranging from extreme elation to severe depression; also known as *manic-depressive disorder*.

black widow spider Poisonous spider that is black with a red hourglass mark on the abdomen.

bladder Organ in the pelvis that stores urine as it is made by the kidneys.

blanket drag Method of moving patient in which the EMT logrolls the patient onto a blanket, sheet, or drape, then grasps a handful of blanket and drags the patient to safety.

blood Made of several types of cells; fluid that carries fuels and wastes around the body for distribution and removal as appropriate.

blood pressure Pressure placed on the walls of blood vessels by the circulatory system.

blood vessels Structures through which blood travels around the body.

bloody show Expulsion of a small amount of bloody mucus from the cervix as the cervix begins to thin in preparation for childbirth.

body language Unspoken message conveyed by body position.

body mass index A clinical classification that takes into account height and weight.

body mechanics The proper or most efficient way to perform physical activities that are safe and energy conserving and help prevent the physical strains that may cause injury.

body substance isolation Protecting oneself from unnecessary exposure to potentially infectious body substances by avoiding direct contact with any body substance that may be infected. Also referred to as *Standard Precautions*.

bowel obstruction Blockage of flow through the intestine that results in proximal distention, abdominal pain, and vomiting.

Boyle's law Scientific principle that explains that the volume of a gas varies indirectly with the surrounding pressure.

bradycardia Decreased heart rate.

bradypnea Slow breathing.

brain contusion Bruising and swelling of brain tissue.

brain laceration Laceration (cut) to brain tissue caused by a penetration in an open head injury or bone fragments in a closed skull fracture.

brainstem The most basic part of the human brain, which acts as a junction box from the body to the rest of the brain structures and back.

Braxton-Hicks contractions Random contractions that occur in the third trimester that are not associated with cervical effacement or dilation; also known as *false labor.*

breach of confidentiality A situation in which a person divulges information about a patient without having the patient's permission to do so.

breech presentation The presentation of the buttocks or a limb instead of the fetal head during birth.

bronchi Cartilaginous tubes that carry air into the lungs; singular: bronchus.

bronchioles Small muscular tubes with cartilaginous rings that carry air from bronchi into smaller air spaces in the lungs.

bronchodilator Medication that specifically opens up narrowed airways.

bronchospasm Constriction of the lower airways in the lungs.

brown recluse spider Poisonous spider that is brown with a classic violin-shaped mark on its back.

burn Injury caused by significant heat applied to the skin.

burnout Condition that exists when an EMT no longer feels able to perform his duties because of the effects of chronic stress.

C

calcaneus The largest bone in the foot, the heel bone.

call sign An identifying name or number assigned to a particular radio or person.

capillaries Tiny blood vessels that receive blood from arteries and pass it into adjacent veins.

capillary bleeding Slow, oozing type of bleeding, easily controlled and usually not life threatening.

capillary refill time The time it takes to see refill (evidenced by a return to normal color) of a capillary bed after blanching (loss of color in area of skin when pressed).

carbon dioxide (CO_2) Gas found in the air and created within the body.

cardiac contusion Bruising of the heart.

cardiac output The amount of blood pumped from the left ventricle in one minute.

cardiac standstill Condition in which the heart lies flaccid and unable to respond to any stimulus.

cardiogenic shock A hypoperfused state resulting from inadequate cardiac pumping, usually due to multiple heart attacks.

cardiopulmonary resuscitation (CPR) Life-preserving technique involving chest compressions and artificial respiration, Which has been widely taught to both civilians and health care providers since the late 1950s.

cardioversion Process of restoring the heart's normal rhythm through controlled electric shock or medication.

caregiver Person who assists in the identification and treatment of an illness and helps to alleviate mental and physical suffering.

carina Point at which the trachea ends and the right and left bronchi begin.

carpal bones The eight bones of the wrist.

carrier Someone who carries an infectious microorganism; a carrier does not necessarily become ill from it, but can transmit it to someone else.

central chemoreceptors Sensors located in the medulla for carbon dioxide levels and the pH of blood.

Centers for Disease Control and Prevention (CDC) U.S. federal agency in charge of monitoring infectious disease outbreaks; typically the CDC provides a supportive role to state and local health departments.

central Directional term used to describe points toward the center of the body.

central nervous system Consists of the brain and spinal cord and is involved in the initiation and transmission of all control-oriented messages throughout the body.

central venous catheter An intravenous tube that may be left in for long periods of time and may be used for intravenous medication administration or blood sampling.

cephalocaudal Head to toe.

cerebellum The part of the brain that controls muscular coordination and complex actions; sometimes called the *athletic brain.*

cerebral circulation Supplies the brain with oxygen and nutrients and removes waste.

cerebrospinal fluid (CSF) The nutrient-rich fluid that bathes and protects the spinal cord and brain.

cerebrospinal fluid shunt A special catheter used to drain excess CSF off the brain and into the abdomen, where it can be easily absorbed.

cerebrovascular accident (CVA) Injury to the brain tissue that occurs as a result of disruption of blood flow to part of the brain; also known as *stroke.*

cerebrum The largest and most highly evolved area of the brain.

certification Recognition of the EMT having attained a certain level of competency as recognized by his or her peers.

cervical dilation Progressive opening of the cervix that occurs as the fetal head descends into the pelvis.

cervical immobilization device (CID) A device intended to assist in maintaining the cervical spine in a natural neutral position.

cervical spine The uppermost section of the spinal column, made up of seven vertebrae in the neck; it protects the cervical spinal cord.

cervix The opening to the uterus at the bottom.

cesarean section The surgical removal of a newborn from the uterus through an abdominal incision.

chain of command Assignment of roles and duties to individuals in a multiple-casualty incident with a specific order of reporting to supervisors.

chain of infection Three essential parts that must exist for an infection to occur: reservoir, transmission, and host.

chain of survival A concept embraced by the American Heart Association that refers to the multiple elements needed in a response system to have a successful resuscitation. As in a chain, each element is connected with the others and the strength of the entire chain depends on the strength of each link.

chemical restraint The use of medications to keep the patient calm or sedated.

Chemical Transportation Emergency Center (CHEMTREC) A 24-hour technical assistance phone number (1-800-424-9300) about hazardous materials.

chemical weapons Poisons that can kill or incapacitate.

chemoreceptors Sensors that measure the chemical changes in the body.

chest thrusts Firm compressions delivered at midchest in an attempt to expel a foreign body from the airway.

Cheyne–Stokes Characterized by periods of shallow, slow breathing increasing to rapid, deep breathing and then returning to shallow, slow breathing followed by a short apneic period.

chief complaint (CC) The patient's main problem and reason for seeking medical services.

child abuse Any act, or failure to act, on the part of responsible adults that results in death, serious physical or emotional harm, sexual abuse or exploitation; or an act or failure to act that presents an imminent risk of serious harm.

childbirth The act of delivering a child.

child neglect When an adult with custodial responsibilities fails to provide legally mandated care for the child.

children with special health care needs (CSHCN) Children who are at risk of having chronic physical, developmental, behavioral, or emotional conditions requiring health and other related services that would not be required by children developing normally.

cholecystitis Infection of the gallbladder often characterized by fever, abdominal pain, and jaundice.

chronic obstructive pulmonary disease (COPD) Group of diseases characterized by chronic airway obstruction and bronchospasm.

chronic stress Repeated stressors that affect an EMT over a period of time.

cilia Hair-like projections from cells lining the airways that keep a thick mucous blanket constantly moving upward and out of the lungs.

Cincinnati Prehospital Stroke Scale A three-item scale used to identify patients with likelihood of stroke.

circulation The action of blood flowing in the circuit of blood vessels and the heart.

clavicle The collarbone; located at the top of the chest, connecting the shoulder to the sternum.

clonic phase The stage in a seizure in which the body paroxysmally stiffens and relaxes.

closed fracture A broken bone in which the bone ends remain roughly in line and do not break the skin.

clothing drag The technique of pulling a patient to safety using the clothing he or she is wearing.

clues Evidence a person was in an area.

coagulation The process of blood clotting.

coccyx The tailbone, or last portion of the spinal column.

cognitive The mental processes of comprehension, judgment, memory, and reasoning.

cognitive impairment Alteration in any of the mental processes of comprehension, judgment, memory, and reasoning.

cold zone Area without any risk of contamination to rescue personnel.

Colles' fracture A broken wrist that is shaped like a silver fork.

command post A centralized location, often off site, where the heads of public safety agencies gather and regulate on-scene operations.

Commission for the Accreditation of Ambulance Services (CAAS) Independent organization that sets minimum standards for ambulance services.

communicable Passed from person to person.

communications center A central dispatch point.

communications specialist (COMSPEC) A specially trained radio operator.

compartment syndrome A buildup of pressure from swelling within muscle cavities.

compassion Ability to be aware of another person's suffering and to have a wish to help relieve it.

compensated shock A hypoperfused state that the body is compensating for by increasing heart rate, increasing respiratory rate, and shunting blood from certain organs.

competent Able to act in a responsible manner and comprehend the decision at hand.

complex partial seizure Begins with a vacant or blank stare, followed by a repetitive, random activity such as lip smacking or chewing.

compress Cotton dressing integrated into a two-tailed bandage.

computer-aided dispatch (CAD) Use of computers to assist emergency medical dispatchers with control and command of emergency services.

concussion Closed head injury caused by blunt force trauma in which mild stretching, tearing, and shearing of brain tissue occurs.

conduction Transfer of heat from a warm object to a cool object by direct contact.

conductor Material that easily carries a current.

confidentiality Privacy; maintaining confidentiality means ensuring that medical information is provided only to the patient's health care providers.

confined space Any area that has limited openings for exit and access and is not designed for worker occupancy.

congenital heart defects (CHD) Structural or functional anomaly of the heart or great vessels present at birth.

congestive heart failure Condition in which the heart does not pump adequately, creating a buildup of fluids in the lungs and eventually the rest of the body.

consensual response Both pupils will have the same response when light is shined in only one of them.

consent A voluntary agreement by a person to allow something to take place.

contagious The state of an illness when the affected person can transmit it to others.

continuing education Training beyond the initial certification requirements.

continuous positive airway pressure (CPAP) Positive pressure applied to the upper airway by machine splinting the airway open and preventing collapse.

continuous quality improvement (CQI) Process by which an organization monitors and addresses areas in need of improvement.

contraindications Reasons why a medication should not be administered.

contusion Bruising of tissue, caused by blunt forces.

convection Heat loss to air currents passing by a warm surface.

coral snake A venomous snake identified by its red and yellow bands directly opposed.

coronary arteries The two arteries that supply blood to the heart muscle.

costal arch The umbrella-appearing arch at the lower portion of the front of the thoracic cage.

costovertebral angle The angle formed by the tenth rib as it meets the thoracic spine.

coup-contrecoup Characterized by damage to brain tissue at the point of the initial impact to the head and also damage on the side opposite point of the initial impact, where the brain impacts the skull on the opposite side.

crackles A popping sound heard in the lungs that is created as tiny air spaces that are stuck together by abnormal fluid accumulation pop open.

cranium The bony skull.

cravat A simple cotton triangular bandage useful in many circumstances.

crepitus The sound of bone ends grinding against one another; the feeling of air under the skin; it feels like Rice Krispies popping under the fingertips.

cribbing Blocks of wood used to stabilize a vehicle.

cricoid pressure A technique of applying pressure to the cricoid ring during ventilation to occlude the esophagus and prevent regurgitation.

critical incident stress debriefing (CISD) Structured sessions facilitated by trained personnel meant to review the incident in detail and encourage the involved group of providers to discuss their experience during and after the incident. Such a debriefing can help participants effectively deal with the stress of the incident.

cross-fingered technique Technique whereby the EMT places the thumb against the upper incisors and the forefinger against the lower incisors to gently force the mouth open in a scissors maneuver.

croup A swelling and inflammation of the larynx, trachea, and to some extent the bronchi, usually caused by a viral infection.

crowing Sound like a crow cawing that occurs when the muscles around the larynx spasm and the opening into the trachea narrows.

crowning The term used to describe the appearance of the fetal head at the vaginal opening when delivery is imminent.

crumple zone Automobile fenders designed to absorb energy while compacting.

crush injury Prolonged pressure on the skin and underlying tissues.

CSF otorrhea Leaking of cerebrospinal fluid from the ear.

CSF rhinorrhea Leaking of cerebrospinal fluid from the nose.

cultural competency The ability to positively interact with—and in the case of an EMT, care for—persons of many cultures.

culture A system of symbols, icons, and activities that is important to a group of people.

current The passage of electricity through an object.

Cushing's reflex Hypertension and bradycardia associated with serious head injury.

Cushing's triad Hypertension, bradycardia, and an altered respiratory pattern seen in serious head injuries.

cyanosis A bluish discoloration to the skin seen with poor oxygen content of the blood.

D

dangerous instruments Things capable of producing death or serious bodily injury when used in certain circumstances.

dead air space Volume of air that stays in the respiratory tract.

dead space The space in the respiratory tract that is not in contact with pulmonary capillaries and cannot participate in gas exchange with the blood.

deadly weapon Any device that, by its nature, is intended to produce death.

deafness Indicates the loss of hearing prior to learning to talk.

debriefing An organized discussion among personnel involved in a difficult situation in an attempt to prevent an unnecessary buildup of stress.

decompensated shock Hypoperfused state for which the body is no longer able to compensate, with resulting hypotension.

decompression sickness A diving injury that occurs during rapid ascent, resulting in expansion of gases that become trapped in tissues; also known as *the bends*.

decontamination Removal of potentially hazardous substances by either chemical or physical means.

decontamination corridor Area where the hazardous materials are cleaned off the rescuers and patients; also referred to as the *warm zone*.

deep Term used to describe an injury that extends far into the injured structure.

defamation Information spoken or written about an individual that can be seen as damaging to that person's character or reputation.

defibrillation Process of applying an electrical shock to the heart to stop an abnormal rhythm, ventricular fibrillation, or pulseless ventricular tachycardia and restore normal rhythm.

deformity Misshapen or not in the usual position.

degloving avulsion The forceful separation of just the skin from an extremity.

dehydration Loss of too much body fluid causing an imbalance of the elements affecting muscle activity and body fluid levels.

delirium Alteration in the level of consciousness exhibited by a sudden erratic change in behavior, usually caused by an acute medical problem.

delirium tremens (DTs) Symptoms associated with the sudden withdrawal of alcohol from an alcohol-dependent person.

deltoid muscle Triangular muscle covering the shoulder and upper arm; a site commonly used for intramuscular injections.

dementia Syndrome characterized by a progressive decline in intellectual function that usually leads to deterioration of occupational, social, and interpersonal functions.

dentures False teeth.

Department of Transportation (DOT) Federal agency responsible for traffic safety; considered the starting point for modern EMS.

dependency The psychological need the person has for a drug.

depression Psychiatric condition characterized by persistent sadness and lack of interest in usual life pleasures.

dermatome An area of movement or sensation that corresponds with a nerve root.

dermis The layer of skin just beneath the surface, or epidermal layer; contains capillaries and specialized nerve endings.

descending corticospinal tract Nerve fiber bundles that send motor instructions to the muscles and organs of the body.

diabetes mellitus Disease in which the pancreas fails to produce insulin.

diabeticcoma Condition of an unconscious, hyperglycemic diabetic patient.

diabetic ketoacidosis (DKA) The result of excessive fat metabolism seen in diabetic patients with hyperglycemia.

diamond stretcher carry A technique in which four EMTs carry a patient on a stretcher, with one EMT at either end and one on each side.

diaphoretic Exhibiting excessive perspiration due to stress or pain.

diaphragm The specialized muscle that separates the chest from the abdomen and is the main muscle of breathing.

diastolic The lower number in the blood pressure; the pressure in the vessels when the heart is resting between contractions.

diastolic blood pressure Pressure exerted on blood vessels when the heart is at rest.

diet-controlled diabetes Condition of a person whose blood sugar is controlled by diet modification.

diffusion Movement of oxygen and carbon dioxide across a membrane from an area of higher concentration to an area of lower concentration.

direct carry Lifting a patient and carrying him a short distance directly to the stretcher.

direct contact Actually coming into contact with the infectious material on a person by touching.

direct current (DC) A unidirectional electrical current.

direct force The transfer of energy to the point of impact of violence.

direct laryngoscopy Use of a laryngoscope to directly visualize the airway structures.

direct pressure Constant firm pushing on the bleeding site.

disease Condition characterized by abnormal symptoms.

dislocation A bone that slips out of joint and out of alignment.

disorder Pathological condition or deficiency of the body or mind.

displacement Avoiding painful emotions by transferring one's emotions to others.

distal Directional term used to describe points farther from the core of the body (trunk).

distracting painful injury A severe injury that occurs when the patient focuses on the injury to the exclusion of everything and everyone else.

diverticula Sac or pouch in the colon that can become packed with fecal matter, causing inflammation.

diverticulitis Inflammatory disease caused by impacted diverticula that may lead to an obstructed colon, perforation, and hemorrhage; often associated with left-side abdominal pain.

domestic terrorists Groups of "nationals," as defined by the U.S. Immigration and Nationality Act, that have disputes with the way the U.S. government is operated or with specific U.S. policies.

domestic violence An act of violence against a partner, spouse, family member, or member of the household.

do not resuscitate order (DNR) A medical–legal order to restrain health care providers from providing invasive procedures and resuscitation such as CPR.

dormant In a state of biological rest.

dorsal Directional term referring to the top or back surface of a structure such as the hand.

dorsiflexion Movement of the toes upward, toward the nose.

dose The amount of a substance; usually refers to the amount of a medication given.

Down syndrome Also known as *trisomy 21*, a disorder caused by the presence of three 21st chromosomes, characterized by similar physical features and varying levels of cognitive impairment.

dressing A sterile absorbent cloth used to cover a wound.

due regard Respect and consideration for others.

duplex A radio that allows the EMT to both speak and listen at the same time, like a telephone.

durable power of attorney-health care (DPOA-HC) A legal document that extends authority of one person to control the legal affairs of another—in this case, the health care issues of a patient.

dura mater (tough mother) Tough, fibrous outer layer of the meninges, lining the cranial vault.

duty to act An obligation to provide care to a patient who requires it.

dysarthria Difficulty speaking resulting in garbled or slurred speech.

dyspnea The feeling or appearance of respiratory distress.

dysrhythmia Abnormal change in the electrical rhythm of the heart.

E

ecchymosis A wider collection of blood under the skin, like a contusion (bruise).

eclampsia A convulsive disorder seen only during pregnancy.

ectopic pregnancy A pregnancy that develops outside the uterus.

edema Fluid seeping out of the bloodstream and into the tissues.

effacement Thinning of the cervix that occurs as a pregnancy nears its conclusion.

elder abuse An act of violence toward or neglect of an elderly person who is dependent on the other person.

electrocardiogram (ECG) A recording of the electrical activity of the heart graphically displayed on an oscilloscope or printed on paper; also abbreviated EKG.

elevate Raising the bleeding site above the level of the heart.

emancipated minor A person who is not the age of majority but who is no longer under the control of a parent or guardian and is legally responsible for his or her decisions and any consequences that result from those decisions.

embolism A physical blockage in the bloodstream.

embolus Debris that travels through blood vessels until it lodges and occludes blood flow.

emergency ambulance A vehicle specifically designed for patient transportation in an emergency.

emergency ambulance service vehicle (EASV) A vehicle used in service to EMS and staffed by EMS personnel.

emergency carry A technique used if the patient must be moved in an emergency over a greater distance.

emergency department (ED) A division or portion of a hospital designated to care for emergency medical problems or trauma; in some countries called an accident room.

emergency dispatch (EMD) A trained person who answers 9-1-1 emergency telephone calls from the public and provides public safety assistance through communication with emergency services such as fire, law enforcement, and EMS.

emergency doctrine A legal principle that allows for emergency treatment of prisoners or children if they are incapable of giving consent.

emergency drag A technique used by a single EMT to move a patient quickly in an emergency.

emergency incident rehabilitation An element of the operational plan that includes rest and rehydration as well as medical monitoring.

emergency medical dispatch (EMD) Specially trained dispatch call takers who are trained to provide specific pre-arrival medical care instructions to callers while emergency crews respond.

emergency medical responder (EMR) Person who has advanced training for first responders, which includes basic assessment, simple airway management, oxygen administration, bleeding control, rescuer CPR, and defibrillation.

emergency medical services (EMS) Coordinated network of professionals whose function is to provide a variety of medical services to people in need of emergency care.

emergency medical services system (EMSS) An organization of equipment such as ambulances, and personnel such as EMTs, which is created to respond to medical emergencies within a community.

emergency medical technician (EMT) Person who has completed the basic entry level of training for prehospital care that includes airway maintenance, oxygen administration, bleeding control, CPR, defibrillation, patient assessment, and limited medication administration.

Emergency Medical Treatment and Active Labor Act (EMTALA) Federal legislation that ensures that patients receive medical treatment regardless of their ability to pay.

emergency move The technique that an EMT uses to quickly remove a patient from danger.

emergency operations plan (EOP) An interagency document that assigns responsibilities to U.S. government departments and organizations, thereby setting lines of command (authority). It describes how emergency responders will protect people and property in the event of a terrorist attack as well as apprehend those responsible.

emergency physician Medical doctor specially trained in rapid assessment and diagnosis of acutely ill or traumatically injured patients.

Emergency Response Guidebook (ERG) A guidebook that provides responders instructions and information on how to handle the first 30 minutes of a hazmat spill.

emergency response team A group of people who arrive and rescue contaminated persons and control, confine, contain, and decontaminate the area.

emergency vehicle operator (EVO) A driver of a vehicle used for emergency service.

emergency vehicle operators course (EVOC) A training course for drivers of vehicles used for emergency service.

EMS director/EMS incident Commander assigning unit leaders for triage, transport, staging, treatment, and morgue.

endocarditis Inflammation of the inside of the heart.

endocrine system Assists the nervous system in maintaining control over the body by producing hormones that act upon certain organs.

enteral Ingested route of medication administration; sublingual, oral.

entrance wound Damage created as an object or electricity enters the body.

environmental assessment An EMT's visual overview of an entire scene while identifying potential hazards.

Environmental Protection Agency (EPA) Federal agency in charge of maintaining the quality of the environment; typically concerned with pollution.

epidermis The outermost layer of skin.

epidural hematoma A collection of blood between the skull and the dura mater, often arterial in nature.

epiglottis Located above the larynx, a cartilaginous structure that protects the trachea from aspiration of foreign bodies.

epiglottitis A bacterial infection, characterized by a swollen, inflamed epiglottis, which can cause upper airway obstruction.

epilepsy A disease characterized by recurrent seizures of a similar nature.

epinephrine A medication that dilates the airways and constricts the blood vessels.

esophageal varices Dilated veins within the lining of the lower esophagus that may bleed profusely if they rupture.

esophagus A collapsible muscular tube that directs food from the mouth into the stomach.

etiology Cause or origin of a disease.

evaporation Transfer of heat into body fluids, such as sweat, for dissipation into the environment.

eversion An outward movement, such as when the foot twists outward and strains the ankle; the opposite of inversion.

evisceration An abdominal wound with abdominal contents protruding through the wound.

excited delirium A state of hyperactive irrational behavior.

exhalation Breathing out.

exit wound Damage created as a foreign object or electricity exits the body.

expected time of arrival (ETA) The anticipated arrival of either the patient or the EMT to the scene.

expiration date The last day that a medication is guaranteed by the manufacturer to be safe and effective as expected.

express consent The act of verbally advising a medical provider to proceed with treatment.

expressive aphasia Difficulty forming words often seen when a stroke affects the brain's speech center.

extension A movement that widens the angle at a joint between two bones; the opposite of flexion.

extremity lift A lifting technique whereby one EMT stands behind a seated patient and grasps him under the shoulders, while a second EMT grasps him under the knees so they can lift and carry him.

extrinsic By external causes.

F

facial droop One-sided facial muscle weakness that indicates focal brain or nerve injury.

fallopian tube Tiny muscular tube that allows an egg to travel from the ovary to the uterus.

false imprisonment The intentional confinement of a patient without the patient's consent and without an appropriate reason.

false motion Movement in the bone where there is not supposed to be movement.

false ribs The eighth through tenth ribs, which are not attached directly to the sternum; rather, they are attached anteriorly to the seventh rib by cartilage.

fasciotomy A surgical procedure whereby skin is cut to relieve pressure.

febrile seizure A seizure that results from a rapid rise in body temperature.

Federal Communications Commission (FCC) Federal agency that regulates radio communications.

federal response plan (FRP) A plan used when state and local authorities are overwhelmed; it brings the immense resources of the federal government to their aid.

feedback A return conversation that helps the EMT ensure that the message sent was correctly understood by the patient.

feeding tube A soft, flexible tube that is placed into the stomach, either through the nose or through the anterior abdominal wall, to allow nutritional supplementation.

femur The single bone in the thigh, the longest and strongest bone in the body.

fetal circulation Temporary circulation between the mother and fetus during pregnancy.

fetus The ovum after it is implanted in the uterine wall.

fibrinolytics (to divide the fibrin) Formerly called *thrombolytics*, is a class of drugs often used in the treatment of AMI.

fibula The laterally placed bone in the lower leg.

field hospital A temporary on-site treatment facility.

fight-or-flight response Describes the reaction of the body to a stressor by preparing to fight to defend itself or to run away.

first responder (FR) The first person who arrives on the scene of an incident; also may refer to the level of medical training provided to persons who expect to be put in this position during their daily routine, such as firefighters, police officers, and security guards. Also referred to as *emergency medical responder* (EMR).

first responder awareness level A person trained to identify and report a hazardous materials incident.

first stage of labor The process of cervical effacement and dilation at the beginning of childbirth.

fixed wing Airplanes.

flail chest A medical condition when a segment of at least two ribs are broken in at least two places.

flail segment Two or more ribs fractured in two or more places where the underlying segment is unstable and moves in a paradoxical motion to the rest of the chest wall.

flat water A body of water without current.

flexible splint Any material that can be formed to fit any angle and then made rigid.

flexible stretcher A lightweight plastic stretcher that may be rolled up when not in use; commonly used in confined space and cave rescue.

flexion A movement at a joint that decreases the angle between the two bones on either side of it; opposite of extension.

floating ribs The last two pairs of ribs in the thoracic cage; they are unattached anteriorly.

flow-restricted oxygen-powered ventilation device (FROPVD) A device that can deliver oxygen to a patient at restricted flow rates.

focused physical examination A physical exam focused upon the medical patient's chief complaint.

fontanel Soft, flexible fibrous region in an infant's skull that allows for skull growth; also known as *soft spots*.

Food and Drug Administration (FDA) Federal agency responsible for drug purity and safety.

footdrop A loss of nervous control that results in a flaccid foot.

foramen magnum Large opening at the base of the skull through which the spinal cord passes.

foreign body airway obstruction (FBAO) Any ingested object that is capable of causing suffocation by blocking the trachea.

Fowler's position Position in which a person is sitting at a 45-degree to 60-degree angle.

fracture A sudden breaking of a bone.

Frank–Starling law (Starling law) Contractility of cardiac muscle relative to the amount of stretch placed on the muscle by additional blood volume.

French catheter A flexible suction catheter meant to suction through endotracheal tubes or via the nasopharynx.

frontal bone The strong anterior-most bone in the skull that makes up the forehead.

frostbite Tissue damage resulting from exposure to freezing and subfreezing temperatures.

frostnip A mild local skin injury resulting from exposure to freezing temperatures.

full-thickness burn A burn that affects all three layers of the skin.

fundus The top of the uterus.

G

gag reflex The protective response that a person has when the back of the throat is stimulated by the presence of a foreign substance.

gallbladder A small pouch-like organ that lies underneath the liver and stores bile to be used in digestion.

gastrocnemius muscle The muscle in the back of the calf that enables a person to stand on his toes.

gastroenteritis A condition characterized by vomiting and diarrhea, usually caused by a viral illness.

gauze dressing Sterile cotton weave cloth.

Geiger counter A device used to detect radiation.

general impression The initial feeling, based on observation, of how seriously ill or injured the patient is.

generalized seizure A seizure that involves the entire brain and results in loss of consciousness; also known as a *grand mal seizure*.

generic name The initial name given to a drug that is shorter than the actual chemical name and is listed in the *U.S. Pharmacopeia*.

geriatrics The study of the diseases of elderly adults.

gestational diabetes A form of diabetes that occurs only in pregnant women and usually only for the duration of the pregnancy.

gestational diabetes mellitus (GDM) Diabetes that occurs during pregnancy, usually disappearing follow birth.

glands Specialized organs that respond to and produce hormones of the endocrine system.

Glasgow Coma Scale (GCS) A scale that is used to quantify a patient's level of responsiveness.

glucose A substance used by the body for fuel.

gluteus muscles Strong muscles in the buttock that are important in allowing proper leg movement.

gonads Organs of reproduction; testes (male) and ovaries (female).

Good Samaritan laws Laws that protect certain classes of people, such as physicians, who volunteer to assist others; laws vary from state to state.

grand mal seizure The old term for a generalized seizure.

gravidity The total number of pregnancies a woman has had.

grunting A noise made on exhalation during periods of respiratory distress.

guardian A person who has authority to act on behalf of another individual and to give consent for medical care.

guarding Muscular tension created by a patient to protect an underlying injury.

guides Instructions for evacuation distance, perimeter boundaries, and potential hazards found in the *Emergency Response Guidebook*.

gunshot wound (GSW) An injury created by a projectile fired by a gun.

gurgling Sound of liquid moving; if heard at the airway, indicates a need for suctioning.

H

hallucination A sensation or perception that has no basis in reality.

halo test Observing for a ring of blood around CSF spilled from the ears or nose in a head-injured patient.

hard of hearing Some hearing ability is present, usually with the use of hearing aids.

hard palate The bony structure that forms the roof of the mouth.

hazardous material Any substance that can cause an exposed person injury or death.

hazardous waste operations and emergency response (HAZWOPER) Legislation that pertains to toxic waste management.

head-tilt, chin-lift Maneuver used to open the airway, involving tilting the head back and lifting the jaw up; used only in non-trauma patients.

health care proxy A person chosen to make medical decisions on behalf of another in the event the person becomes incapable of making such decisions.

Health Insurance Portability and Accountability Act (HIPAA) An act of Congress that protects health insurance coverage for workers and their families when they change or lose their jobs; regulates national standards for electronic health care transactions and the security and privacy of health data.

hearing impairment Reduction in the ear's responsiveness to loudness and pitch.

heart Four-chambered muscular organ that pumps to provide the body with nutrient-rich blood.

heat cramps Painful, involuntary muscle spasms caused by dehydration and exposure to heat.

heat exhaustion The mildest form of generalized heat-related illness, characterized by multiple symptoms and often by dehydration.

heat stroke A life-threatening form of heat illness that involves a rise in body temperature and altered mental status.

heavy rescue The use of special vehicle extrication equipment.

Heimlich maneuver A series of forceful upward abdominal thrusts that force air out of the lungs and the trachea.

hematochezia Passage of bright red blood from the rectum.

hematoma An accumulation of blood.

hematemesis Vomitus that consists mostly of blood.

hemoglobin Protein molecule found on the surface of red blood cells responsible for carrying oxygen in blood.

hemoglobin saturation Amount of oxygen-rich hemoglobin in the blood.

hemophilia Rare, inherited bleeding disorder in which there is a deficiency or absence of specific clotting factors preventing blood from clotting normally.

hemoptysis Spitting up or coughing up blood.

hemorrhage Medical term for bleeding.

hemorrhagic shock A hypoperfused state resulting from loss of blood.

hemorrhagic stroke Injury to brain tissue as a result of rupture of a vessel that supplies it with blood.

hemostasis The process of controlling bleeding.

hemostatic dressing Contains powders or substances that promote blood clotting when placed on an open wound.

hemothorax Bleeding between the lung and the chest wall.

hepatitis B virus (HBV) The virus responsible for hepatitis B infection, which attacks the liver.

high-altitude cerebral edema (HACE) Swelling of the brain as a result of hypoxia at high altitudes; characterized by altered mental status, difficulty walking, and decreased level of consciousness.

high-altitude pulmonary edema (HAPE) Pulmonary edema as a result of hypoxia at high altitudes; characterized by dry cough and dyspnea on exertion.

high-efficiency particulate air filter (HEPA) A filtration device intended to remove very small airborne contaminants.

high index of suspicion Based on the noted mechanism of injury, the feeling that there is a high likelihood of injury.

high-Fowler's position Position in which a person is sitting upright at a 90-degree angle.

history of present illness (HPI) An account of the course of an illness; typically done as a narrative from witnesses such as family members.

homeostasis The body's ability to maintain a steady optimal state for growth and development and to resist any influence, internal or external, that would upset this balance.

hormones Chemicals that are excreted into the bloodstream by specialized organs called glands.

hospice A facility with a team of health care professionals who care for dying patients.

host The target of an infection.

hot zone The immediate vicinity of the hazardous material spill that is considered contaminated and a risk to rescue personnel.

human immunodeficiency virus (HIV) The virus that causes AIDS (acquired immunodeficiency syndrome).

humerus The single long bone of the upper arm.

humidification The process of adding moisture to the inspired air.

hyperbaric chamber A device that creates a simulated dive to allow for recompression of air in a diver suffering from decompression sickness or other diving-related illnesses.

hypercarbic High carbon dioxide.

hyperemia Increased blood flow.

hyperextension Excessive backward bending.

hyperflexibility Loose-jointedness.

hyperflexion Excessive forward bending.

hyperglycemia A high amount of sugar in the blood.

hyperosmolar hyperglycemic non-ketonic coma (HHNK) Condition of diabetes that can lead to coma; different from keto-acidosis.

hypertension Abnormally high blood pressure.

hyperthermia Overall heat gain greater than heat loss, resulting in a rise in body temperature.

hyperventilate To breathe faster and more deeply than usual.

hyphema A collection of blood in the anterior part of the eye.

hypoglycemia A condition of low blood glucose levels.

hypoperfusion Inadequate supply of oxygenated blood to a tissue or organ.

hypopnea Slow, shallow breathing.

hypothermia Condition in which the body temperature drops below 95 degrees Fahrenheit.

hypotonia Low muscle tone.

hypoventilation Breathing more slowly than normal or less effectively than usual.

hypovolemia A state of decreased blood volume.

hypovolemic shock A hypoperfused state resulting from low fluid levels.

hypoxemia Insufficient oxygen in circulation blood for perfusion.

hypoxia Lack of oxygen in the body.

hypoxic drive Process of respiration to increase oxygen levels, not to reduce carbon dioxide levels.

I

idiopathic Unknown etiology or cause for an illness or disease.

iliac bones The main component of the bony pelvis, the hip bones, sometimes described as "wings" because of their shape.

illiteracy The inability to read or write or understand the spoken word.

immunity Insusceptibility to a specific illness, usually as a result of prior exposure or immunization.

immunization The process of exposing the body to or inoculating it with weakened pathogens to allow it to create specific antibodies.

immunocompromise Lack of disease resistance.

impaled object A foreign object embedded in the skin.

implied consent The legal presumption that a patient who is unable to verbally express agreement to treatment would agree to be treated in certain circumstances.

Incident Command System (ICS) A system of command and control that defines operation and management components and the structure of incident management organizations throughout the incident.

incident commander (IC) The person in command who has overall responsibility for the entire incident.

incision A cutting of the skin.

incontinence Loss of bowel and/or bladder control.

indication The reason to use a drug to treat a specific condition.

indirect contact Exposure to an infectious agent that is on a nonhuman surface.

indirect force A transfer of energy as a result of violence away from the point of impact.

infarction Death of cells as the result of prolonged lack of oxygen.

infection control Taking preventive measures to lessen the likelihood of disease transmission.

infection control officer Designated officer of a company or department that is assigned to monitor infection control practices and act as a liaison to the hospital's infection control department.

inferior Lower than the reference point.

Infirmity Patient incapacitated by infection.

inflammation The body's attempt to prevent infection and begin healing.

informed consent Consent given following explanation of the risks and benefits of treatment.

initial assessment The first evaluation performed on every patient to address life-threatening problems. Also referred to as *primary assessment*.

initial report The first emergency responder's first radio report of scene conditions; includes hazards, number of patients, and requests for additional resources.

innervate Nerves that connect to muscles and organs of the body.

inspiration Breathing in.

insulin A hormone produced by the pancreas that allows glucose utilization by the body.

insulin-dependent diabetes A condition for which the diabetic patient must inject insulin into the body to survive.

insulin shock Condition resulting from low blood sugar due to either too much insulin or too little sugar.

integumentary system The skin and skin structures that cover and protect the body.

intercostal muscles Muscles between the ribs.

intercostal retraction A retraction of skin and muscle between the ribs with each breath, as seen in a child with respiratory distress.

intermammary line The imaginary horizontal line that runs between the nipples.

international terrorists Terrorist groups that cross over national borders and often have subgroups, called cells, in other countries to perform terrorism.

International Association of Fire Fighters (IAFF) An international group representing more than 263,000 firefighters in more than 3,500 communities in the United States and Canada.

intervertebral disk The fibrous pad that cushions each vertebra from the others.

intonation Changes in pitch, volume, and cadence of voice.

intracranial pressure (ICP) The pressure within the skull.

intramuscular Referring to administration of medication into the muscular layer under the subcutaneous layer of soft tissue.

intravenous (IV) Referring to administration of medication into the veins.

intrinsic By internal causes.

inversion Turning something inward; opposite of eversion.

irreversible shock Hypoperfusion that has progressed to a point where survival is highly unlikely.

ischemia Injury of tissue resulting from a blockage of the vessel that normally supplies that tissue with blood.

ischemic stroke Injury to brain tissue as a result of blockage of the vessel that supplies it with blood.

ischium The portion of the bony pelvis that supports body weight while in the sitting position.

J

jaundice A yellow discoloration of the skin caused by excess bilirubin in the bloodstream.

jaw thrust A technique that lifts the mandible and tongue up and away from the pharynx, often effective in opening the airway; is used on trauma patients with suspected spinal injury.

jugular vein A large vein in the side of the neck that is situated rather close to the surface of the skin.

jugular venous distention (JVD) Bulging veins in the side of the neck.

JumpSTART Triage A triage system that uses the specific assessment techniques for infants and children to differentiate them from adults.

K

keto-acid An organic acid that is the by-product of ineffective metabolism; also called *ketone*.

kidney A solid organ in the retroperitoneal space that filters toxins from the blood and makes urine to dispose of such toxins and excess salts or water.

kidney stone Particulate material crystallizes in the urine, resulting in a formed piece of solid material.

kinematics of trauma Science of analyzing the mechanism of injury.

kinetic energy The energy possessed by a body because of its motion.

kinetics The mechanics dealing with the motions of material objects.

knee The joint that joins the upper leg and the lower leg.

Kussmaul's respiration Deep, almost sighing, respiration.

kyphosis Severe outward curvature of the upper back.

L

labor The childbirth process by which the uterus expels the fetus and placenta.

laceration A type of wound characterized by a full-thickness tear in the skin.

landing zone (LZ) An area intended for the purpose of landing and taking off in a helicopter.

lap belt syndrome A phenomenon in which a misplaced seatbelt causes liver and spleen injuries.

large intestine Hollow digestive organ that encircles the abdominal cavity and receives digested food from the small intestine.

laryngoscope A tool that is used to view the lower airway structures during endotracheal intubation.

laryngoscopy The use of a laryngoscope to view the lower airway structures.

larynx A cartilaginous structure in the midline of the neck that contains the vocal cords and is the beginning of the trachea or windpipe.

lateral Directional term used to describe the side of a structure; points farther from the midline.

lateral bending Forced sideways motion.

law enforcement officer (LEO) The broad category including police officers, state police, deputy sheriffs, FBI agents, and DEA agents, who have the responsibility to uphold the law.

leadership Quality of causing others to follow in one direction to accomplish a goal.

left lateral recumbent position Position in which the person is lying on his or her left side; also known as the *recovery position*.

legal duty to act The requirement that an EMT respond to calls whether as an employee under contract or as a volunteer.

liability The legal responsibility for one's own actions.

libel Statement that makes a false claim, expressively stated or implied to be factual, that may harm the reputation of an individual.

ligament Connective tissue that connects bone to bone.

light-emitting diode (LED) An electronic device that shines light using small amounts of electricity.

linear A straight course.

liters per minute (lpm) A measurement of the rate of flow of a liquid.

litter A stretcher or other means of patient conveyance that does not have wheels and must be carried.

liver Large, solid organ in the right-upper abdomen that creates bile for digestion, produces special factors to help in blood clotting, and filters blood from the intestines to rid the body of specific toxins.

living will A document signed by a patient that informs the reader of what types of treatment and under what conditions that patient would want or would not want medical treatment.

loaded bumper A vehicle's front or rear bumper that, when compressed and locked, is able to suddenly and unexpectedly spring forward.

locked A bone that is unable to return to its natural position.

lower extremities Term used to refer to the legs.

lumbar vertebrae The five vertebrae that make up the lower back and support the weight of the entire upper body.

lumen Hollow center of blood vessels.

lymph Straw-colored fluid similar to plasma that carries white blood cells.

lymph node Solid gland-like bodies, such as the tonsils, where white blood cells destroy microorganisms.

lymphatic system Part of the immune system that carries microorganism-laden white blood cells in a fluid, called lymph, to lymph nodes for removal. Also assists the circulatory system by draining the body's tissues of excess fluids and returning that fluid to the central circulation.

LZ officer A designated person on the scene of an incident responsible for choosing a landing zone (LZ) for the helicopter and ensuring its safety.

M

malaise Feeling of weakness or exhaustion.

malfeasance Action or failure to act that causes intentional damage.

malleolus Bony prominences at the medial and lateral aspects of the ankles.

malpractice Act or omission by a health care provider that deviates from accepted standards of practice in the medical community and that causes injury to the patient.

mandated child abuse reporter Individuals within certain groups such as daycare providers, educators/teachers, law enforcement, and EMTs, who are required to report suspected child abuse.

mandated reporter Individual who comes into contact with certain situations, such as child abuse, and is required by law to report these situations to the proper authorities.

mandible Bony lower jaw.

manubrium Upper section of the bony sternum.

mass Weight of an object.

mastoid process Bony prominence behind the ear.

material safety data sheet (MSDS) Reference list of the health and safety information for a chemical substance.

maturation Positive mental, physical, or psychosocial growth or change.

maxilla One of the two fused bones that form the upper jawbone; plural, maxillae.

mechanical ventilator Machine that provides artificial ventilation for a patient who cannot breathe effectively on his or her own.

mechanism of action How a drug works on the body.

mechanism of injury (MOI) The instrument or event that results in harm to a patient.

meconium Fetal stool.

med channel Radio frequency used by paramedics and EMTs to speak to base hospital physicians.

medial Directional term used to describe points closer to the midline of the body.

medial malleolus Bony prominence on the tibia side of the ankle.

mediastinum Hollow area between the right and left lungs that houses the trachea.

MedicAlert Emergency medical information service that provides a directive worn on the patient's body.

medical direction Advice provided by a higher medical authority, usually a physician.

medical director A physician who acts as a medical expert, consultant, and educator.

medical protocols Set of written regulations that specify the proper procedures for patient care.

medically necessary restraint Used when a patient must be confined to prevent him or her from harming himself or herself or others.

megahertz (MHz) Frequency band of radio wave transmission.

melena Dark, tarry stool containing digested blood caused by bleeding in the upper gastrointestinal tract.

meninges The three membrane layers covering the brain, brain stem, and spinal cord.

meningitis An infection and inflammation of the lining around the brain and spinal cord.

menstruation Monthly flow that rids the uterus of its lining when fertilization of an egg does not occur.

mental illness Any disorder that impairs the brain's function and that is without a firm physical (organic) cause.

metabolism Chemical and physical reactions taking place within the cells.

metabolites Small molecules left over from chemicals after the cells have reacted with them.

metacarpals The five bones that connect the carpal bones in the wrist to the phalanges in the fingers.

metered dose inhaler (MDI) Handheld device that carries a form of medication that may be aerosolized on discharge of the inhaler device.

microorganism Tiny living creature visible only by microscope.

midaxillary line Imaginary line drawn from the center of the armpit down the side of the chest.

midclavicular lines Imaginary lines drawn from the middle of each clavicle, or collarbone, down the front of the chest.

midline Imaginary line drawn down the center of the body, splitting it equally into a right half and a left half.

miles per hour (mph) Measurement of the speed of a vehicle.

military anti-shock trousers (MAST) Device that is inflated over the lower extremities and pelvis to attempt to increase blood flow to the core organs; also called *pneumatic antishock garment (PASG)*.

millimeters of mercury (mmHg) The measurement of the height of mercury that is an indirect measurement of a pressure, such as blood pressure.

minimum data set The specific pieces of information required on a patient care report.

minute volume Amount of air breathed in and out in one minute.

miscarriage Spontaneous, unintentional termination of a pregnancy.

misfeasance Performing the duty inadequately or poorly.

mitral valve Bicuspid valve that prevents blood flow backward from the left ventricle into the left atrium.

mobile radio Radio unit mounted inside a vehicle.

mobile work stations Computerized device in emergency vehicles that communicates with a central dispatch or communications center.

modified Trendelenburg Position in which a person is lying supine with legs elevated 12–16 inches; also known as *shock position*.

morbidly obese Patients with potentially life-threatening weight-related health problems.

morgue An area set aside for the collection of the deceased.

motion artifact A false ECG reading created by vibration.

motor nerves Nervous tissue that carries impulses that initiate muscular contraction.

motor neurons Nerve cells that control voluntary muscle movement.

motor vehicle collision (MVC) Formerly referred to as a car accident; when a vehicle forcefully strikes another vehicle or object, often leading to trauma.

mottling Skin discoloration similar to cyanosis but in a blotchy pattern.

mucous membrane Porous tissue lined with blood vessels, which creates a liquid that serves to wash away the surface of the respiratory and gastrointestinal tracts that are regularly in contact with the outside environment.

multiagency coordination system Defines operating characteristics, management components, and the organizational structure of supporting organizations.

multi-drug resistant organism Pathogens that have adapted to and developed the ability to resist antibiotics that would normally be prescribed to treat them.

multiparous Term used to describe a woman who has previously given childbirth.

multiple-casualty incident (MCI) Incident involving multiple injured patients, often overwhelming the initial responding units.

multiplex radio Multiple-channel radio that allows for complex data such as ECGs and spoken messages to be transmitted simultaneously.

Murphy eye Opening on the side of the distal end of the endotracheal tube.

myocardium Heart muscle.

N

Nader pin Case-hardened pin designed to prevent the vehicle door from springing open in a motor vehicle collision.

Narcan (naloxone) Reduces the effects of a narcotic, as seen with heroin overdose.

nasal cannula (NC) Device placed in the patient's nose to deliver between 24 percent and 44 percent oxygen.

nasal flaring Widening of the nostrils during breathing; a sign of increased respiratory effort commonly seen in children.

nasogastric tube Small-diameter, flexible plastic tube placed through the nose and the esophagus and into the stomach.

nasopharyngeal airway (NPA) A flexible tube that may be passed through the nose into the pharynx that can help to hold the tongue off the back of the throat and keep the airway open; also called a *nasal airway*.

nasopharynx Back of the throat immediately behind the nose; the nasal passage.

National Association of Emergency Medical Services Physicians (NAEMSP) National organization of physicians and EMS professionals dedicated to providing leadership in EMS and promoting excellence in EMS care.

National Association of Emergency Medical Technicians (NAEMT) National organization that represents EMS practitioners to the public and government.

National EMS Education Standards Broad educational statements that state the objective of EMS education and recognize that EMS is a rapidly changing profession that requires flexibility within limits.

National Fire Protection Agency (NFPA) Advisory board of fire service experts who publish standards and advocate for improved emergency services.

National Highway Traffic Safety Administration (NHTSA) Division of the U.S. Department of Transportation that has taken a leading role in establishing standards for training for emergency services.

National Incident Management System (NIMS) Management criteria enabling all responding agencies to work together when disaster incidents occur.

National Institute of Occupational Safety and Health (NIOSH) Federal agency charged with studying causes and prevention of work-related illness or injury.

National Registry of EMTs (NREMT) National EMS certification organization that provides a valid, uniform process to assess the knowledge and skills required for competent practice required by EMS professionals throughout their careers and maintains a registry (list) of certification status.

nature of the illness (NOI) Explanation of the character and history of an illness, analogous to MOI in trauma.

near-drowning Water submersion that does not result in death within a 24-hour period.

nebulizer Device that creates a fine mist of a liquid medication so that it can be inhaled.

necrosis Tissue death.

necrotic Dead tissue.

necrotizing fasciitis "Flesh-eating disease," an aggressive soft tissue infection associated with streptococcal bacteremia.

negative pressure ventilation Change of pressure inside the lungs compared to the pressure outside the atmosphere.

negligence Delivery of care in a manner considered to be below the accepted standard.

neonatal Life from birth to the end of the first month.

neonate Newborn infant up to 1 month old.

nephrons The functional parts of the kidney.

nerve roots Where nerves enter and exit the spinal column between the spinal vertebrae.

nervous system Body system made up of the brain, spinal cord, and nerves, which controls and coordinates all body functions.

neurogenic shock Hypoperfused state resulting from injury to the spinal cord and generalized vasodilation.

neutral inline alignment Natural anatomical position of the neck.

NFPA 704 symbol Diamond-shaped warning sign with four more diamonds inside designating the presence of hazardous material on a truck or tank.

9-1-1 Three-digit phone number for accessing emergency services in the United States.

nitrogen dioxide (NO_2) Airborne pollutant that can cause severe respiratory irritation.

nitrogen narcosis Reversible condition caused by the anesthetic effect of nitrogen at high partial pressures seen in divers at depth; commonly referred to as *the bends*.

nitroglycerin Medication that dilates, or opens, blood vessels.

nonfeasance Failure to perform the duty at all.

non-insulin-dependent diabetes Condition of a diabetic patient whose blood sugar is controlled by diet or drugs and not by insulin injections.

noninvasive blood pressure monitor (NIBP) Mechanical blood pressure device that automatically obtains serial blood pressures.

non-rebreather mask (NRB) Device that when used with oxygen at 10–15 lpm can deliver up to 100 percent oxygen.

nonverbal information Information gathered through observation, including body language and position.

normal saline solution (NSS) Commonly used intravenous solution that consists of 0.9% sodium chloride.

normal sinus rhythm (NSR) Predominant natural pacemaker of the heart.

nothing by mouth (NPO) Prohibition against ingestion to prevent aspiration secondary to vomiting; acronym stands for the Latin *nil per os*.

nuchal rigidity Stiff and painful neck condition.

nuclear dispersion device (NDD) Conventional bomb that spreads radioactive material across a wide area.

O

objective information Obtained by the EMT through direct observation or assessment.

obsessive-compulsive disorder (OCD) Psychiatric disorder characterized by repetitive behaviors.

obstetrics (OB) Medical practice involving pregnancy and childbirth.

occipital bone The most posterior bone in the skull.

occlusion Blockage.

occlusive dressing Bandage secured on three sides that allows air to escape from the open wound but prevents air from entering the open wound.

Occupational Safety and Health Administration (OSHA) Federal organization that regulates safety requirements for businesses.

off-line medical control Concept that physician does not have to be physically present while the EMT is caring for a patient but, through protocols and procedures, has control over each patient's care.

onboard oxygen Large oxygen tank kept on an ambulance for purposes of administering oxygen to a patient in the ambulance.

ongoing assessment Continuing observation of the patient throughout contact. Also referred to as *reassessment*.

on-line medical control Direct communication between the EMT and physician while care is being rendered in the field.

open fracture Broken bone in which the bone ends erupt through the skin.

open-ended questions Questions that cannot be answered with simple yes or no or automatic answers.

operations level responder Person expected to minimize the spread of a hazardous materials spill and to prevent further injuries.

OPQRST Abbreviation used to prompt questions related to a patient's complaint: onset; provocation; quality; region, radiation, relief; severity; time.

oral Route of medication administration by the mouth.

orbit The bony cavity that houses the eyeball.

organophosphates (OP) Class of chemicals used to make fertilizers and chemical weapons.

oropharyngeal airway (OPA) Plastic device that may be placed in the mouth to assist in keeping the tongue off the back of the throat and keeping the airway open; also called an *oral airway*.

oropharynx Section of throat that is visible from the mouth.

orthopedic "scoop" stretcher Stretcher that splits in two halves and can be placed under the patient one half at a time.

orthopedics Study of the musculoskeletal system.

orthostatic vital signs Heart rate and blood pressure measured in different positions, usually lying, then standing.

osteopenia Loss of bone mineral density.

osteoporosis Progressive loss in the calcium content of the bones seen commonly in elderly women.

out-of-hospital DNR Do not resuscitate order that is binding in the prehospital setting in specifying that lifesaving measures should not be started.

ovary Primary female gonad, located in the pelvis; produces female sex hormones.

overdose Intentional exposure to, usually ingestion of, a potentially harmful substance.

over-the-counter (OTC) Nonprescription medication self-administered by the patient and readily available at a pharmacy.

overtriage Use of a resource based on set criteria when the end result is not as severe as initially predicted.

ovulation Release of an egg from the ovary.

ovum Female egg released from the ovary.

oxygen Colorless gas the body needs in adequate amounts to function normally.

oxygenation Amount of available oxygen in a medium, such as the air.

P

pallor Pale skin color.

palmar Directional term used to describe the palm of the hand.

palmar method Method of determining the percentage of burned skin using the patient's palm.

palpate To feel with one's hands.

pancreas Organ located in the retroperitoneal space that produces both digestive enzymes and hormones such as insulin.

pancreatitis Inflammation of the pancreas characterized by abdominal pain and often vomiting.

pandemic Global disease outbreak.

panic stop Emergency stop for an unexpected obstacle.

paradoxical motion Movement of a flail chest segment in a direction opposite to that of the rest of the chest wall.

paralysis Inability to move a limb.

paramedic Highest level of EMS provider; paramedics are typically educated in rigorous college-level courses covering comprehensive patient assessment, advanced airway management, intravenous access techniques, expanded medication administration, and cardiac arrest management.

paraplegia Paralysis of the lower extremities, typically due to a spine injury below the cervical spine.

parenteral Inhaled or injected route of drug administration.

paresis Muscular weakness.

paresthesia Decreased ability to feel in extremities.

parietal bone The largest of the bones in the skull, located in the lateral part of the cranium.

parietal pain Localized, intense, sharp, constant pain associated with irritation of the peritoneum; also called *somatic pain*.

parietal pleura The thin covering adhering to the inside of the chest wall.

parity Total number of children born to a woman.

partial seizure Malfunction in the brain isolated to a small portion of the brain; formerly known as *petit mal*.

partial-thickness burn Burn that affects the epidermis and dermal layers of skin.

passive rewarming Treatment geared toward preventing any further body heat loss.

patella Small bony island over the knee joint, known as the kneecap.

pathogenesis The beginning and progression of disease.

pathogens Microorganisms or agents that cause disease, including bacteria, viruses, and fungi.

pathology Study of disease.

pathophysiology Study of the functional changes associated with or resulting from disease or injury

patient care report (PCR) Document on which an EMT records the evidence of the patient encounter.

patient history Detailed investigation of the present illness or injury and the patient's current health status and pertinent past medical history.

patient refusal form Specific form a patient must sign if he or she refuses to allow care or transport.

patient's bill of rights The rights and privileges to which a patient is entitled.

pattern of injury Injuries characteristic of a particular mechanism of injury.

pectoralis major muscles Muscles that cover the upper part of the anterior chest and help to lift the sternum and upper ribs.

Pediatric Assessment Triangle (PAT) A quick look assessment tool used to assess the patient's appearance, work of breathing, and circulation to the skin to help form a general impression.

Pediatric Glasgow Coma Scale (PGCS) Adult assessment tool modified for assessing the neurological status of infants and children.

pelvic girdle The bones of the pelvis and the attached legs.

penis Male organ that serves as a conduit for the passage of urine and semen.

perfusion Supply of oxygenated blood to an organ or tissue throughout the body.

pericardial tamponade Blood within the pericardial sac around the heart.

perimeter Imaginary boundary created, which divides safe areas from dangerous areas.

peripheral Directional term used to describe points farther from the core of the body (trunk).

peripheral nervous system Composed of nerves that originate in the spinal cord and transmit messages to and from the body's organs and tissues.

PERRL Acronym to report an eye exam: pupils equal, round, and reactive to light.

personal flotation device (PFD) Device that has positive buoyancy such as a life jacket or life preserver.

personal protective equipment (PPE) Gear that may be used by a health care provider to protect against exposure or injury.

personal safety The assurance that no hazards are present that might endanger the EMT.

pertinent negatives When the patient denies the specific signs and symptoms that could normally be seen with the condition the patient is experiencing.

pertinent past medical history Relevant information concerning past illness or injuries the patient has experienced that are pertinent to the current condition.

petechiae Small pinpoint hemorrhages under the skin.

petit mal seizure The old term for a partial seizure.

phalanges Fingers and toes.

pharmacology The study of medications and their interactions.

pharynx The back of the throat.

photophobia Abnormal sensitivity to light.

phrenic nerve Located in the third, fourth, and fifth cervical segments of the spinal cord.

physical restraint Restriction of a patient's freedom of movement by use of ties, cravats, or other means.

physician's assistant (PA) An allied health care professional, sometimes referred to as a *mid-level provider*, who generally has authority to write medical orders that are later reviewed by a physician.

physiology Study of the function of an organism.

pia mater Innermost membrane covering the spinal cord and brain.

pit viper Venomous snake that can be recognized by characteristic pits in front of each eye.

placard Sign established by the U.S. Department of Transportation (USDOT) to identify the presence of a hazardous material.

placenta Interface between the uterus and the fetus.

placenta previa Condition in which the placenta grows over the cervical opening.

placental abruption Condition in which the placenta prematurely detaches from the uterine wall.

plantar Directional term used to describe the bottom surface of the foot.

pleural cavity/potential space Tiny space between lungs and chest wall.

pneumatic anti-shock garment (PASG) Another name for military anti-shock trousers (MAST), a device that is inflated over the lower extremities and pelvis to attempt to increase blood flow to the core organs.

pneumatic lift pads Airbag lift devices.

pneumatic splint Splint that conforms to the shape of the injury by either inflation or vacuum.

pneumothorax Air in the pleural space potentially causing collapse of the lung.

pocket mask Dome-shaped plastic tool used as a barrier device for artificial ventilation.

point tenderness Finite area that is painful when pressed.

poison A potentially deadly substance, solid, liquid, or gas, that is detrimental to an individual's health or causes death.

poison control center Regional center that serves as a resource for laypeople and health care providers on poisons and the management of the poisoned person.

poisoning Exposure to a substance that results in illness.

polypharmacy Use of multiple medications by a single patient.

portable radio Small handheld radio unit that typically has power output of 1–5 watts.

portal of entry Route an organism uses to enter the body.

position of function Natural relaxed position of a hand or foot.

positional asphyxia Suffocation that results from the patient's inability to take a deep breath when in a particular position.

positive pressure ventilations (PPV) Method of artificial ventilations by forcing air into the lungs.

posterior Directional term referring to a location toward the back.

posterior tibial pulse Easily palpable pulse created by blood flow through the posterior tibial artery behind the medial malleolus of the ankle.

postictal phase Recovery period immediately after a seizure.

post-traumatic seizure Seizure that may occur after head trauma.

post-traumatic stress disorder (PTSD) Psychiatric disorder that is the result of mental shock to the patient (e.g., witnessing a horrific trauma).

postural hypotension Drop in blood pressure associated with a change in position, usually from lying to standing.

pounds per square inch (psi) Measurement of pressure applied to a surface.

power of attorney (POA) Designated person who makes decisions on behalf of another who is incapacitated.

pox Small blisters filled with virus.

precipitous delivery Occurs when the birth of the fetus takes place less than three hours after labor begins.

prefix Complements a root word; placed at the beginning of the root and adds meaning to the word.

prehospital health care team Multidisciplinary team composed of medical personnel, firefighters, and police officers who care for patients before their admittance to the hospital.

preload Volume of blood returning to the heart.

premature delivery Delivery that occurs prior to 36 weeks of gestation.

premature ventricular complex (PVC) A small group of irritated cells in the ventricles that fire earlier than expected.

preoxygenation Providing high-concentration oxygen to a patient for a period of time before a procedure, such as endotracheal intubation or suctioning, is performed.

preplan Agreed-on response that is planned before an emergency occurs.

pressure points Specific areas over major arteries where if compressed, bleeding from that artery can be halted.

preventive maintenance (PM) Program of replacing and repairing vehicles or equipment before they fail.

priapism A painful, sustained erection that is the result of spinal cord injury.

primary assessment Rapid, systematic assessment and management of life-threats to the patient, his/her mental status, airway and breathing, and circulatory status. Also referred to as *Initial Assessment*.

primary brain injury Direct trauma to the brain and associated vascular structures.

primary spinal cord injury Spinal cord injury that occurs at the time of the trauma.

professional conduct Behavior demonstrating a caring, confident, and courteous demeanor; expected from all health care providers.

prognosis Expected or predicted outcome of a disease.

projection When one person attributes his or her thoughts or feelings to another.

prolapsed umbilical cord Presentation of the umbilical cord prior to the infant, resulting in compression of the cord.

pronation Action of turning something, such as the hand, downward.

pronator drift A test of neurological function that involves raising both arms straight out in front of the body, palms up, eyes closed; a positive test involves one arm drifting and indicates weakness in that arm.

prone Position in which a person is lying face down.

prophylaxis Doing something to prevent an unwanted outcome.

prostate gland Male organ that produces a fluid that assists in the transport of sperm.

protected health information (PHI) Personal patient information protected from accidental disclosure or discovery by HIPAA.

provocation Aggravating or making the pain, discomfort, or condition worse.

proximal Directional term used to describe points on the body that are closer to the core of the body (trunk).

psychiatry The medical study of mental illness.

psychogenic shock (vasovagal shock) Form of neurogenic shock in which the vagal nerve is stimulated (by sudden fright or severe pain), resulting in a quick dilation of the peripheral blood vessels, causing a sudden loss of consciousness.

pubis The front of the bony pelvis.

public access defibrillation (PAD) Public training in the use of an AED.

public address system (PA) An electronic device designed to project a voice loudly.

public information officer (PIO) An individual designated by the incident commander to meet with the media and report the state of affairs at the incident.

public information systems Procedures, processes, and systems required for communicating timely and accurate information to the public during a disaster or emergency situation.

public safety access point (PSAP) A local dispatch office that receives 9-1-1 calls from the public. A PSAP may be local fire or police department, an ambulance service, or a regional office covering all emergency services.

pulmonary artery Large artery that transfers blood from the right ventricle to the pulmonary circuit for oxygenation.

pulmonary circuit Blood vessels that pass through the lungs and allow oxygenation and removal of carbon dioxide.

pulmonary circulation Circulation of blood through the lungs for gas exchange.

pulmonary contusion Bruising of the lungs.

pulmonary edema Swelling of the pulmonary blood vessels.

pulmonary embolism Occurs when the blockage breaks free from a lower extremity and lodges in the arteries of the lungs.

pulmonary embolus Blockage in the pulmonary arterial circulation resulting in an area of lung that does not allow alveolar capillary gas exchange.

pulmonary valve A semilunar valve that prevents the backflow of blood from the pulmonary artery back into the right ventricle.

pulmonary vein The large vessel that takes oxygenated blood from the pulmonary circuit and delivers it to the left atrium.

pulse The palpable feeling of blood flow through a superficial artery; count of the heartbeat.

pulse, movement, sensation (PMS) Assessment of distal neuro-vascular function to assess for injury.

pulse oximeter Tool that allows noninvasive measurement of the blood's oxygen saturation.

pulse pressure The difference between systolic and diastolic blood pressures.

pulseless electrical activity (PEA) Situation in which a pulse is not created but the ECG will show a rhythm.

puncture A hole created in the skin by a sharp, pointed object.

pupil The black center of the eye.

Purkinje fibers Specialized cardiac conduction fibers within the ventricles.

pursed lip breathing Exhaling past partially closed lips.

pyelonephritis A urinary tract infection (UTI) that involves the kidneys.

Q

quadriceps muscle The strong muscle in the anterior thigh that permits leg extension.

quadriplegia Paralysis of all four extremities, typically caused by high cervical spine injury.

quality assurance (QA) A review of care to ensure minimum standards are met.

R

raccoon's eyes Bruising around the eyes that may be indicative of a skull fracture.

radiation The transfer of heat from the warm body into the cooler environment just by the fact that a temperature gradient exists.

radiation pager A portable device that clips to the belt and measures radiation in the environment, alarming the wearer when dangerous levels of radiation are present.

radio head The main section of a mobile radio, often located in the driver's compartment of the vehicle.

radius The more lateral of the two bones in the forearm.

rales A bubbly or soft crackling sound, like hair rubbed between the fingers next to the ear.

range of motion (ROM) The movement that a bone or limb is allowed in a joint.

rapid extrication Technique for quickly removing an unstable potentially spine injured patient.

rapid physical examination A quick head-to-toe examination done on a patient who is unable to provide a history owing to a decreased level of consciousness.

rapid trauma assessment A quickly performed head-to-toe examination of a seriously injured trauma patient to discover hidden or suspected injuries.

rationalizations Patient developing a logical explanation to events in order to avoid dealing with painful emotions.

receptive aphasia Inability to comprehend language, often seen when a stroke affects the speech center in the brain.

recovery position Position in which the patient is on the side so that secretions may spontaneously drain from the airway; also known as the *coma position* or *left lateral recumbent position.*

rectum End of the large intestine where stool is stored before it is eliminated via the anus.

red blood cells Hemoglobin-carrying blood cells whose function is to deliver oxygen to tissues.

Reeves stretcher Commercially available, long, flat litter with handles on all corners that can be wrapped around the patient; allows for easy movement of the patient who has not suffered a spinal injury.

referred pain Pain felt in a body part away from the point where the pain originates.

refusal of medical assistance (RMA) When a patient refuses medical care and understands the risk and possible consequences of such action; generally there is not a great risk for loss of life or limb.

regulator Device placed on an oxygen tank to regulate the flow of the gas; also called a *flowmeter.*

reinforce Brace or strengthen a bandage.

remission Nonactive state.

renal stone The accumulation of solid material in the kidney that may become lodged in the ureter during passage to the bladder.

repeater Radio receiver/transmitter that picks up the signal from a mobile unit and increases or boosts the signal to the base station receiver.

rescue Helping another person who is incapable of freeing himself or herself from confinement.

rescuer assist The use of one EMT on one side of a walking patient for assistance with walking.

respiration The exchange of gases, such as oxygen and carbon dioxide, at the capillary level.

respiratory rate Number of breaths in one minute.

respiratory syncytial virus (RSV) Infectious form of bronchiolitis seen more commonly in children than adults.

responsive to painful stimuli Term used to describe the mental status of a patient who is aroused only by uncomfortable action of touch.

responsive to voice Term used to describe the mental status of a patient who is aroused by verbal stimuli but is not spontaneously awake and interactive.

resuscitate To attempt to revive a patient by way of medical therapies.

retroperitoneal cavity The most posterior section of the abdomen, containing organs such as kidneys, pancreas, and aorta.

return of spontaneous circulation (ROSC) Pulses returning with just CPR or defibrillation.

revised trauma score Standard method of trauma scoring that uses results of the Glasgow Coma Scale and the patient's respiratory rate and systolic blood pressure, assigning a number to each element.

rhonchi Coarse sounds that are heard over the lungs when mucus or other foreign material accumulates in the larger airways.

rhythm A regularly repeating ECG pattern.

rib cage Bony ribs that surround the organs of the chest like a protective cage.

right-of-way Privilege of proceeding ahead of others on a roadway.

rigid splint Any firm material that can provide support for a limb.

rigor mortis Generalized stiffening of the body following death.

riot gas (CS) Noxious gas used to disperse crowds.

risk factors Predisposing factors that can make a person more susceptible to disease.

risk management Actions geared toward protection from hazard.

Risk Mitigation Process of identifying hazards and ensuring protection.

risk profile Likelihood of the presence of a disease in a person or group of people.

roller bandage Cotton cloth rolled into a cylinder for easier control when unwrapping.

rolling the dash Pulling the vehicle's dashboard off the patient.

rollover protective structure (ROPS) A protective bar or canopy that prevents the driver from being crushed under the weight of the tractor.

rotor wing Helicopters.

route Where a drug is administered, i.e., enteral (ingested, sublingual and oral) and parenteral (inhalation and injection).

rule of nines Formula to determine the percentage of burnt skin.

Ryan White law Regulation that states that a hospital is required to notify an EMS agency if its staff identifies an infectious illness to which the agency's employees may have been exposed.

S

sacral vertebrae Five strong bony vertebrae that close the pelvic ring posteriorly.

safety corridor Zone of protection, created by a barrier, that permits the EMT to work safely.

safety glass Piece of glass sealed between two sheets of plastic designed to remain in one piece if damaged.

safety officer (SO) Designated person who is charged with knowledge of relevant regulations and standards regarding responder and patient safety.

saliva Normally occurring secretions from the mouth.

SAMPLE Acronym to remember the most important basic history questions: signs and symptoms, allergies, medications, past medical history, last oral intake, events leading up to the incident/illness.

scalene muscles Responsible for lifting the sternocleidomastoid muscle.

scanner Electronic device that may be used to listen to various radio frequencies.

scapulas Strong bony prominences on the back, also known as the *shoulder blades*.

scene survey Procedure used to initially evaluate a situation for potential dangers.

sciatic nerve The primary sensory and motor nerve of the legs.

scope of practice Legal description of the limits of care that an EMS provider can offer to a patient.

scrotum Externally located sac that encloses the male testes.

search and rescue (SAR) Organized and disciplined approach to the rescue of injured, ill, or lost persons.

seat carry Technique of carrying a conscious patient in which two EMTs join arms and allow the patient to sit on their arms as if they formed a seat.

second stage of labor Phase of childbirth that begins when the cervix is completely dilated and ends with the delivery of the infant.

secondary brain injury Extension of the primary brain injury, such as hypoxia and hypotension.

secondary device Explosive device intended to harm emergency services responders and delay emergency operations.

secondary spinal cord injury Spinal cord injury that occurs after the trauma, often as a result of mishandling.

seizure Event that begins within the brain and results in involuntary movements and sometimes loss of consciousness.

self-contained breathing apparatus (SCBA) Equipment that permits the wearer to have an independent air supply; used in hazardous environments.

self-splint When a patient uses his or her body to protect and stabilize a limb.

Sellick maneuver Cricoid pressure.

sensory nerves Nervous tissue that carries impulses of feelings such as pressure or pain.

septic shock Hypoperfused state resulting from overwhelming infection and generalized vasodilation.

sexual abuse Any sexual activity with a child in which consent is not or cannot be given.

sexual assault Physical and psychological trauma of a sexual nature.

sexual molestation Form of sexual abuse that is performed for the sexual gratification of the parent or caregiver.

shaken baby syndrome Shaking an infant violently and causing a head injury.

sharps Instruments with a sharp point, such as needles, syringes, and sharp blades.

sharps container Puncture-proof container used to dispose of needles and other sharp instruments; the container is usually red with a biohazard label on the side.

shingles Adult chicken pox.

shipping papers Paperwork that accompanies hazardous material while in transit; it contains the chemical name of the materials, as well as the U.N. designation of the substance being transported.

shock State in which the body is hypoperfused, resulting in inadequate oxygenation of cells, tissues, and organs.

shock position Position in which the body is hypoperfused, resulting in inadequate oxygenation of cells, tissues, and organs.

short spine immobilization device (SSID) Interim device used to stabilize a patient's spine while transferring him or her to a long backboard.

shoulder dislocation Separation of the scapula and the humerus.

shoulder dystocia Shoulders become wedged against the pubic bone and sacrum during birth.

shoulder girdle The scapula, clavicle, and attached arms.

side effect Effect of a medication that was not the intended effect.

sign Something the examiner can objectively see.

signs of circulation Responsiveness, breathing, coughing, and movement.

silent myocardial infarction Death of heart tissue, which occurs without the patient experiencing classic cardiac symptoms such as chest pain.

simple partial seizure Seizure in which the patient is awake but experiencing jerky movements, usually in only one area of the body, which are not controlled.

simplex A type of radio that can only receive or transmit at one time; allows only one-way communication.

sino atrial (SA) Point at the top of the heart, at the atria, where a collection of nervous tissue is found; this nervous tissue is the primary pacemaker of the heart.

sinoatrial (SA) node Specialized cardiac conduction fibers that serve as the primary pacemaker of the heart.

siren mode Characteristic patterns of sound to alert motorists of the vehicle's presence.

size-up Rapid determination of the situation, including hazards, at the scene of an emergency.

slander False statements spoken with malicious intent or reckless disregard, which injure a person's reputation or good name.

sling A loop of webbing used to help balance the load when carrying a litter or a basket.

sling and swathe (S/S) The use of a cravat and a triangular bandage to splint a limb.

slippery sheets Specially coated sheets that reduce friction between the patient and the bed and allow for an easier transfer.

slow-moving vehicle (SMV) Any vehicle, typically farm machinery, that is incapable of maintaining posted highway speeds.

SLUDGEM Characteristic symptom pattern seen with nerve agents; acronym represents salivation, lacrimation, urination, defecation, GI distress, emesis, and muscle contractions.

small intestine Long, hollow organ that takes up much of the abdominal cavity and is responsible for much of the absorption of nutrients from food.

small volume nebulizer (SVN) Methods of delivering humidified oxygen.

snoring Sound made when a partial upper airway obstruction, such as the tongue, exists in the supine patient.

special incident report (SIR) Specific document upon which the EMT writes the details of a defined special incident, such as equipment failure.

sperm Male reproductive material responsible for fertilization of the female egg.

sphygmomanometer A device that is used to measure blood pressure; a blood pressure cuff.

spinal canal Passageway in the vertebrae through which the spinal cord passes.

spinal column Series of bones that support the back and protect the spinal cord.

spinal cord The collection of nerves that run from the brain through the spinal column and branch out as peripheral nerves to body organs and tissues.

spinous process The centrally palpable posterior element of each vertebrae.

spiral bandage A roller bandage wrapped around a limb.

spleen Solid, highly vascular organ, located in the left-upper quadrant of the abdomen that serves to store blood, destroy old red blood cells, filter foreign substances from the blood, and produce lymphocytes.

spontaneous abortion Loss of a pregnancy, also known as *miscarriage*.

spontaneous reduction A bone that returns to its natural position, within a joint, without assistance.

sprain A stretch of a ligament or tendon beyond its range of motion, resulting in tissue injury.

sputum Secretions formed in the airway.

staging Designating a specific area for emergency vehicles and providers entering a scene.

staging area An off-scene location where personnel and vehicles assemble and await assignment.

staging officer A manager of an area who assembles and assigns equipment and personnel to specific duties or tasks.

stairchair A specially designed chair that has handles on the back and on the front that a patient may be secured into and then carried down a flight of stairs by two EMTs.

stand by Radio terminology meaning "hold on a minute."

standard anatomical position Facing forward, legs slightly apart, with feet pointing forward, arms straight and extended a few inches away from the side, with palms facing forward.

standard comfort measures Treatments that are provided to ease suffering but that do not include resuscitation of a patient.

standard of care Level of care recognized as being appropriate for a particular level of training and certification.

standard precautions Refers to the personal protective equipment used routinely in certain circumstances.

standing orders Off-line medical control consisting of procedures that are to be followed by the EMT for specific injuries or illness.

standing takedown Technique in which rescuers use a rigid backboard to gently move a patient from the standing upright position to a horizontal supine position.

START Triage System Standardized system for triage; acronym stands for simple triage and rapid treatment.

status epilepticus One continuous seizure or one or more seizures without an intervening period of consciousness.

stenosis Constriction or narrowing of a duct or passage, such as a vessel or valve; a stricture.

sterilization Thorough cleaning of an item so that all microorganisms have been completely removed.

sternal angle The bony ridge where the manubrium meets the body of the sternum; also called the *angle of Louis*.

sternal body The largest center piece of the bony sternum, or breastbone.

sternal retraction Sternal depressions with each breath seen in a child with severe respiratory distress.

sternal rub Technique used to assess a patient's response to a painful stimulus; with this technique the knuckles are rubbed against the patient's sternum.

sternocleidomastoid muscle Important accessory muscle of respiration and the main muscle that moves the head; a triangular muscle that connects the sternum with the clavicle and mastoid process; also called the *strap muscle.*

sternum The bony island in the center of the chest, also known as the *breastbone.*

Stokes basket Type of basket stretcher that allows complete immobilization and protection of the patient during a move over rough terrain.

stoma Surgically created hole at the base of the neck to allow breathing in patients with severe upper airway diseases.

stress Physical, emotional, and behavioral response of the body to changing external conditions.

stress management program Means of dealing effectively with acute and chronic stress.

stressors Events that trigger stress.

stridor Harsh, high-pitched sound heard during inspiration characteristic of an upper airway obstruction due to swelling in the larynx.

stroke Injury to brain tissue that occurs as a result of disruption of blood flow to part of the brain; also known as a *cerebrovascular accident.*

stroke volume Amount of blood the heart pumps out with each beat.

subarachnoid space Space between the dura mater and arachnoid layers of the meninges, filled with cerebrospinal fluid.

subcutaneous Space just under the skin, made up of fat and tiny blood vessels.

subcutaneous emphysema Air under the skin and above the chest wall.

subcutaneous tissue The fatty tissue beneath the dermis of the skin; connects the skin to the underlying muscle.

subdural hematoma A collection of blood between the surface of the brain and the dura mater, often venous in nature.

subjective information Information the patient or family members tell an EMT.

subjective, objective, assessment plan (SOAP) A system of organizing medical information, called charting, into an organized and coherent document.

subjective, objective, assessment plan, intervention, evaluation (SOAPIE) Additional EMS-specific information added to the SOAP format of charting.

sublingual Under the tongue.

subluxation Partial dislocation at a joint.

substance abuse Misuse of a drug to alter perception or mood.

sucking chest wound Wound on the chest through which air can enter the pleural space, making a sucking sound.

sudden cardiac death (SCD) Death of a patient early in the course of a heart attack, usually due to an arrhythmia.

sudden infant death syndrome (SIDS) The sudden, unexplained death of an infant in the first year of life.

suicide Voluntary taking of one's own life.

superficial Term used to describe something at or close to the top or surface.

superficial burn A burn affecting only the uppermost layer of skin.

superior A directional term referring to a location toward the top of an object.

supination The action of turning something, such as the hand, upward.

supine Position in which a person is lying face up with the spine to the ground.

supine hypotensive syndrome Compression of the vena cava when a pregnant woman lies flat, resulting in a loss of blood pressure.

suprasternal notch The notch formed where the clavicles meet the manubrium.

surrounding area The space above and around the touchdown site where a helicopter will land.

suspension A powder suspended in a liquid so that it may be more easily ingested.

sutures Immovable joints, composed of connective tissue, in the skull where the cranial bones meet; these joints begin to fuse as a child gets older and are completely fused in an adult.

swelling An increase in soft tissue size due to inflammation.

swift water A rapidly moving body of water.

symbiotic A mutually beneficial relationship between a microorganism and its host.

symphysis pubis The joint at the center of the front of the pelvis where the two pubis bones meet.

symptom Sign of illness or injury reported by a patient or discovered on examination.

syndrome Group of features, including certain signs, symptoms, and characteristics that occur together.

systemic circulation Supplies blood to the organs of the body's systems.

systemic vascular resistance (SVR) Resistance to flow that blood must overcome to move through the circulatory system.

systolic The top number in a blood pressure; refers to the pressure in the vessels when the heart is contracting.

systolic blood pressure Pressure exerted against the vessel walls when the heart contracts.

T

tachycardia Increased heart rate.

tachypnea Respiratory rate faster than normal.

tactile hallucination A false perception of a sensation of the skin; a false feeling.

takedown procedure Planned orderly restraint of a patient for a medical purpose.

target organs Specific organs upon which hormones are intended to work.

tarsals Small bones within the foot, corresponding to the carpal bones of the wrist.

tattooing A peppering of gunpowder to the skin.

teachable moment Ability to affect the patient's behaviors in the future because the patient's mind is receptive to suggestion today.

tear gas (CN) Noxious gas used to disperse crowds.

technical rescue Complex rescue operations performed by highly trained technicians using specialized equipment.

telemetry Sending an ECG rhythm strip to the base hospital for physician interpretation.

temporal bone Cranial bone that forms the base of the skull, behind and at the sides of the face.

tender Referring to an area that is sensitive or painful upon palpation.

tendon The connective tissue that attaches the muscle to the bone.

tension pneumothorax Air in the pleural space under tension, causing complete collapse of the affected lung and shift of the heart and other intrathoracic structures.

teratogens Chemicals that affect fetal development in the womb.

terminal A patient who is at the end of a disease that will result in death.

terminal bronchioles The smallest tubular airways leading to the alveoli.

terrorism The unlawful use of force against persons or property to intimidate or coerce a government, the civilian population, or any segment thereof, in the furtherance of political or social objectives.

testes Male gonads.

therapeutic communications Communication techniques demonstrating compassion and caring, which can have positive effects on the patient's health.

therapeutic effect Desired effect the drug was administered to achieve.

thermoregulation Attempt to balance the amount of heat lost and heat gained to maintain a constant body temperature.

third stage of labor Final stage of labor during which the placenta is delivered.

thoracic cavity The space enclosed within the rib cage, bordered inferiorly by the diaphragm; otherwise known as the *chest cavity*.

thoracic vertebrae The twelve vertebrae that are found below the cervical spine and above the lumbar spine; these are attached to the twelve sets of ribs.

thrombus An accumulation of platelets and other blood components that locally occlude a vessel; a blood clot.

tibia The larger of the two bones in the lower leg; the shinbone.

tidal volume Volume or amount of air inhaled and exhaled in one breath.

tilt test Test for hypovolemia that is considered positive if the heart rate goes up by 10–20 beats per minute and the systolic blood pressure drops by 10–20 mmHg with a change of position from sitting or lying to standing.

tonic phase The stage in a seizure in which the entire body stiffens.

tonsils Pillars of soft tissue on each side of the back of the throat.

topical On the surface; refers to administration of medication by placing it on the surface of the skin so it can be slowly absorbed.

tort law Area of law involving civil wrongs against another and a finding of liability in a civil case, typically only resulting in the award of monetary damages.

tourniquet (TK) A tight, constricting band that stops blood flow to a limb.

toxic organic dust syndrome (TODS) Special respiratory hazards caused by organic dust that can be inhaled, leading to fever, headache, and malaise.

toxic substance Any substance that is poisonous to the human body.

toxicology The study of toxins, antidotes, and the effects of toxins on the body.

toxin Any drug or substance poisonous to the human body that can affect cellular respiration by internal and external means, causing a decline in health and ultimately leading to death.

TRACEM Mnemonic used to indicate the threats created by a terrorist attack; T stands for thermal harm, R for radiation harm, A for asphyxiation, C for corrosive chemicals, E for etiologic, and M for mechanical.

trachea The cartilaginous tube that is the passageway for air to get from the upper airway to the lungs; also known as the *windpipe*.

tracheal deviation Movement of the trachea from the mid-line.

tracheostomy The surgical creation of a hole in the anterior neck into the trachea to allow more effective ventilation in patients with upper airway problems or chronic lung disease.

tracheostomy tube Rigid tube placed into a tracheostomy to maintain a patent airway.

traction The application of a steady pull in line with an axis.

traction splint A splint that provides a continuous pull along the axis of the bone.

trade name The brand name given to a medication by the manufacturer.

transfer sheets Special heavy-duty vinyl sheets reinforced with webbing to carry extra weight.

transient ischemic attack (TIA) Temporary disruption of blood flow to part of the brain that results in signs and symptoms of a stroke, yet resolves within minutes to hours.

transmission The transfer of an infectious agent from one source to another.

transportation officer The individual responsible for the overall movement of patients from the scene to appropriate hospitals.

trapezius muscle Triangular muscle that covers the upper back and helps to lift the shoulders.

trauma Physical injury or wound caused by external forces.

trauma center A specially designated hospital that is experienced in and capable of caring for patients with severe injuries.

trauma dressing A large cotton dressing placed over a major open wound.

traumatic asphyxia A crushing blow that forces air and blood out of the chest.

traumatic brain injury (TBI) Injury to the brain due to a direct cause (penetrating trauma), indirect cause (blow to the skull), or secondary cause (hypoxia).

treatment officer The person responsible for setting up the field hospital.

trend Identification of a pattern over a period of time.

triad Three signs that are characteristic of a disease.

triage A system of distribution of patients into treatment classifications according to their injury severity.

triage officer The individual responsible for the distribution of patients into treatment classification according to their injury severity.

triage tag A special document that is used in multiple-casualty incidents to indicate the priority of each patient.

triangular bandage A 36-by-42-inch triangular piece of muslin cloth.

triceps muscle The muscle in the back of the upper arm that allows elbow extension; antagonist to the biceps muscle.

tricuspid valve The three-cusped valve between the right atrium and right ventricle that prevents backflow of blood.

tripod position The three-legged position maintained by a person with severe difficulty breathing; with the upper body leaning slightly forward, arms straight, and hands supporting the upper body by resting on the upper legs.

true ribs The first seven pairs of ribs, which attach directly to the sternum anteriorly.

tuberculosis (TB) The bacterium responsible for the disease tuberculosis, which typically attacks the lungs.

tunica adventitia Outer layer of blood vessels' walls made of white fibrous connective tissue.

tunica intima Inner layer of the walls of blood vessels.

tunica media Smooth muscle middle layer of the walls of blood vessels.

tunics Layer or coats of vessel walls.

twelve-lead ECG tracing the heart's electrical activity from twelve different views.

twisting force Turning force of violence.

two-way radio Wireless electronic device that permits the transmission of messages to distant radio receivers as well as receipt of signals from those distant radios.

U

UHF Ultrahigh frequency radio signal.

ulcer Erosion of the lining of the stomach that can lead to pain and/or bleeding.

ulna The more medial bone in the forearm.

undertriage Failing to use a resource based on set criteria when the end result is more severe than originally predicted.

unilateral Directional term used to describe a point on only one side of the body.

unipolar traction splint A traction splint with a single shaft.

United States Fire Academy (USFA) The federal training organization for firefighters.

universal dressing A 9-by-36-inch gauze dressing.

unresponsive Term used to describe the mental status of a patient who cannot be aroused with verbal or even painful stimuli.

unstable angina Injured heart muscle that creates pain, generally due to a narrowing of the coronary artery.

upper extremities Term used to refer to the arms.

ureters Muscular tubes that carry urine from the kidneys to the bladder.

urticaria Raised, red rash that results from localized dilation and leaking of blood vessels resulting in red, warm swelling to the surface of the skin; also known as *hives*.

U.S. Pharmacopeia The national drug reference that includes drug indications, contraindications, and side effects.

uterus Muscular chamber that holds the products of conception; also known as the *womb*.

uvula Small piece of tissue that is seen hanging off the roof of the mouth in the pharynx.

V

vagina Part of the female genitalia that allows passage of menstrual flow or a baby during labor and serves as the conduit for the acceptance of the male penis during coitus.

vallecula Space posterior to the base of the tongue, anterior to the epiglottis.

veins Vessels that carry blood back to the heart, usually with deoxygenated blood.

velocity Speed.

vena cava The largest vein in the body.

venous bleeding Bleeding from the oxygen-poor veins; can be severe and life threatening.

ventilation The process of moving air into and out of the lungs; breathing.

ventral Directional term referring to points located in the front of the body.

ventricles Primary pump chambers of the heart.

ventricular fibrillation Uncoordinated and spontaneous contraction of individual heart muscle fibers.

ventricular tachycardia A cardiac event in which a small group of irritated cells in the ventricles start to fire automatically at rates of 100–250 beats per minute (bpm).

ventriculo-peritoneal (VP) A shunt that diverts extra cerebrospinal fluid from the brain to the abdomen, thereby preventing increased intracranial pressure.

venules Tiny vessels that connect the capillaries and veins.

verbal communication Communication through the use of speech.

verbal report A spoken account of the patient encounter given to the accepting health care provider.

vertebrae Individual bones of the spine.

vertebral foramen A canal, formed by a ring of bone that houses the spinal cord.

VHF Very-high-frequency radio signal.

vial of life Complete patient history documented and stored in a designated spot marked in a patient's home.

visceral pain Poorly localized, intermittent, crampy, dull, or achy pain originating with an organ.

visceral pleura The membrane lining the surface of the lungs.

visual hallucination False perception of the sensation of the eyes; a false visualization.

W

weapons of mass destruction (WMD) Weapons created to indiscriminately kill or maim large numbers of civilians and to disrupt normal government operations.

wheezing High-pitched expiratory sound heard when lower airway narrowing exists.

white paper Detailed or authorization report on any subject; the National Academy of Sciences' article titled "Accidental Death and Disability: The Neglected Disease of Modern Society," written for President Kennedy, laid the groundwork for EMS legislation.

window punch A special tool for breaking window glass.

withdrawal symptoms The unpleasant physical and/or psychological effects experienced by a drug-addicted patient when the drug is kept from him or her.

wound Damage to the skin as a result of trauma.

X

xiphoid process The inferior portion of the sternum.

Y

Yankauer A rigid suction catheter that has a curvature meant to follow the pharyngeal curve and a large open suction tip.

Z

zygomatic bones The facial bones that extend anteriorly from the temporal part of the skull on each side to form the prominence of the cheeks.